Patients and Purse Strings
Patient Classification and Cost Management

Franklin A. Shaffer, Editor

Pub. No. 20-2155

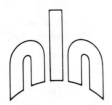

National League for Nursing

ISBN 0-88737-263-5

The views expressed in this publication represent the views
of the authors and do not necessarily reflect the official views
of the National League for Nursing.

Many of the papers in this volume were presented at the Northwestern
Memorial Hospital Conference on "Patients and Purse Strings: Patient
Classification and Cost Management," Chicago, Illinois, December 12–
13, 1985.

Contents

iii

3. New Uses for Patient Classification

4. Afterword

Preface

> If we nurses criticize DRGs as incomplete definitions, it is up to us to fine tune the data bases so nurses' contributions to patient care, to costs, and to revenues are apparent. Having a data system at hand gives us the opportunity to learn exactly how nursing works [Thompson & Diers, 1985, p. 438].

Patients and Purse Strings is a book about "how nursing works." It provides specific, practical information on the development and use of patient classification systems for nursing that will allow us to determine resource use and thus evaluate both the efficiency and quality of the care we provide.

The first section of this volume lays some groundwork for consideration of the state of the art in patient classification research. The authors of these papers present different conceptual approaches. They review some of the basic concepts, trace the process of developing a system, highlight the problems encountered, and explain how instruments can be made more rigorous. As Giovannetti (1985) has pointed out, while the growing computerization of the hospital has greatly facilitated the implementation of patient classification systems and their integration with other hospital data, the responsibility to ensure that these systems are reliable and valid and are used accurately "cannot be passed on to the machine." In this section on Developing and Testing Patient Classification Systems, Dijkers, Paradise, and Maxwell examine some of the pitfalls that result when what systems are expected to measure differs from what they actually assess, while Kaspar treats critical reliability and validity issues.

The second section groups studies that relate patient classification systems to DRGs and nursing costs. In the three-plus years since the Medicare prospective payment system came into effect, it has become apparent that nursing holds a crucial place in the new health care system's struggle to provide quality services in an atmosphere of cost-cutting and increased concern for efficiency. Nursing managers are more eager than ever to cost out nursing per case, to link nursing classification criteria to hospital cost-accounting systems, and to bill patients for nursing care. Many of the seminal studies in this area were reported in *Costing Out Nursing: Pricing Our Product* (Shaffer, 1985); and studies in the second section of this volume, such as those by Harrell, Wolf and Lesic, Lucke and Lucke, Bailie, and Martin and Kelly continue the work that has been done in this area to devise methods of measuring, analyzing, and predicting nursing costs.

In other responses to the new cost-conscious climate in health care, nursing managers have challenged the age-old assumption about the percentage of the patient's bill that nursing charges represent in an effort to have the nursing department considered as a profit center within the hospital—showing that nursing constitutes less than 20 percent of total hospital charges (Dahlen, 1985; Mitchell, Miller, Welches, & Walker, 1984; Riley & Schaefers, 1983; Walker, 1983). And, they have performed studies, many of which are represented in this volume, showing the variable relationship between DRG classification and consumption of nursing resources.

The DRG system under which hospitals are reimbursed today is not the same system put into place in October 1983; it is different still from the system that will be in effect in 1989 or 1995. In the last several years we have seen a freeze on Medicare reimbursement rates that was lifted only with the Consolidated Omnibus Budget Reconciliation Act of May 1986; a Medicare freeze on physicians' fees and charges; changes in Medicare reimbursement for capital costs, for graduate medical education, and for hospitals that serve large numbers of indigent patients; and changes in the rate of the transition to nationwide prospective system rates.

We are also seeing the beginning of prospective payment systems for long-term care, outpatient care, home care, and other services. Thus, the final section of this book, New Uses of Patient Classification Systems, represents some of the first attempts to devise classification systems to help address the effects prospective payment is having outside the hospital. In addition to systems devised specifically for home care, these authors discuss the development of patient classification systems for groups that have special requirements, such as maternity service patients.

Recent studies commissioned by the Health Care Financing Administration (HCFA) and the Prospective Payment Assessment Commission (ProPAC) have examined the relationship between nursing care, nursing costs, and prospective payment. A project undertaken by the American Nurses' Association for HCFA studied the relationships between DRG rates and nursing costs for patients classified in 21 DRGs (*DRGs and Nursing Care*, 1986). The study showed a strong statistical correlation between DRG weights and consumption of nursing resources for most of the DRGs studied. The exceptions, however, included some of the most common DRGs, including DRG 127, heart failure and shock. The researchers also found, moreover, that within some DRGs patient care needs vary widely from one patient to another.

This study confirmed the findings of Sovie, Tarcinale, VanPutte, and Stunden (reported in this volume) in a major study covering 459 of the DRGs and 93 percent of the patients in one hospital over a period of a year that "DRGs, as a case-mix profile, do not predict individual patients' needs." This conclusion is also supported by the studies reported here by Buck; Atwood, Hinshaw, and Chance; Bailie; and Wolf and Lesic. It is clear from this research that nursing costs cannot be predicted from DRG assignment alone. The problem with using DRGs as a measure of nursing care—and thus nursing costs—is, as many authors have pointed out, "that DRGs do not take into account the significant criteria for determining nursing workload levels, namely, patients' physical and emotional states" (Giovannetti, 1985). Moreover, as Giovannetti (1985) points out, and Wolf and Lesic show in their paper in this volume, the demand for nursing care varies over the course of a hospital admission, and the pattern is different for different DRGs.

Yet, many of these same studies suggest that DRGs can be used in combination with nursing classification systems to more accurately predict patients' needs, as well as length of stay and hospital costs (Lucke & Lucke, this volume). Thus, it is the attempt to link DRGs with nursing measures of patients' needs for nursing care that constitutes the next wave of nursing research. If a hospital were able to devise a computer system that could link a nursing measure, such as nursing diagnoses or one of the measures of nursing intensity discussed here, and nursing care plans with cost accounting, it would go a long way toward documenting variances in patient charges. Such systems might pave the way toward greater integration of nursing charges into DRG weights.

In its 1985 annual report, ProPAC recognized that there may be inaccuracies in the nursing weights used by Medicare to assign costs per DRG. A recent study commissioned by ProPAC explored the nursing literature on patient classification in order to provide background information on what systems were available, their validity and reliability, and the problems involved in measuring nursing acuity (Health Economics Research, 1986a, b). The report points out certain problems inherent in any attempt to quantify nursing care: because of their origins as nurse staffing systems, most nursing patient classification systems are necessarily task oriented and thus do not measure many of the most important dimensions of professional nursing, such as assessment and evaluation. Some of the studies in this volume begin to address this lack. Bailie, for example, reports a study using Reitz's Nursing Intensity Index, which is based not on discrete nursing tasks, but on the nursing process, and includes planning, evaluation, psychosocial interaction, and patient education.

The ProPAC report concludes, however, that existing nursing classification systems are measures of nursing quantity, not quality. Yet, with the focus on cutting costs, increasing productivity, and reducing patients' length of stay, concerns about quality are mounting. To measure the quality of patient care, three "vaguely defined" but "crucial" variables must be considered: "(1) the assessment and evaluation of patient need; (2) the delivery of appropriate care; and (3) the outcome of these efforts from the perspective of the patient" (Health Economics Research, 1986b, p. 2-3). ProPAC's investigators caution that as efforts are made "to increase the productivity and efficiency of nursing care delivery . . . the possibility that cost-savings will be achieved at the expense of quality cannot be ruled out" (Health Economics Research, 1985b, pp. 2-3–2-4). Edwardson addresses this problem in this volume, reviewing strategies that can be used to make gains in productivity without trading off on quality. Thus, oversight of quality is rapidly becoming the major health issue today.

In our efforts to justify the importance, cost-effectiveness, and high quality of the care we provide, we may lose sight of the fact that the classification systems we use were originally derived as a means of estimating staffing needs. As Giovannetti notes in her assessment at the end of this book, the meaning, use, and validity of a patient classification system depend in large part on its intended purpose. Many studies published over the past several years have linked patient classification to costs per patient, costs per DRG, costs of an all-RN staff, or to nursing diagnosis or some measure of nursing quality. These preliminary studies are the first efforts at making the leap toward real, justifiable measures of nursing effectiveness and quality. The studies in *Patients and Purse Strings* continue in this vein nursing's efforts to "fine tune the data bases" to reveal nursing's contribution to patient care.

—F. A. S.

REFERENCES

Dahlen, A. J., & Gregor, J. R. (1985). Nursing costs by DRG with an all-RN staff. In F. A. Shaffer (Ed.) *Costing out nursing: Pricing our product* (pp. 113–122). New York: National League for Nursing.

DRGs and nursing care (1986). Kansas City, MO: American Nurses' Association.

Giovannetti, P. (1985). DRGs and nursing workload measures. *Computers in nursing, 3*(2), 88–91.

Health Economics Research (1986a). *An evaluation of Medicare's current method of allocating nursing costs and an examination of alternative approaches.* Unpublished report (Contract No. T-31415512 RFP-01-85-ProPAC), Prospective Payment Assessment Commission, Washington, D.C.

Health Economics Research (1986b). *Summary critique of literature related to allocating nursing costs, nursing skill level and quality of care, and the relationship between nursing intensity and patient's severity of illness.* Unpublished report (Contract No. T-31415512 RFP-01-ProPAC) Prospective Payment Assessment Commission, Washington, D.C.

Mitchell, M., Miller, J., Welches, L., & Walker, D. D. (1984). Determining cost of direct nursing care by DRGs. *Nursing Management, 15*(4), 29–32.

Riley, W., & Schaefers, V. (1983). Costing nursing services. *Nursing Management, 14* (12), 40–43.

Shaffer, F. A. (Ed.). (1985). *Costing out nursing: Pricing our product.* New York: National League for Nursing.

Thompson, J. D., & Diers, D. (1985). DRGs and nursing. *Nursing & Health Care, 6*(8), 434–439.

Walker, D. D. (1983). The cost of nursing care in hospitals. *Journal of Nursing Administration, 13*(3), 13–18.

Part 1
Developing and Testing Patient Classification Systems

Pitfalls of Using Patient Classification Systems for Costing Nursing Care

Marcel Dijkers, Teri Paradise, and Marylou Maxwell

Patient classification systems were developed for one primary purpose: staffing. As such, they are used to assign float personnel to the units most in need of staff or to admit new patients to the most overstaffed (or, more commonly, the least understaffed) units. A secondary traditional use of the information produced is for preparing budgets for the nursing department; the number of staff needed as well as the staffing mix is determined based on the expected census and patient mix. Additional uses have been suggested or implemented in selected hospitals: quality assurance, management reporting, charging for nursing care, and utilization review.

With the arrival of diagnosis related groups (DRGs), the interests of nursing managers have focused on determining the cost of nursing care. Nursing represents about 20 percent of the operating budget of the average hospital and an estimated 50 percent of "routine care" costs (Mason & Daugherty, 1984). Thus, the importance of a correct cost-finding methodology for nursing care hardly needs to be stressed. Nursing administrators and directors have been urged to develop mechanisms to determine the average cost per DRG in order to be better prepared to make decisions on what type of services the hospital should offer for what type of patients (Mason & Daugherty, 1984; Riley & Schaefers, 1983).

Several authors have suggested that a patient classification system offers a quantification of nursing care needs and as such is a natural starting point for determining cost of nursing care by DRG (Curtin, 1983; Nyberg

& Wolff, 1984). The method they propose is, in general, as follows: Determine the total direct cost of nursing care; allocate it to patients on the basis of their scores in the classification system—for example, patient care units (PCUs)—accumulated over their total length of stay; and add indirect ("overhead") cost (for example, for nursing administration), allocated on the basis of patient days or PCUs. The result is total nursing care cost by stay, which then can be averaged by DRG (Curtin, 1983; Staley and Luciano, 1984). A simplified example of this approach is presented in Table 1. (For applications of such a methodology, see Lagona & Stritzel, 1984; McClain & Selhat, 1984; Riley & Schaefers, 1983; Sovie, Tarcinale, VanPutte, & Stunden, 1985.)

Table 1
Calculation of Mean Cost of Nursing Care, by DRG:
Simplified Example of General Approach

Patient	PCUs on Day									Total PCUs	Total Days
	1	2	3	4	5	6	7	8	9		
A	15	20	23	19	19	16	14	5	—	131	8
B	13	25	24	20	18	16	10	8	4	138	9
C	8	14	10	5	—	—	—	—	—	37	4
D	7	15	11	12	7	4	—	—	—	56	6
Total										362	27

Total direct cost of nursing care	= $1,200	Direct cost per PCU:	$1,200 ÷ 362 =	$ 3.31
Total indirect cost of nursing care	= 500	Indirect cost per day:	$ 500 ÷ 27 =	$18.52
Total cost of nursing care	= $1,700			

	Direct costs	+ Indirect costs	= Total costs
	Total PCUs × Cost per PCU	Total Days × Cost per Day	
DRG I			
A	131 × $3.31 = $433.61	8 × $18.52 = $148.16	$ 581.77
B	138 × $3.31 = $456.78	9 × $18.52 = $166.68	623.46
Total			$1,205.23
Mean			$ 602.62
DRG II			
C	37 × $3.31 = $122.47	4 × $18.52 = $ 74.08	$ 196.55
D	36 × $3.31 = $185.36	6 × $18.52 = $111.12	296.48
Total			$ 493.03
Mean			$ 246.52

It would seem that these authors have overlooked several potential pitfalls that may result in erroneous cost data. There are two major problems: First, many patient classification systems do not really quantify the amount of nursing care needed by the patients being rated. Second, a properly designed patient classification system determines the amount of nursing care a patient *should* have, while costs ought to be based on the amount of care the patient *has* received or is likely to receive. Whenever there is a discrepancy between the two, patient classification cannot be used to estimate costs, unless one is willing to make some special assumptions.

We will discuss these and other problems connected with the use of patient classification information for costing and make suggestions on how the various pitfalls can be avoided in developing a costing method. Although all our hypothetical examples refer to estimating cost per DRG, the same issues have to be dealt with in developing estimates of cost per case by any other factor, such as third-party payer.

VARIETIES OF PATIENT CLASSIFICATION SYSTEMS

A patient classification system is a method of quantifying the need for nursing care required by individual patients. Patient classification means the "categorization of patients according to some assessment of their nursing care requirements over a specified period of time" (Giovannetti, 1979). Other terms used are "acuity system" and "(nursing) workload measurement system"; the latter is preferable as it clearly reflects the goal of the system. However, we will use the customary term, patient classification, in this paper.

Since the Joint Commission on Hospital Accreditation made patient classification a requirement in 1979 a virtual deluge of systems have been developed and presented in the literature. It seems that every hospital feels compelled to develop its own. Not surprisingly, there is great variation in approach and quality. Problems of reliability and validity have been addressed by others and will not be discussed here. With respect to the issue at hand—estimation of nursing care cost—the following two extreme types of classification systems may be distinguished:

1. Systems that only *rank order* patients with respect to the degree of care required, such as the Montefiore system (Jackson and Resnick, 1982). These are, in the most common terminology, "subjective" systems or "prototype evaluation" (Giovannetti, 1979).

2. Systems that directly *measure* nursing care needs in terms of hours of care required. These are the "objective" systems or "factor evaluation," such as GRASP in its many varieties (Meyer, 1978, 1981).

For those who remember their nursing research course, these two types correspond, respectively, to the ordinal and ratio scales of measurement. There are many systems that offer partial quantification and should be classified between these two extremes. The two types of classification systems and their implications for cost estimation are discussed in detail in the following sections.

Rank Ordering with Respect to Care Requirements

At the simplest level, the rank-ordering classification systems work as follows:

- Profiles are developed of three or more "typical" patients who differ in their nursing care needs, which range from minimal through maximal. Each profile mentions characteristics, such as the patient's capacities for activities of daily living, need for treatments and medications, and emotional and behavioral state. The profiles are numbered from 1, signifying the lowest level of need, through the number indicating the highest level in that system, commonly 4 or 5.

- Nurses are required to classify their patients by determining which of the profiles each patient most resembles. The number of the profile selected is taken to express the need for nursing care.

- The numbers of the profiles selected are added across all patients on a unit to determine the need for nursing staff compared to other units. Staff is assigned to units proportionally to each unit's summative scores.

The basic problem with such a system is that the numbers assigned to patients do not indicate absolute amounts of care required. Although a level 3 patient needs more care than a level 2 patient, there is no information about whether they need 6.6 hours and 4.4 hours, respectively, or 7.3 and 4.1 hours. As such, these systems are not suitable even as a basis for staffing decisions. Assigning hours of care to each level on the basis of expert judgment and/or time studies of samples of patients in each category, as is commonly done (see, for example, Burgher & Hanson, 1980; Johnson, 1984), improves the situation, but only marginally.

For an analysis of the cost of nursing, a system based on rank order has the same disadvantages as it has for staffing; if the relationship between level and hours of care is undetermined, then the relationship between level and cost of care is undetermined. Even if a realistic number of hours are assigned, the disadvantage remains that these classification systems generally use too few categories. A range of four or five categories is too limited to reflect the variability in intensity of care required by patients. Distortion will occur, especially at the upper extreme. Most systems group together in the highest category patients requiring anywhere from 12 hours through 24 hours of care per day, thus compressing the high range.

The problem of reducing variation is solved by systems that require the nurse to rate separately, by means of a profile, the need for each of several elements of care: diet, medications, behavior, and so forth (see, for example, Des Ormeaux, 1977). For each element, a range from 1 (minimal care) to 3 or 4 or 5 (maximum care) is possible. The subscores are added to obtain a total score. For instance, in a system that requires rating of six elements of care on a scale ranging from 1 (minimum) to 5 (maximum), the lowest possible score is 6, and the highest is 30.

Classification systems of this type still only rank order patients, however, and by themselves do not indicate the absolute amount of nursing care needed. In addition, the advantage of greater possible variation in scores is often negated by grouping, or categorizing, scores. That is, once scores have been assigned, they are categorized into a limited number of classes or levels, often indicated by roman numerals. For example, patients with 6 to 11 points are grouped into level I; those with 12 to 19 points into level II, and so on (Des Ormeaux, 1977). Other drawbacks are that all areas of care have the same weight (a score of 1 on diet is supposed to represent the same need for hours of care as a score of 1 on elimination), and that the maximum score in each area is the same. Thus, the most labor-intensive task in the area of elimination, for example, is assumed to take the same time as the most burdensome task in the area of treatment.

Some more sophisticated systems of the rank-order variety do use unequal weights for the elements of care and/or more variegated rankings within areas of care, which more faithfully reflect the hours of care required (Burgher & Hanson, 1980). As such, they begin to shade over into the second group of classification systems, those that actually measure hours of care.

Direct Measurement of Hours of Care

At the simplest level, the "factor evaluation" systems, such as GRASP methodology systems (Meyer, 1978, 1981), work as follows:

- The most frequently provided and/or the most time-consuming (direct care) nursing tasks are identified.
- The time needed, on the average, to perform each task is determined (by means of expert judgments, time studies, or other means).

- Time needed is multiplied by frequency of the task to obtain the total time per day or shift for each task.

- A "menu" is developed, listing these nursing activities and their duration, expressed in points, with each point representing a certain number of minutes (points are used in most systems to simplify the necessary arithmetic.)

- The nurse is required to classify her patients by determining which tasks on the "menu" each patient requires during that shift or day. The points for the items selected are added to obtain a total score.

- Scores are added across all patients on a unit to determine the need for nursing staff compared to other units. Staff are assigned to units proportionally to each unit's summative scores.

The nursing tasks that are not on the menu because they are required infrequently or take up minor amounts of time are assumed to be (for every patient) directly proportional to the tasks on the menu. In many systems, these "other" activities are taken into account in determining the points assigned to each task. Similarly, indirect care time is accounted for in some way. Consequently, in these systems the point total for every patient directly reflects the time units of nursing care the patient needs. At least in theory, a patient could receive no points, indicating that he or she needs no nursing care at all; at the other end of the spectrum, a point score indicating the need for 24 hours of continuous care per day should be possible. Because they measure directly hours of nursing care required, these systems are useful for staffing and also may be used for cost analysis.

The advantages of such direct measurement systems are also frequently thrown away by categorizing the scores into a limited number of levels. This is done to simplify the totaling of scores across patients for an entire unit. This manipulation undoes, to some degree, the link between point score and nursing care hours required and reduces the variability between patients. With computers more available to nursing units, and sometimes used directly for classification (by means of a screen providing the menus of nursing activities), this simplification should not be needed anymore. Even a simple calculator may be adequate to handle the numbers.

Our conclusion is that various types of patient classification systems vary in their usefulness for cost analysis of nursing care. Rank-ordering systems require additional studies or estimates of hours of care required by each rank, and are characterized by a restriction of variability that may be unacceptable in determining cost of nursing care. Direct measurement of hours of care provides ideal information, provided that the usefulness of this information is not reduced by categorization. Table 2 provides an example of the mean hours of care for one day for two DRGs, as determined by various hypothetical systems. The hours of care for DRG I vary from 69 to 80 percent of those of DRG II. Estimated *costs* should vary even more than suggested by these figures, given the fact that patients with a high acuity score generally require relatively more care from RNs, who are the more costly nursing resource (Meyer, 1981, p. 88).

CARE REQUIRED VERSUS CARE RECEIVED

A patient classification system used for staffing should quantify the amount of nursing care patients should be given to receive optimal care for their physical, emotional, and spiritual needs, in accordance with the standards of care of the hospital. When such a system is utilized for staffing or admitting, the aim is to use the total scores of nursing units to assign patients or personnel in such a way that all units have the same ratio of nursing care required to nursing care available. In this way, the burdens of understaffing and the joys of overstaffing are equally divided.

Understaffing seems to be the more common situation. In patient classification systems that directly measure hours of care required, there is a need to continuously remind the nurses doing classification that they must determine the nursing care the patients *need*, not the care they are likely to *get* because of lack of staff. Under conditions of understaffing, classifying according to the care the patient is likely to receive results in continued understaffing of the unit, because it affirms the status quo. Similarly, nursing administration has to guard against floor nurses "over-classifying" patients, as this falsifies the competition between units for additional personnel and exaggerates the gap between nursing resources available and required.

Although staffing should be determined on the basis of care needed, determination of the cost of nursing care should be based not on the care *needed*, but on the care actually *rendered*. If, over the course of a hospital stay, a patient is classified to require a total of 220 hours of care, but only receives 170 hours as a result of understaffing, then hours of care required are an inadequate basis for an estimate of actual cost. If understaffing is uniform across units or patient diagnoses, a simple adjustment can be made to arrive at accurate cost-of-care estimates. If understaffing is not uniform—that is, the ratio of care required to care available differs between patients in two different DRGs—care required is not an adequate basis for estimating nursing care costs. Most authors who propose using a patient classification system to derive cost estimates

Table 2
Mean Hours of Nursing Care for Two DRGs as Determined by Various Patient Classification Systems

Patient	Simple Ranking System[a]	Assigned Hours of Care[b,c]		Complex Ranking System[d]	Assigned Hours of Care[e]	Categories 1[f]	Assigned Hours of Care[g]	Categories 2[h]	Assigned Hours of Care[i]
		1	2						
DRG I									
A	1	2.25	3.25	8	2.66	I	3.20	I	2.80
B	1	2.25	3.25	10	3.33	I	3.20	I	2.80
C	2	4.90	6.15	18	6.00	II	6.50	III	8.20
D	3	7.25	7.50	27	9.00	III	10.70	IV	10.15
E	3	7.25	7.50	24	8.00	III	10.70	IV	10.15
F	3	7.25	7.50	30	10.00	III	10.70	V	13.20
G	2	4.90	6.15	20	6.66	II	6.50	III	8.20
H	1	2.25	3.25	9	3.00	I	3.20	I	2.80
Total	—	38.30	44.55	—	48.65	—	54.70	—	58.30
Mean	—	4.79	5.57	—	6.08	—	6.84	—	7.29
DRG II									
I	2	4.90	6.15	20	6.66	II	6.50	III	8.20
J	2	4.90	6.15	23	7.67	II	6.50	IV	10.15
K	3	7.25	7.50	30	10.00	III	10.70	V	13.20
L	4	11.30	8.75	32	10.67	III	10.70	V	13.20
M	3	7.25	7.50	27	9.00	III	10.70	IV	10.15
N	2	4.90	6.15	21	7.00	II	6.50	III	8.20
Total	—	40.50	42.20	—	51.00	—	51.60	—	63.10
Mean	—	6.75	7.03	—	8.50	—	8.60	—	10.52
Mean of DRG I as a percentage of mean of DRG II		71	79		72		80		69

[a] Simple ranking system, four categories ranging from 1, minimal nursing care needs, to 4, very high needs.

[b,c] Hours of nursing care required by each category (a) assigned by expert judgment:

Category	Hours—1	Hours—2
1	2.25	3.25
2	4.90	6.15
3	7.25	7.50
4	11.30	8.75

[d] Complex ranking system, scores ranging from 8 (score of 1 in eight areas) to 32 (score of 4 in eight areas).

[e] Hours of nursing care required assigned by expert judgment: 20 minutes per point in the complex ranking system (d).

[f,g] Categories derived from total point score in complex ranking system (d) with three categories. Hours of care required assigned by averaging hours assigned in (e) over patients classified in category.

Points	Category	Hours
8–16	I	3.20
17–23	II	6.50
24–32	III	10.70

[h,i] Categories derived from total point score in complex ranking system (d) with five categories. Hours of care required assigned by averaging hours assigned in (e) over patients in category.

Points	Category	Hours
8–12	I	2.80
13–17	II	5.35
18–22	III	8.20
23–27	IV	10.15
28–32	V	13.20

seem to overlook this issue, with the exception of Curtin (1983) and Grimaldi and Micheletti (1982). The discrepancy between care needed and care received is even more important in instances where the classification system is used as a basis for billing for nursing care, as has been proposed and implemented in a few instances (see, for example, Ethridge, 1985).

The significance of the discrepancy between hours of care needed and hours of care provided, and the resulting problems of cost allocation, depend on the nature of the discrepancy (shortfall or oversupply of staff), its relative size, and especially whether it is constant across patients. If there is *more* staff than needed, the patient presumably will receive the care needed and not more. (It would do the patient no good, for example, to be catheterized every two hours and might do him or her some harm). In this instance, the cost of *necessary* care can be determined by multiplying hours needed by cost per hour. (The *actual* cost to the hospital is higher: the cost of the surplus personnel carried should be accounted for, and probably should be allocated to the cost of individual stays in some fashion.)

If there is *less* staff than needed, using the classification system's points or PCUs to determine nursing care costs would result in an overestimate of costs. Corrections for this could be made easily, provided that it can be assumed that the nursing care hours shortfall is distributed equally over all patients. However, we do not have the facts to support this assumption.

Limited research information is available on what actually happens if there is less staff than needed. What nurses say is that some tasks are dropped (charting, teaching, certain observations deemed not essential), and that others are curtailed by providing just the physical care and not the emotional care or social support called for in the hospital's standards of nursing care. One study (Chagnon, Audette, Lebrun, & Tilquin, 1978) provides data supporting the notion that in case of a staff shortage, low-priority tasks are dropped. It is unclear what the result is in terms of nursing care hours received by various categories of patients. Is the amount of care given to each patient reduced by the same percentage, so that everybody gets 75 percent or 83 percent of the care needed? Or is the care reduced by a fixed number of hours, so that everyone gets 0.75 or 1.33 hours less than required? Alternatively, it is possible that care is reduced by a fixed or proportional number of hours, with a limit as to the minimum number of hours each patient gets. Reality may be even more complex, with different "floors" used for patients who need varying qualities or quantities of nursing care.

All these possibilities of bridging the gap between hours of care needed and hours available have different implications for cost estimates, as illustrated in Table 3. This example assumes that on a given day, the available full-time equivalent staff are only 80 percent of the staff actually needed. Depending on the patient's acuity and on which scheme for distributing available nursing care is found to be operating, nursing care given as a percentage of care required varies from 62 to 87 percent. DRGs vary in their average length of stay and in the mean quantity of nursing care required per day. Consequently, a deficit of nursing care hours available cannot be assumed to leave analysis of cost per DRG unaffected.

Only if it can be assumed that in case of staff shortages the amount of care given to *all* patients is reduced by the *same* percentage is a discrepancy between care needed and care rendered unimportant for purposes of cost analysis. In all other approaches for dividing scarce nursing resources over patients, disregarding the gap between hours available and hours needed results in distortions of cost estimates. How large these distortions are depends on the size of the discrepancy.

TYPES OF NURSING PERSONNEL

Most patient classification systems do not consider the level of preparation of the nurse providing the care. A few systems do assign tasks to an RN, LPN, or nursing aide or require the person doing classification to specify the level required for each particular task for a certain patient. These systems, such as the Providence Hospital System (Meyer, 1981, p. 62), provide a numerical indication of the need (by patient or by nursing unit) for each of the three types of personnel. Alternative approaches are possible, for example, deriving required numbers of personnel of each skill level from tabulation of the total number of patients in each acuity level by means of conversion tables (Torrez, 1983). And of course, with all-RN staffing the issue does not present itself.

Most systems disregard the preferred or required level of preparation of the nurse, because it would make the system too complicated, or because staffing decisions cannot take the results into account. It is difficult to assign .47 RN, .38 LPN, and .29 nursing aide from floating staff; most hospitals will assign one RN or LPN, if available.

Disregarding the type or level of personnel may have serious implications for cost finding, however. Most units do not have the same staffing mix, and experience indicates that not all patients on a particular unit receive their needed care from the same mix. Generally, the higher the acuity score, the more hours of RN care, absolutely and relatively, the patient requires. For instance, intensive care units often are staffed entirely by RNs. There may be factors other than acuity that determine skill mix—for example, the need for specialized nursing expertise. It is

Table 3
Nursing Care Actually Given as a Percentage of Required Care under Four Schemes for Distributing Available Nursing Personnel in Case of Short Staffing

Patient	Hours Required per Day	Scheme 1: Equal Percentage		Scheme 2: Equal Amount of Time		Scheme 3: Equal Percentage, with Floor		Scheme 4: Equal Amount of Time, with Floor	
		Actual Hours [a]	% of Required Hours [b]	Actual Hours [c]	% of Required Hours	Actual Hours [d]	% of Required Hours	Actual Hours [e]	% of Required Hours
A	3.45	2.75	80	2.14	62	3.00	87	3.00	87
B	6.50	5.18	80	5.19	80	5.14	79	5.02	77
C	4.95	3.95	80	3.64	74	3.92	79	3.47	70
D	8.15	6.50	80	6.84	84	6.45	79	6.66	82
E	4.30	3.43	80	2.99	70	3.41	79	3.00	70
F	8.35	6.66	80	7.04	84	6.61	79	6.87	82
G	9.45	7.53	80	8.14	86	7.48	79	7.97	84
Total	45.15	36.00	80	36.00	80	36.01	80	35.99	80
Mean	6.45	5.14	80	5.14	80	5.14	80	5.14	80

[a] Hours of nursing care delivered, if only 80 percent (36 out of 45 hours) of the nursing care required is available, and each patient's care is reduced by the same percentage.

[b] Percentage of care required that is made available under Scheme 1.

[c] Hours of nursing care delivered if only 80 percent of the nursing care required is available, and each patient's care is reduced by the same amount of time (1.31 hours).

[d] Same as Scheme 1 (a), but no patient receives less than 3.00 hours of care.

[e] Same as Scheme 2 (c), but no patient receives less than 3.00 hours of care.

worth investigating whether skill mix varies among patients and if it is related to acuity or other factors that vary with DRG classification (Vanderzee & Glusko, 1984).

Table 4 gives an example of the cost of nursing care per patient per day for two DRGs, determined with and without differentiation of the cost of levels of care. For those patients (or groups of patients, such as those assigned to the same DRG) who receive care from a skill mix that is similar to the skill mix of the unit or department (here 30 percent RN, 30 percent LPN, and 40 percent aide), method does not make much of a difference, as can be seen with patients G and K in the table. The more the skill mix for a patient (or for a DRG) differs from the skill mix on the unit, the larger the discrepancy between the cost of care as calculated according to the two methods.

The issue of skill mix is important to the degree that (1) labor costs of RNs, LPNs, aides, and other nursing personnel vary from one to another; and (2) the skill mix of caregivers varies among patients and is related to DRG.

DIRECT AND INDIRECT COSTS

Another factor determining the importance of a staff shortage for nursing costs is the ratio of direct to indirect costs. Indirect costs refer to the costs of tasks performed by nursing department personnel that are not assignable to a particular patient (Riley & Schaefers, 1983). This includes activities such as nursing administration, staff development, and recruiting at the department level and activities of head nurses and unit secretaries or clerks at the unit level. Direct costs are the costs associated with services to a particular patient, whether it is direct care (hands-on contact with the patient) or indirect care.

The ratio of direct to indirect costs may vary from one hospital to another. It depends on how patient care is organized as well as a number of other factors. Riley and Schaefers (1983) calculated the following percentages of total costs (for a tertiary teaching hospital):

Direct costs:	60 percent
Indirect costs—unit level:	30 percent
Indirect costs—department level:	10 percent

The larger the proportion of the total costs that is indirect, the less important is the discrepancy between hours of care needed and available. However, the larger the proportion the indirect costs constitute, the more important the proper allocation of these indirect costs becomes for accurate cost finding.

Three different methods of allocating indirect costs are possible, and

Table 4
Mean Nursing Cost for Two DRGs, with and without Differentiation of Skill Level of Nursing Staff

Patient	Hours of Care Provided	RN		LPN		Aide		Total Cost[c]	Cost Based on Average Hourly Rate[d]	Ratio of Costs[e]
		Hours[a]	Cost[b]	Hours[a]	Cost[b]	Hours[a]	Cost[b]			
DRG I										
A	4.15	0.83	$ 11.93	1.04	$ 10.76	2.28	$ 18.55	$ 41.24	$ 44.30	93
B	6.80	2.04	29.33	2.04	21.17	2.72	22.10	72.59	72.59	100
C	5.30	1.06	15.24	1.33	13.75	2.92	23.68	52.67	56.58	93
D	9.10	3.64	52.33	3.19	33.04	2.28	18.48	103.85	97.14	107
E	8.10	3.24	46.58	2.84	29.41	2.03	16.45	92.44	86.47	107
F	10.70	5.35	76.91	4.28	44.41	1.07	8.69	130.01	114.22	114
G	7.55	2.27	32.56	2.27	23.50	3.02	24.54	80.60	80.60	100
Total	51.70	18.43	$264.86	16.97	$176.04	16.31	$132.50	$573.40	$551.90	104
Mean	7.39	2.63	37.84	2.42	25.15	2.33	18.93	81.91	78.84	104
DRG II										
H	4.75	0.95	$ 13.66	1.19	$ 12.32	2.61	$ 21.23	$ 47.20	$ 50.71	93
I	3.15	0.32	4.53	0.63	6.54	2.21	17.92	28.98	33.63	86
J	5.30	1.06	15.24	1.33	13.75	2.92	23.68	52.67	56.58	93
K	3.05	0.92	13.15	0.92	9.49	1.22	9.91	32.56	32.56	100
L	2.80	0.28	4.03	0.56	5.81	1.96	15.93	25.76	29.89	86
Total	19.05	3.52	$ 50.60	4.62	$ 47.91	10.91	$ 88.66	$187.17	$203.36	92
Mean	3.81	0.70	10.12	0.92	9.58	2.18	17.73	37.43	40.67	92

a It is assumed that the percentage of care provided by each level of nursing personnel varies by patient acuity, as follows:

Hours of Care Required	Percentage of Care Provided		
	RN	LPN	NA
2–4	10	20	70
4–6	20	25	55
6–8	30	30	40
8–10	40	35	25
10–12	50	40	10

b Salary and fringe benefits (25 percent of salary) of each level of personnel:

RN: $11.50 + $2.88 = $14.38
LPN: 8.30 + 2.08 = 10.38
NA: 6.50 + 1.63 = 8.13

c Total of costs for RN, LPN, and aide. Represents cost of care determined while differentiating skill mix.

d Assuming a skill mix on the unit of 30 percent RN, 30 percent LPN, and 40 percent nursing aide, the average salary and fringe benefits can be calculated at $10.675 per hour. This column represents cost of care as calculated based on the average cost of nursing care per hour, without skill mix differentiation.

e Ratio of cost of care calculated with skill mix differentiation to cost calculated with average cost per hour figure (without skill mix differentiation).

a hospital may decide to use one, two, or all of them, for the total of the indirect costs or for its various parts: (1) divide indirect costs equally over all admissions; (2) allocate indirect costs in proportion to length of stay; and (3) allocate indirect costs in proportion to classification scores or nursing care hours received, cumulated over the entire stay.

Costs that are more or less the same for each patient, independent of length of stay or intensity of care, such as the cost of the admitting kit, may be divided equally over admissions. Most or all personnel costs would more appropriately be allocated on the basis of the patients' total days in the hospital and/or the total nursing care hours received (direct costs). For example, the unit clerk performs many functions for all patients on a unit as a group, such as totaling classification points to determine hours of care needed for the unit as a whole. Other tasks are done, more or less in proportion to direct care hours, for a particular patient—for example, processing laboratory orders; the higher a patient's acuity score, the more orders have to be processed for him or her. The costs of these activities are best allocated on the basis of PCUs or patient care hours needed.

Table 5 gives a hypothetical example of the effect on the total nursing care costs of allocating indirect costs in relation to days or hours. (It is unlikely that a substantial part of indirect costs will be allocated according to stays). These figures indicate that choice of method can make a substantial difference in cost estimates. The effects are most pronounced for patients and groups of patients with extremely high and extremely low average nursing hours per day.

If and when it is decided that part or all of the indirect costs are best allocated based on the direct care costs, the issue of distortions of cost finding due to understaffing or overstaffing becomes prominent once more, because a larger percentage of the total nursing department costs are allocated based on erroneous assumptions.

CONCLUSION

It is very attractive to nursing administrators to use an existing system—patient classification—as the basis for estimating costs of nursing care. It saves the time and expense of developing and implementing a special mechanism for costing information. In addition, the results can be used to justify costs, on the basis of care needed. The importance of an accurate and valid system for allocating nursing costs is obvious: about 20 percent of the average hospital's operating budget is spent on nursing care, and the need for care varies greatly between categories of patients. Within general units, the most labor-intensive patients may require five

Table 5
Mean Nursing Care Cost for Two DRGs Using Two Methods of Allocating Indirect Costs

Patient	Length of Stay (days)	Hours of Nursing Care	Hours of Nursing Care per Day	Direct Costs[a]	Indirect Costs Allocated in Proportion to:[b]		Total Costs Based on Allocation to:[c]		Ratio of Total Costs[d]
					Length of Stay	Hours of Care	Length of Stay	Hours of Care	
DRG I									
A	4	20.5	5.1	$ 218.74	$ 111.36	$ 93.74	$ 330.10	$ 312.48	95
B	5	67.5	13.5	720.23	139.20	308.67	859.43	1,028.89	120
C	6	24.5	4.1	261.42	167.04	112.04	428.46	373.45	87
D	13	96.4	7.4	1,028.59	361.93	440.82	1,390.52	1,469.41	106
E	8	60.5	7.6	645.54	222.73	276.66	868.26	922.19	106
F	9	44.3	4.9	472.68	250.57	202.58	723.25	675.26	93
Total	45	313.7	—	$3,347.18	$1,252.83	$1,434.51	$4,600.01	$4,781.68	104
Mean	7.5	52.3	7.0	557.86	208.81	239.08	766.67	796.95	104
DRG II									
G	4	27.5	6.8	$ 293.43	$ 111.36	$ 125.75	$ 419.18	$ 419.18	104
H	3	11.8	3.9	125.91	83.52	53.96	209.43	179.87	86
I	5	17.7	3.5	188.86	139.20	80.94	328.06	269.80	82
J	6	22.1	3.7	235.81	167.04	101.06	402.85	336.87	84
K	5	21.2	4.2	226.20	139.20	96.94	365.41	323.15	88
Total	23	100.3	—	$1,070.20	$ 640.33	$ 458.66	$1,528.86	$1,528.86	89
Mean	4.6	20.1	4.4	214.04	128.07	91.73	342.10	305.77	89
Grand total	68	414.0	—	$4,417.38	$1,893.16	$1,893.16	$6,310.54	$6,310.54	100
Grand mean	6.2	37.6	6.1	401.58	172.11	172.11	573.69	573.69	100

a Using a cost per hour (including fringe benefits) of $10.67.

b Indirect costs of $1,893.16 (assumed to be 30 percent of total costs) are allocated to patients or DRGs in proportion to length of stay in days and hours of nursing care received, respectively.

c Total cost calculated as sum of direct costs (d) and indirect costs, (e) or (f).

d Ratio of total costs, calculated using allocation in proportion to length of stay, to total costs, calculated using allocation in proportion to hours of nursing care received.

times as much nursing care as those with the lowest acuity; the ratio becomes even larger if intensive care unit patients are considered too.

It should be realized, however, that not all patient classification systems are appropriate for the purpose of estimating costs, and some are not even appropriate for staffing. In addition, certain assumptions are made, knowingly or unknowingly, with respect to what happens if there is a shortage of nursing staff. Depending on the size of the shortage and the realism of the assumptions made, cost estimates derived from a classification system may have systematic errors that limit their usefulness.

Given the correct data on cost of direct care per hour, indirect costs, hours of care required by each patient, total hours of care rendered by the unit or department, and so forth, it is possible to explore the implications of different assumptions. Various allocation schedules can be compared to determine whether a particular assumption makes a significant difference in estimated costs. Microcomputer spreadsheet programs are an ideal tool for exploring the implications of various assumptions and estimating the impact on mean cost by DRG. If the differences in costs are relatively minor, it does not matter which scheme is used, and the assumptions that result in the simplest method of estimating costs should be used. If there are significant differences, research can be done to determine which assumption reflects most closely the actual state of affairs in the hospital involved.

The tables included in this paper presented not extreme situations, but not unrealistic ones that might occur in an average hospital. An issue not explored is whether the various potential distortions of costs will tend to cancel one another out or build upon one another, although we have pointed out where the issues are related. Further explorations of these and other pitfalls in using patient classification systems for costing nursing care are needed.

REFERENCES

Burgher, D., & Hanson, R. L. (1980, May–June). Patient classification for nurse staffing in rehabilitation. *Association of Rehabilitation Nurses Journal*, 5(3), 16–20.

Chagnon, M., Audette, L. M., Lebrun, L. G., & Tilquin, C. (1978, June). Validation of patient classification through evaluation of the nursing staff degree of occupation. *Medical Care*, 16(6), 465–475.

Curtin, L. (1983, April). Determining costs of nursing services per DRG. *Nursing Management*, 14(4), 16–20.

Des Ormeaux, S. P. (1977, April). Implementation of the C.A.S.H. patient classification system for staffing determination. *Supervisor Nurse*, 8, 29–35.

Ethridge, P. (1985, August). The case for billing by patient acuity. *Nursing Management, 16*(8), 38–41.

Giovannetti, P. (1979, February). Understanding patient classification systems. *Journal of Nursing Administration, 9*(2), 4–9.

Grimaldi, P. L., & Micheletti, J. A. (1982, December). DRG reimbursement: RIMs and the cost of nursing care. *Nursing Management, 13*(12), 12–22.

Jackson, B. S., & Resnick, J. (1982, December). Comparing classification systems. *Nursing Management, 13*(1), 13–19.

Johnson, K. (1984, June). A practical approach to patient classification. *Nursing Management, 15*(6), 39–46.

Lagona, T. G., & Stritzel, M. M. (1984, May). Nursing care requirements as measured by DRG. *Journal of Nursing Administration, 14*(5), 15–18.

Mason, E. J. & Daugherty, J. K. (1984, September). Nursing standards should determine nursing's price. *Nursing Management, 15*(9), 34–38.

McClain, J. R., & Selhat, M. S. (1984, October). Twenty cases: What nursing costs per DRG. *Nursing Management, 15*(10), 27–34.

Meyer, D. (1978). *GRASP: A patient information and workload management system.* Morgantown, NC: MCS Publications.

Meyer, D. (1981). *GRASP TOO: Applications and adaptations of the GRASP nursing workload management system.* Morgantown, NC: MCS Publications.

Nyberg, J., & Wolff, N. (1984, April). DRG panic. *Journal of Nursing Administration, 14*(4), 17–26.

Riley, W., & Schaefers, V. (1983, September). Costing nursing services. *Nursing Management, 14*(12), 40–43.

Sovie, M. D., Tarcinale, M. A., VanPutte, A. W., & Stunden, A. (1985, March). Amalgam of nursing acuity, DRGs and costs. *Nursing Management, 16*(3), 22–42. Reprinted in this volume, pp. 121–148.

Staley, M., & Luciano, K. (1984, October). Eight steps to costing nursing service. *Nursing Management, 15*(10), 35–38.

Torrez, M. R. (1983, May). Systems approach to staffing. *Nursing Management, 14*(5), 54–58.

Vanderzee, H., & Glusko, G. (1984, May). DRGs, variable pricing, and budgeting for nursing services. *Journal of Nursing Administration, 14*(5), 11–14.

The Credibility of Patient Classification Instruments

Deborah Kaspar

The term patient classification has been tossed around by many disciplines and used for very diverse purposes. For the purpose of nurse staffing, patient classification can be defined as the grouping of patients into a predetermined number of separate and identifiable groups that are homogenous with respect to their requirements for nursing care. Patient classification instruments have become one of the most frequently used vehicles for explicating the nursing costs per patient; it is important, therefore, to explore the credibility of these instruments. Two issues of primary importance are the extent to which we have evidence of the instruments' reliability and validity.

Terms such as *direct costs*, *indirect costs*, *reducing*, *relating*, and *comparing costs* pepper the vocabulary of nursing today, but are we talking the same language? This emphasis on costs draws us naturally to the bottom line and allows us to assume that we can talk about nursing costs generically. This assumption is unwise, since too many differences in meaning and too many problems in measurement remain. This paper will identify some of the differences in meaning and offer practical solutions to some of the problems in measurement. If such differences can be clarified, we will be able to make more meaningful cost comparisons and proceed to identify more efficient and effective means of satisfying patients' care requirements.

There are literally hundreds of patient classification systems in use today. The majority of patient classification instruments are derivations of either prototype or factor-type evaluation systems (Giovannetti, 1979).

Prototype systems rate patients on an ordinal scale by level of care required, while the factor-type systems list specific elements of care on which to base patients' rating. Many nursing departments are inclined to choose between the two types based on the proclaimed merits of one or to avoid past problems associated with the other. Neither type has proven to be more effective; the choice appears to be a matter of preference. Not infrequently, the selected tool is customized for a particular institution or individual nursing unit through modification in format or content. The result has been a proliferation of patient classification instruments. Since the instruments generate the data used to direct nurse staffing decisions and calculate nursing costs, some fundamental questions must be raised regarding their degree of reliability and validity.

RELIABILITY

Reliability is an estimate of the consistency or repeatability of a measure. The reliability of a patient classification instrument is a measure of the consistency of the instrument in grouping patients with similar requirements for nursing care time. There are many types of reliability and various statistical approaches for the measurement of each type. Every measurement has an error component that "may be due to numerous factors, such as those associated with the subjects themselves (e.g., fatigue), the instrument (e.g., poor wording of items), and/or the administration of the measure (e.g., unclear instructions or unrealistic time constraints)" (Goodwin & Prescott, 1981, p. 324). The goal of instrument development is to minimize error.

Interrater reliability is used whenever ratings or judgments are made about the activities or behaviors of subjects. Since patient classification instruments for nurse staffing require the use of raters or judges, the measurement of interrater reliability is important. The percentage of agreement among raters is a frequently used statistical approach that is especially suited for determining the interrater reliability of categorical data (Goodwin & Prescott, 1981). This approach expresses reliability as the number of times the raters or judges agree compared to the total number of observations made:

$$\frac{\text{Number of agreements}}{\text{Total number of observations}}$$

Agreement in this approach is an absolute; ratings are either in agreement or disagreement (Tinsley & Weiss, 1975). The advantages of percentage of agreement as an approach to reliability include ease of calculation and interpretation. Disadvantages include the all-or-none fashion of measuring agreement and the fact that it ignores chance agreement. The kappa statistic, K, may be more appropriate because it corrects for chance (Tinsley & Weiss, 1975). K is calculated as follows:

$$K = \frac{P_0 - P_C}{1 - P_C}$$

where P_0 is the proportion of ratings in which the two judges agree, and P_C is the proportion of ratings for which agreement is expected by chance. A K of 0 indicates that the observed agreement is exactly equal to the agreement that could be expected by chance. A negative value of K between -1.0 and 0 indicates the observed agreement is less than the agreement expected by chance, and a K of $+1.0$ indicates perfect agreement between raters. There seems to be a consensus among researchers who use percentage of agreement that 65 percent represents minimum acceptable agreement. (Guttman, Spector, Sigal, Rakoff, & Epstein, 1971). This author finds 85 to 90 percent agreement by category a more acceptable standard.

There are several other approaches for assessing interrater reliability, including correlational techniques, comparisons of means, and generalizability theory techniques. A researcher should select or use the approach that will yield the amount and type of information considered appropriate to measure the interrater reliability of an instrument. Irrespective of the particular statistical approach used, a reliability coefficient for an instrument is specific to a particular group of subjects and a given set of conditions. The reliability estimate obtained in one study does not apply to all uses of an instrument and does not remain stable over time (Goodwin and Prescott, 1981). Therefore, interrater reliability must be measured on an ongoing basis. It is for this reason in particular that the percentage of agreement method is commonly employed. The approach is readily understood and easily performed. It can be checked and rechecked on a regular basis, monthly or at least quarterly. The accuracy of the final outcomes (in this case, accuracy of nursing costs) depends heavily on the credibility of the measures used.

VALIDITY

Another measure of equal importance to reliability in determining the credibility of a measure is the measurement or assessment of validity. Validity addresses the question of whether a classification instrument accurately measures what it is intended to measure. This question must be separated into two components: (1) the component that classifies the patient, and (2) the component that assigns hours of care to each category (Chagnon, Audette, Lebrun, & Tilquin, 1978). Each has its own validity requirements.

Too often, as various classification instruments are obtained and evaluated for use within an institution, questions of validity remain unchecked. Often this lack is based on certain erroneous assumptions; for example, that if an instrument looks impressive in terms of format or appears to include the necessary or relevant items it can accurately classify patients; that altering an instrument's format, indicators, or the wording of indicators does not affect the overall functioning of the instrument; or that if an instrument was used elsewhere, then it must "work." Moreover, additions, modifications, and deletions often are made in an instrument so that, in the user's eyes, it more accurately reflects the kinds of patients found on a particular unit and the kinds of activities that occupy nurses' time. However, if evidence of the validity of the instrument was demonstrated when it was first developed (and frequently validity has not been tested), such subsequent changes could invalidate it.

How then can the validity of an instrument's indicators and scheme (patient categories) be determined? Cronbach and Meehl (1955) divide validity studies into four different categories: predictive validity, concurrent validity, content validity, and construct validity. Concurrent validity is the approach used most often to evaluate a classification scheme (Chagnon et al., 1978). For example, the categorization of a sample of patients according to one classification instrument can be compared with the categories obtained by using another classification instrument with the same patients. This approach is not as easy as it appears, however, because the tool used for comparison must itself have initially been validated.

Another approach is to compare the categorization of a sample of patients obtained from an instrument with the subjective opinions of experienced nurses. The nurses are asked to identify groups of similar patients on a continuum from "minimal care" to "complete care." A comparison is then made between the classifications of patients subjectively rated as needing minimal, moderate, or complete care and the classifications resulting from the instrument in question. Subjective classification, however, has not proven to be very reliable (Giovannetti, Mainguy, Smith, & Truitt, 1970).

Finally, a panel of experts could be asked to evaluate the instrument and a comparison could be made of the categories they identify with those determined by the instrument. This approach takes a certain amount of time and money, depending upon how much agreement there is between the experts' responses and the groups specified by the instrument.

Although user acceptability is an important criterion for patient classification instruments, this explanation of the need for evidence of validity should serve as a deterrent to the endless unvalidated revisions that are made on such instruments. Research studies have identified critical indicators that can be used to distinguish between groups of patients. Using these research findings and previously validated instruments, validational studies could be performed across hospitals using just a few instruments, such as a prototype and a factor type. Time and money could then be spent on the second component of the validity question regarding the assignment of hours of care to each category. Hours of care represent the nursing hours required to care for each category of patient each shift. The hours of care per category multiplied by the number of patients in each category provide the basis for staffing decisions. How well the actual staffing matches the hours of care required indicates how an institution will be able to manage the cost-containment efforts it needs to see it into the future.

HOURS OF CARE

The rhetoric of the 1970s was "cost containment," while the reality of the 1980s is "margin." Dollars must be available after expenses in order to fund the future. Consequently, one issue paramount to nursing in the 1980s is productivity—labor productivity, to be more exact. Productivity can be simply defined as the relationship between inputs, outputs, and quality. Therefore, an improvement in productivity is any action that favorably affects the ratio of inputs to outputs while maintaining or improving quality.

The inputs for nursing are usually defined in terms of nursing hours, while the outputs are generally considered patient days, admissions, adjusted admissions, or diagnosis related groups (DRGs). It is important to note that inputs represent resources, not expenses, and outputs represent services, not revenue. Dollars place a *value* on a resource or service, and value is not considered in the productivity equation. The use of nursing care patient classification data creates a further level of detail that makes the analysis of the input-output equation more meaningful, as shown in the following equation:

$$\frac{\text{Actual nursing hours}}{\text{Patient classification hours of care}}$$

$$+ \frac{\text{Patient classification hours of care}}{\text{DRG}} = \frac{\text{Actual nursing hours}}{\text{DRG}}$$

The ratio of actual nursing hours to patient classification hours of care is a measure of *efficiency*—how closely the actual nursing hours worked correspond to the nursing hours required according to the patient classifications. This measure reflects the manager's ability to adjust staffing according to the fluctuations in patients' requirements for nursing care.

The ratio of patient classification hours of care to DRG is a measure of *effectiveness*. This ratio shows the relationship between an input (patient classification hours of care) and an output (DRG). A manager might be very efficient at ensuring that the actual nursing hours worked correspond to those required by the patient classifications, but the hospital's viability might still be threatened because the nursing hours exceed the revenue allocated per DRG.

The ratio of actual nursing hours to DRG, a resource measure, is the most encompassing productivity measure, because it relates an input (nursing hours) to an output (DRG) that has value. It is important that the inputs and outputs have value, even though value is not considered in a productivity analysis. Value is considered later in a financial analysis, however, when dollars are attached to inputs or outputs in order to determine the "bottom line" or "margin" for an institution.

The hours of care per category of patient are influenced by many factors, such as types of patients, nursing care delivery styles, physician practice patterns, plant layout, and ancillary support systems to mention only a few. Therefore, the hours of nursing care assigned to each category cannot be transferred from one institution to another (Giovannetti, 1979). Thus, institutions that adopt standards developed in other institutions have no evidence of the validity of their system. Yet these systems are used to generate data for allocation of staff, budgeting, productivity monitoring, and cost accounting. Each institution must address the validity of the system used to calculate hours of care per category of patient. The decision regarding which approach to use to calculate hours of care and provide an analysis of nursing activities is usually based on such factors as time, cost, level of confidence required, user acceptability, and compatability with professional nursing practice. Several approaches and combinations of approaches are used today, although they are basically of three types: negotiation, standardization, and observation.

Standards established through negotiation are either based on the intuitive judgments of professionals or are derived as ratios from budget figures. Both methods lack a statistical basis for making inferences. Use of standardized data violates the basic premise that hours of care are not transferable. The remaining approach is the observational study, of which there are primarily three types: time-and-frequency studies, work-sampling studies, and direct patient care sampling studies.

Time-and-frequency studies identify the tasks nurses perform, the frequency with which they are performed, and the time it takes to perform each task. Since nurses frequently perform more than one task or activity at a time and usually do not have the prerogative of distributing these required tasks evenly over the course of a shift, the work-sampling approach is often considered more representative than the time-and-frequency approach. Direct patient care sampling studies involve periodic observations of patients to record whether or not staff are present. These studies are used to determine the average minutes of direct care per category of patient per shift.

WORK SAMPLING:
THE SAN JOAQUIN METHODOLOGY

Research conducted at San Joaquin General Hospital in Bakersfield, California (Murphy, Dunlap, Williams, & McAthnie, 1978) serves as one model of the work-sampling and direct care care types of studies. These approaches involve recording observations of patients and staff at specified intervals to determine the average minutes of direct care provided to patients and the percentage of staff time spent in direct care, indirect care, unit-related activities, and personal activities. The average minutes of direct care per patient category per shift are divided by the percentage of staff time spent in direct care on each shift in order to derive the staffing coefficients or hours-or-care standards.

The San Joaquin methodology for quantifying the patient classification system has been replicated by many institutions and consulting firms and is considered by many experts as a state-of-the-art approach. However, various loopholes in the validity of the methodology have been created as it has been adapted and used by others.

For example, the direct patient care sampling approach captures the amount (average minutes) of direct care provided to various categories of patients. Underlying this approach is the assumption that the nurses are providing the care that patients require. A Unit Staffing/Care Evaluation Questionnaire is utilized to check that assumption by eliciting the head nurse's perception of the adequacy of staffing for a given workload (patient mix) on each shift of data collection. However, although what a professional nurse does for or with a patient is a good indicator of a patient's requirements for care, it is important to recognize that the time it takes the nurse to deliver that care is a function of his or her efficiency. The nurse's knowledge, skill, energy (physical, mental, and emotional), motivation, and self-directedness all contribute to his or her efficiency (Hanson, 1982). The perception of staffing adequacy elicited by the Unit Staffing/Care Evaluation Questionnaire is only a reflection of the staff's perception of their ability to provide services under differing conditions.

The quality of care provided and the effectiveness and efficiency of staff are not accounted for in the San Joaquin methodology or in any other methodology per se.

Although these issues have been considered important, the impetus to address them did not exist until now. We cannot continue thinking that "what is" is "what ought to be." We cannot set standards based on "what is" without critical analysis of the efficiency and effectiveness of the nursing care provided. The attempt of the Unit Staffing/Care Evaluation Questionnaire to supplement otherwise quantitative measures with a measure of professional judgment is credible, but further steps must be taken. A solution might be to identify the major staff activities—those requiring the most time or those perceived as most important to the customer (physician, health maintenance organization, patient, and so forth). The efficiency and effectiveness of those activities could then be evaluated prior to work sampling and the necessary changes instituted, or they could be evaluated following work sampling and productivity-related adjustments made in the data obtained. Either approach relies on other fields, such as management engineering, industrial engineering, and quality assurance, for evaluation techniques. The data collected cannot be used as if it were empirical evidence since it quantifies only part of the input-output equation.

A second potential loophole in the validity of the San Joaquin methodology is the combination of predictive patient classification and actual measurement of required hours of care. The nursing staff classify patients by predicting or anticipating each patient's nursing care time requirements for the following shift. The predicted classification of a patient is then entered on the data collection tool and the actual care received is recorded. This provides the average minutes of care per category of patient. This technique appropriately tests the ability of the tool to group patients based on predicted requirements for care. However, using it to measure the mean care time per category of patient introduces more variance than if the staff were to classify the patient at the end of the shift, retrospectively. The author has compared predictive and retrospective classifications, and the results were similar enough to use for staffing allocation (given that the precision with which we can respond is measured in whole persons or at best half-shifts of persons). However, it is preferable to use retrospective classifications for the quantification studies.

Sampling is another area of concern. According to the San Joaquin methodology, "for either work sampling or direct patient care sampling a period of 80 hours of observation over 10 days by the observer team will provide a reliable sample of data for a unit under most circumstances. These 80 hours of observation should cover the day, evening and night shifts (Murphy, Dunlap, Williams, & McAthnie, 1978, p. 10). It is suggested that 15 to 25 patients be observed on each unit and patients be chosen on a stratified sampling basis according to classification. Several problems may arise in attempting to replicate this method. First, the recommended sample size was based on a four-category patient classification system. If additional categories are used, the sampling requirements change. Second, 80 hours of observation is sufficient if there is a fairly even distribution of patients in all categories. If one or more categories are underrepresented, insufficient data may be collected to accurately estimate the average care times of patients in those categories. Third, this sampling distribution was used in conjunction with a specific patient classification instrument at San Joaquin General Hospital which grouped patients into four separate and identifiable groups that were homogenous with respect to their requirements for nursing care time. If the data obtained using a different instrument are less homogenous and more variable than the San Joaquin data, the sample size of 80 hours may again be insufficient. A cost-benefit analysis must be performed if any of these qualifying conditions are present, as more extensive work sampling may be prohibitively expensive. In that case, a lower level of confidence might be accepted for the least-used patient categories.

Two final reliability and validity issues associated with work sampling involve the use of data collectors. The San Joaquin methodology required about five to seven hours for orientation, practice, and testing of data collectors. Training included "dry-run" practice with recording, onsite practice followed by comparisons of agreement in actual observations, and paper-and-pencil exams. Groups of two or three observers made simultaneous, independent observations of the same event, and results were compared. Ninety percent agreement was considered acceptable. However, interrater reliability may be more effectively tested using a videotape, since real-life situations cannot be played back for discussion or reevaluation. San Joaquin observers were also instructed to make "instantaneous observations" every 10 minutes for the direct care study and every 15 minutes for the work-sampling study. Observers were told to vary the starting point of their rounds and record the "first activity seen." However, keeping observations "random" is difficult at best. A more formal plan is necessary to maintain the random nature of observations. A scheme should be laid out ahead of time using a table of random numbers to determine the starting time or starting place for each round.

The use of patient care classification data as a means of budgeting, monitoring of productivity, and nursing cost accounting is appropriate, but the meaningfulness of comparisons among institutions is diminished by the lack of reliability and validity of the patient classification instruments and quantification methodologies utilized. Specific problem areas have been identified and some alternative approaches have been offered. These issues should be considered not from an academic perspective but from an operational perspective. With this understanding, fewer patient classification instruments should be developed; more time and energy should be diverted to measurement of the reliability and validity of the tools now in existence; and more information should be available to nursing administrators in language they can understand regarding the advantages and disadvantages of the various methodologies available for quantifying patient classification data.

REFERENCES

Chagnon, M., Audette L., Lebrun, L, & Tilquin, C. (1978). Validation of patient classification through evaluation of the nursing staff degree of occupation. *Medical Care, 16*(6), 465–475.

Cronbach, L., & Meehl, P. (1955). Construct validity in psychological tests. *Psychology Bulletin, 52*.

Giovannetti, P. (1979). Understanding patient classification systems. *Journal of Nursing Administration, 9*, 4–9.

Giovannetti, P., Mainguy, J., Smith, K., & Truitt, L. (1970). *The reliability and validity testing of a subjective patient classification system.* Research report. Vancouver, British Columbia: Vancouver General Hospital.

Goodwin, L., & Prescott, P. (1981). Issues and approaches to estimating interrater reliability in nursing research. *Research in Nursing and Health, 4*, 323–337.

Guttman, H., Spector, R., Sigal, J., Rakoff, V., and Epstein, N. (1971). Reliability of coding affective communication in family therapy sessions: Problems of measurement and interpretation. *Journal of Consulting and Clinical Psychology, 37*, 397–402.

Hanson, R. (1982). Managing human resources. *Journal of Nursing Administration, 12*.

Murphy, L., Dunlap, M., Williams, M., & McAthnie, M. (1978). *Methods for studying nurse staffing in a patient unit—A manual to aid hospitals in making use of personnel* (DHEW Publication No. HRA 78-3). Washington, D.C.: U.S. Department of Health, Education and Welfare.

Tinsley, H., & Weiss, D. (1975). Interrater reliability and agreement of subjective judgments. *Journal of Counseling Psychology, 22*(4), 385–376.

Developing a Patient Classification System: A Case Study

Karole Schafer Heyrman and Kathleen M. Nelson

Significant technical and economic changes in the institution of health care have resulted in a rise in overall acuity of both inpatient and outpatient populations and a reduced length of hospital stay. These changes have altered the structural arrangement of professionals' work in acute-care settings. Professional nursing has expanded its focus to include more assessment, evaluation, and complex treatment activities. These activities must be purchased with a shrinking health care dollar. Consequently, nurses in acute-care settings must justify their utilization of resources and rely on improved systems for planning care in a shortened time frame.

How do nurses obtain objective data to respond to the changing demands for service? Research-based instruments such as patient classification tools have been in existence since the late 1950s. Few were designed to collect the comprehensive information required to project the character of changes associated with trends in demand. Most tool formats classify patients' general health status, in a range from ambulatory to critical, rather than the specific nursing care patients require. These instruments were developed to dictate allocation of existing departmental resources.

The authors wish to acknowledge efforts of the clinical staff of the Department of Nursing, University of Illinois Hospital, the administrative support of Jacqueline Miller, Associate Director, and the contribution of Sharon Day, Assistant Director of Nursing.

Nurses at the University of Illinois Hospital have, over a five-year period, developed a system that provides administrative and clinical information. They have designed, pilot tested, and implemented a generic tool as part of a workload estimate completed for all adult medical-surgical and critical care patients units. The tool provides a mechanism for comprehensive documentation of nursing care delivered as well as a mechanism to predict nursing care needed during the next eight hours. The unit of measure is temporal. The resulting data bank can be used for short-term and long-term resource allocation, trend reports, clinical research, quality management, dynamic care planning, and utilization review. Behavioral, obstetric, pediatric, ambulatory, and perioperative tools are in various stages of development. The availability of these tools facilitates the task of documentation, since the clinician chooses a tool based on type of service rather than the patient's location.

This paper focuses on the process of developing and implementing the University of Illinois Hospital's patient classification system, rather than simply presenting outcomes. Ideally, then, administrators and clinicians who must construct their own plan for a patient classification system can better gauge the resources needed.

PHASE I
ASSESSMENT AND PLANNING

In November 1981, the Nursing Executive Council at the University of Illinois Hospital approved a proposal to implement a patient classification system. New clinical cost centers had been created as a result of a move to a new hospital building. This reorganization, coupled with the technical and economic changes in the health care system, emphasized the need for information on the nursing services being provided and future services for which to plan. At the same time, the hospital was beginning to discuss the imposition of prospective payment systems for reimbursement. The tool selected for use was a modification of a prototype format developed by St. Luke's Hospital of Phoenix, Arizona. The Department of Nursing had prior experience with a factor type of classification system that had fallen short of expectations. The format of choice was a prototype tool that was ratio based and used a temporal dimension of measurement (minutes of direct care).

A task force was appointed in December and met monthly until July. The functions of the task force were to further modify the St. Luke's tool, identify all direct nursing activities, select pilot units, and educate strategic members of the department. The following fall, a patient classification committee was convened to continue modification of the tool and staff education. The committee members were selected to be representative of the clinical and administrative staff of the entire department.

During the initial phase of the patient classification project, the committee conducted an assessment of internal and external sources of information on patient classification and its application in the modern health care industry. Assessment of external sources included an exhaustive literature review as well as site visits to similar institutions. These activities provided an opportunity to understand the historical development of patient classification to gain insight into the logic and hidden assumptions of these systems, including much of the industrial engineering work (time-and-motion studies) of the 1950s that underlies existing classification tools.

Internal assessment led the committee to outline several institutional considerations. First, the patient classification project had to promote professional practice that was consistent with the university's missions of service, education, and research, as well as with the Department of Nursing's policies and procedures. Second, in response to the introduction of prospective payment systems, the institution's managers required a clearer articulation of the allocation of nursing resources. Third, we had to take into consideration the response of nursing staff to the measurement and documentation of work. This concern was heightened by the well-documented negative reaction of workers to computer measurement of output since the computerized information system was the intended medium, for the tool.

Fourth, any new system had to be consistent with the hospital's current priorities. A major goal of the project was to build on the institutional strengths (such as an operative computer information system) as well as the organizational strengths (for example, its clinical experts). Finally, for the patient classification system to achieve its purposes, the design had to move from the administrators' drawing board to the clinicians' bedside clipboard. Design of the tool had to address both documentation of care given on the present shift and care predicted for the following shift. To this end, project activities were kept highly visible and open to review by hospital and departmental committees.

Pilot Testing

Once the patient classification committee had completed its external assessment, internal assessment, and modifications of the St. Luke's tool, it planned a pilot test. The committee had constructed separate medical-surgical, critical care, and behavioral tools. These tools, known collectively as the Illini tool, would be compared to control tools that had already been validated for use on an inpatient unit. At this time the long-term goals of patient classification included using the tools to document actual direct care given and to assist in evaluating short-term (next shift) staffing needs. Direct care was defined as all patient-focused activity done at the bedside.

The pilot plan included criteria for selecting representative pilot units and personnel. The medical-surgical tool was tested on a 29-bed surgical unit specializing in the care of patients with disorders of the eye and a 62-bed adult general medical unit. Both units used similar acuity formulas for staffing determinations. The surgical unit was already on-line to the computer information system and used the computer system to complete both the experimental and the control tools. The medical unit used paper tools in both cases and completed them manually. This arrangement met a project goal of developing both computer screens and manual back-up material.

The critical care tool was tested in the 15-bed organ transplant unit. The behavioral tool was tested in the 22-bed closed psychiatric unit. Both these units used the computer information system to complete the experimental and control tools.

The control tools were selected for several reasons. First, they were factor tools, and although the committee's assessment had led us away from this format, it was essential to verify our assumptions in a controlled manner. Second, the factor tools had been tested for validity, were frequently used in inpatient settings, and were easily used to determine user reliability. The control tool selected for use on the medical-surgical and critical care units is one in common use, called the Public Health Tool. The behavioral tool used as a control on the psychiatric unit was the Menninger tool.

Criteria for selecting staff to serve as subjects for the pilot test reflected each unit's 24-hour staffing pattern. The unit's natural organization was followed to improve evaluation results pertaining to the staff's proficiency in completing the tools. All staff on the pilot units were oriented to the project.

Each participant was asked to complete one copy of both the control tool and the experimental tool for each patient assigned to them during a two-week period. A communication log was placed on each of the pilot units. Project staff made daily rounds to check for feedback and comments and collected, reviewed, and hand coded the tools on a daily basis. The unit manager (head nurse) was responsible for the compliance of participating staff. The effectiveness of the unit manager's role was noted early in the project and has been reinforced and relied on throughout the life of the project.

Pilot testing of the patient classification tool was completed in January 1983, approximately one and one-half years after the initial proposal.

In this first phase of the project, testing focused on whether the prototype format was the method of choice for documenting direct nursing care services. The limited human resources available to complete the coding process dictated the choice of several key variables. Data were coded by patient care unit, work shift, acuity as indicated on the control tool, and the categories on the experimental tools. This approach to coding allowed the reviewer to examine the total range of direct nursing services in each of six major categories for each patient over a period of 24 hours. These findings were also compared with the measurements of acuity on each of the control tools.

Information gleaned from communication logs and daily round observations were focused on project protocol. No problems arose in following directions or comprehending definitions on the experimental tools. Staff expressed negative feelings about the control tools, especially regarding the limited selection of activities available on the factor-type tools. Two major categories typically relied on as predictors of patient acuity on the control tools were "IV treatment" and "activity level." Experienced clinicians noted that these predictors were obsolete in present health care. Maintaining an individual's activity at the maximum possible level is a primary goal of professional nursing. Intravenous therapy is only one of a large range of interdependent and independent nursing services provided to a client. Being ambulatory or without an IV does not vitiate the need for intensive professional nursing assessment and observation.

Despite information given to staff during their orientation to the pilot study about the scope of the tool, staff members repeatedly expressed concern that much of their time was spent in tasks that did not appear on the tool. However, these tasks were generally outside the scope of direct care.

The results of the initial study indicated that the control tools were not sensitive to patients' nursing care needs. For example, in critical care, 90 percent of the patients scored in the lowest two acuity levels. In contrast, the Illini tool differentiated critical care patients from medical-surgical patients. The control tools represent an assessment of patient acuity based on a dated functional approach. They do not help to gather data on direct nursing services by provider skill level. The factor-type control tools do not provide a data bank for nursing research and evaluation.

As a prototype tool, however, the Illini tool provided a mechanism for establishing baseline information about direct nursing care. Although further revision and testing were necessary, the direction was set for the development of a tool that would be more complete than simply comprehensive. The object of analysis was not patient acuity but rather the nurses' work. For example, the work schedules of a primary and associate nurse on the surgical unit who were both participants in the pilot test would naturally complement one another to provide continuity of care for their patients. As a result, the Illini tool provided a profile of the nursing services delivered to a single patient over a three-day surgical hospitalization. This incidental finding encouraged further investigation of patterns of work and profiles of patients by service category and skill level.

Based on findings of the pilot study, recommendations for further action included: (1) revision and expansion of tool content; (2) establishment of standardized times for each item; (3) testing of the Illini format in additional clinical areas; (4) development of methods for measuring nurses' work not accounted for on the tool; and (5) directing project activities in concert with other institutional work related to prospective payment and utilization review systems. To achieve these aims, the Department of Nursing devoted one full-time position to the project, filling it with two clinical nursing consultants who served as project coordinators. In addition, money was dedicated to pursue technical assistance and external validation of the Illini tool.

PHASE II
TOOL VALIDATION AND WORKLOAD ESTIMATE

The confirmation that a prototype tool format would be most useful and the need for a more comprehensive method to measure work dictated the objectives for phase II of the project.

In April 1983, a preliminary report that outlined the project's activities and recommendations up to that point was circulated within the Department of Nursing. The written report provided an excellent opportunity to educate nurse managers and engage them in the developmental process. Project coordinators found this medium of communication useful throughout the project. These written reports included definitions to establish a common vocabulary among project consultants and departmental leadership and to avoid possible confusion in meanings. This was especially important in developing the methodology for measuring work. Description of activities and recommendations were kept brief to encourage staff to read the reports. Appendixes included revised tools, definitions, evaluation forms, and tables of results. Later in the project, reports were used to establish a prospective plan of action. Great care was taken to enumerate assumptions about subsequent steps to be taken and resources needed, and to develop an approximate calendar of events.

External Consultants

The summary reports and formative plans of action were invaluable when external consultants became involved to provide technical assistance and external validation of the Illini tool. Much literature exists on the role and function of consultants. Although the consultants' tasks would appear to be peripheral to the project activities, the role of the external consultant is pertinent to a consideration of the developmental process. The consultants were already at the hospital as part of a larger project with the university. The Department of Nursing requested and was granted authorization to capitalize on that arrangement to provide validation of the work already in progress. At that point, the project needed consultation in obtaining computer hardware and software and designing forms as well as a cross-institutional perspective.

The status of the consultants while on site is an important consideration. Frequently, consultants are placed in the role of rescuer. To make effective use of an external consultant who is scheduled to be on site for a limited time, it is necessary to integrate them into departmental and project activities rather than to abandon staff efforts and encourage dependence on the consultants. At the University of Illinois Hospital, the external consultants worked with and reported to the project coordinators (internal consultants) who remained responsible to the associate director and responsible for project administration. The project coordinators consulted with the unit nurse managers, who remained responsible for unit personnel. This structure served to ensure accountability, maximize the quality of feedback, and keep work focused.

It was imperative that the project coordinators maintain their active role while the external consultants engaged in data analysis. During the evaluation phase, project staff reviewed and analyzed the results at each step of data reduction. Assumptions made during the collapse of information were articulated in accord with professional standards and project activities, allowing a more meaningful interpretation of what conclusions would and would not be made, based on data collection. Departmental staff worked actively with the external consultants until the consultants wrote their final report and recommendations. The managers were then in a position, with the aid of an internal consultant, to call on the external consultants to defend their findings. Without the active role of the project coordinators all along, such a challenge would not be possible, nor could the coordinators defend those findings to others.

Tool and Definition Development

During this second phase of the project, the patient classification committee met bimonthly and changed from a working committee to a reviewing committee. Time was an essential consideration since the external consultants were present for a limited period and departmental staff had other major administrative and clinical responsibilities. The project coordinators assessed the particular tasks and the personnel needed to achieve the principal objectives. Nurse managers were asked to dedicate individual staff members to the project for tool and definition development and to release them from work responsibilities for a portion of their shift. Subcommittees were appointed for each tool.

In preparation for work with the external consultants, the project coordinators and subcommittee members reviewed project goals to ensure that any tool development was consistent with the desired outcomes. This was invaluable because the project goals were different than any the external consultants had previously encountered. The consultants suggested a factor-type format to predict nursing service. They discouraged the prototype format as a method of documenting both actual nursing service and predicted nursing service because of the problems associated with constructing a tool to document as nearly as possible 100 percent of direct nursing service. The most direct nursing care measured by any tool they were aware of was roughly 80 percent. As noted, however, factor-type tools with ordinal-scale acuity systems had already been rejected, and the tools were intended to document actual care given. For these two reasons the tools had to be more than comprehensive; the activity accounted for on the tools had to be complete.

The medical-surgical and critical care subcommittee began revising the medical-surgical and critical care tools in September 1983. A member of the consulting firm also met with them initially to advise them of potential pitfalls in tool construction generally and definition writing in particular. Since times ultimately would be assigned to each item on the tool, items and their definitions had to be mutually exclusive. The following is an example of a category, its items, and the corresponding definitions:

Vital Signs

    Simple: T (oral/rectal/axillary); P (radial/brachial/apical); R (ventilator/ nonventilator); and BP. Frequency: every 4 to 8 hours.

    Intermediate: T (oral/rectal/axillary); P (radial/brachial/apical); R (ventilator/nonventilator); and BP ($\bar{c}$ or $\bar{s}$ arterial line). Frequency: every 2 to 3 hours.

    Complex: T (oral/rectal/axillary/core); P (radial/brachial/apical); R (ventilator/nonventilator); and BP ($\bar{c}$ or $\bar{s}$ arterial line). Frequency: every one hour or more often.

As the subcommittees began their work on revision and expansion of the tool content, they noted some unacceptable deviations from existing policy and procedure. The subcommittees agreed that the Department of Nursing's "Policy and Procedure Manual" was the standard from which to define activity. A mechanism was established for regular communication with the chairperson of the policy and procedure committee.

It was imperative to adhere to the department's philosophy that standards guide practice, practice does not dictate standards. For this reason also, it was not necessary to define procedures separately. Consequently, treatment and procedure items do not have corresponding definitions.

Project coordinators also found that the medical-surgical and critical care tools were becoming more similar. Distinctions between the two tools and among the units were usually related to unit and individual behaviors rather than different nursing practice. This experience of finding overall similarity among different tools occurred repeatedly as new tools developed. However, the project coordinators found it valuable to allow the process of development to take its natural course. As each new specialty or division in the department was approached for tool development, administrative and clinical staff at first maintained that a unique tool was essential. When project coordinators requested specific feedback about which aspects of the existing tool were not acceptable and what was missing, they found that only minor changes in items and definitions and the addition of a few treatments and procedures were necessary. Moreover, because the computerized information system accommodates a number of different tools and is accessible wherever a terminal is available, a nurse can use a menu of tools to choose the one suitable for the type of nursing care delivered in a particular case rather than being limited to the tool designed for a particular geographic location.

As a result of the effort to meet individual unit and project needs, a generic patient classification tool design was selected, combining the medical-surgical and critical care tools, and a process of review of content was instituted. This made possible the establishment of a common language for specialists to use in activities such as interunit patient transfers and nursing consultation. Thus, after the subcommittee completed the generic medical-surgical/critical care tool and its definitions, a subcommittee of psychiatric nurses revised the generic tool to accommodate psychiatric patients' nursing care and the milieu on a closed unit. The full patient classification committee approved both tools for the second round of pilot testing. The external consultants assigned a time to each item in each category on the tool using standardized times (a form modified from GRASP/PETO). The subcommittee reviewed the standardized times for each item and negotiated changes based on members' experience.

Workload Estimate

Once a methodology for measuring work became concrete, definitions of the work of nursing personnel were formalized. The three key terms, *direct care, indirect care,* and *personnel fatigue and downtime,* are fairly standard in the literature, and were defined for the project as follows:

Direct Care: Activity that is hands-on, generally occurring inside the patient's room. ("Client" includes patient and family or significant other.)

Indirect Care: Activity in support of direct care, generally occurring outside the patient's room. Indirect care is either variable or invariable.

Variable: Activity that does *not* occur on a regular, planned, or predictable basis (e.g., charting, order transcription).

Invariable: Activity that occurs on a regular, planned, or predictable basis (irrespective of patient acuity or census) or on which data can be gathered historically (e.g., staff meetings, performance appraisals, meals, breaks).

Personnel Fatigue and Downtime: Activity of nursing service personnel that does not contribute to direct or indirect care, exclusive of meals and breaks. Downtime may be forced or voluntary.

Forced: Occurs when the skill mix of staff is mismatched to the clients' need for nursing service.

Voluntary: Occurs when personnel elect not to engage in direct or indirect care.

A workload estimate, then, is a quantitative estimate of direct care, indirect care, and personnel fatigue and downtime. Three methods of measurement were used: patient classification, self-recording, and work sampling. Patient classification is a method of documenting the actual and predicted direct nursing care given to patients. Self-recording is a method by which personnel document, in a predetermined manner, the activities they perform and the frequency of the activity (indirect variable activity). Work sampling is intermittent direct observation of direct care and personnel activity. The frequency of observed activity was compared to the direct care documented by the patient classification tool and the self-reporting tallies.

Thus, direct care was measured by using the patient classification instrument (the Illini tool). Indirect care and personnel fatigue and downtime were measured by using self-reporting and work-sampling methods. This conceptual framework for a method of measuring the work of nursing personnel constitutes patient classification at University of Illinois Hospital. Although patients are never "classified," the misnomer has been retained because the term has credibility and political value outside the Department of Nursing.

Clinical Test of Revised Tool and Workload Methodology

The same four clinical sites used for pilot testing in the initial phase of the project were used for testing in phase II. These units had achieved good participation by both administrators and clinicians in phase I and staff were already familiar with patient classification activities. Also, the patient case mix on these units was representative of the general patient population at University of Illinois Hospital, and the general patterns of patient acuity derived from the control and experimental tools provided baseline information for comparative analysis.

The project coordinators met with the head nurse of each pilot unit and negotiated tools, the process and timing of data collection, and dates for the clinical testing to minimize disruption of unit activities and improve staff participation. Project staff began meeting with unit nursing staff on all three work shifts once the head nurse gave approval.

One week of training sessions was set up to provide staff with specific information about the data-collection process, including a detailed, written set of instructions for both direct and indirect data collection. Staff also practiced classifying assigned patients using the Illini tool. Head nurses and project coordinators reviewed the tools completed by staff during the training period to improve accuracy.

Four work-sampling workshops were conducted by the external consultants. Work samplers were staff nurses, nursing administrators, or senior nursing students. No one was assigned to observe their home unit. The personnel costs of conducting work sampling on four units for 20 hours a day for seven days were very high. One advantage of the open communication practiced during the project was the response to a call for volunteer work samplers. The head nurses of units not participating in the testing were asked to release staff from unit assignments whenever possible, so overtime expense was not necessary.

Data on direct care was collected before data on indirect care to minimize confusion of staff over what activities fit into each of these categories. Because direct care was clearly defined in the tool, once they had collected data on direct care, staff were better able to differentiate it from indirect care. Staff were instructed to complete a patient classification tool for each patient they were assigned to for a period of seven days. Concurrently, a sample of approximately ten patients per unit was observed by work samplers. Patient rooms for work sampling were selected by using a random number table to pick ten room numbers per unit. Each day the room numbers were advanced by one, using unit-approved bed lists. Observations were conducted at 10 to 15 minute intervals, and randomness was achieved by the natural irregularity of nursing activity and by varying the starting points of observational tours.

Time spent in direct care as measured by the work samplers' observations of the sample patient population was compared with the total actual cumulative time spent in direct care as documented on the tool for each patient in the sample population. The results of this comparison, coupled with a list of direct care services not accounted for by the tool, would measure the validity of the patient classification tool.

Once the week of direct care data collection was completed, nursing staff were directed to collect information about indirect care for the next seven days (24 hours a day). Data for the indirect care component included results of the personnel work sampling completed the previous week, a list of invariable indirect activities completed by unit-based administrative nurses, and activity cards or logs completed by staff. A daily census for each unit was documented throughout the 14-day data-collection period and used to calculate patient care days.

The workload estimate was completed on schedule. Staff completed the patient classification tool for 97 percent of the 464 patients. Compliance in the area of self-reporting was less successful. According to the external consultants, this was due to staff members' inability or unwillingness to interrupt daily routine to make notations. The poor self-reporting could be controlled for by interpretation of work-sampling data.

Findings

Results of the direct care data collection indicated that the Illini patient classification tool accounted for approximately 97 percent of all direct nursing care delivered on the pilot units. An example of activity that work samplers documented that did not appear on the Illini tool was transporting a patient, a task that occurs by necessity but is not part of the nurse's expected activities.

Once it was established that the tool items were complete, the second analytical task was to validate approximate times for each tool item. Standardized time estimates are used to see that assigned times correspond to the actual average times for each task when the cumulative time is inspected for a given work shift, clinical area, or location. Actual rather than projected care measured by the tool was used to compare with work samplers' observations. The validity of the assigned times used in the tool was tested using a linear regression between direct care work sampling and actual care measured by the tool for a given unit by both 8-hour (work shift) and 24-hour (patient day) time frames.

Results from the three pilot units using the medical-surgical/critical care tool indicated that the tool was valid in measuring the direct nursing services provided for a full range of patient needs. In the data-collection process on the psychiatric unit, however, work samplers apparently measured patient activity rather than direct nursing care for the sample group. Therefore, the data for direct care tool sampling had to be deleted from the study. However, the personnel work-sampling forms provided some information concerning direct care activities for this analysis. The external consultants recommended that the behavioral tool be put into use with careful auditing for the first few months and, if necessary, that part of the work-sampling process be repeated.

Results of the indirect data collection were coded and analyzed by the external consultants. These results will be used as part of the workload measurement that is a component of a staffing formula.

Tasks completed in phase II were validation of two patient classification tools and testing and approval of a technique for completing workload estimates. The next step was to take the information gained in the pilot test and apply it to the same process in the entire medical-surgical and critical care areas.

Based on the findings in phase II, the recommendations for phase III included: (1) completion of inpatient unit tool design, testing, and implementation; (2) evaluation of implementation; (3) investigation of project work in an ambulatory care setting; and (4) ensuring that project activities remain consistent with goals of departmental and hospital activities.

PHASE III:
IMPLEMENTATION AND EVALUATION

Once the generic patient classification tool was validated, the overall goal for the third phase of the project was implementation and evaluation of a patient classification system throughout the department. The specific objectives were (1) adaptation of the generic tool to the various clinical areas, (2) commencement of tool usage, (3) completion of workload estimates, and (4) initiation of a fully operative system. The process of evaluation is implicit in these implementation activities.

Once nursing management approved the goals and objectives of the third phase, 17 adult medical, surgical, and critical care inpatient units were targeted as a priority for implementation of the system. The choice was essentially one of economy. Adaptation of the generic tool in these areas was expected to be an easy task, given the previous experience with the process. Also, these 17 units represent a major portion of the department's budgeted human resources. Concurrent developmental work was planned on tools for the family centered (obstetric), pediatric, and perioperative areas.

Based on experience in the earlier phases of the project, the project coordinators and unit managers prepared a checklist of tasks necessary to ready the units for implementation of the tool. Modifications in the process and time frames were negotiated for particular units. At all times the project coordinators adhered to their own advice on the role of the consultant. The unit manager was responsible for activities to further agreed-upon unit objectives. The project coordinators made weekly rounds and modified time frames accordingly. Any delay was seen as requiring a new agreement. Unit managers were encouraged to contact managers of pilot units for information.

Adapting the Tool

Each unit designated approximately three experienced staff nurses to review the generic tool items and definitions. As mentioned earlier, the initial response of most of the nurses was that a unique tool would have to be created and that there was nothing generic about professional nursing. The project coordinators did not attempt to impose the generic tool, allowing staff effort to be constructively channeled into disproving their own position. By-products of this process were thorough assessment of the tool for usefulness, identification of minor changes and updates, and the education of staff in the process of tool construction and revision. Acceptance of the tool content was never a problem.

Project coordinators oriented staff in groups to the patient classification project and to the specific tools. The unit manager was responsible for scheduling and attendance at these sessions.

The last activity in adapting the generic tool for each unit was determining the proficiency of staff in completing the tool, or user reliability. This was done through an audit of the nurses' skill in completing the "actual care given" column of the Illini tool, since this focused on the user's knowledge and application of definitions without the variable of prediction. A compliance rate was calculated by dividing the total number of correct entries on the tool made by the user by the total number of correct tool entries as indicated by the auditor. A unit compliance rate was calculated by averaging the rates of personnel audited during the orientation. No unit moved to the next stage of implementation without reaching an 80 percent user compliance rate.

Using the Tool

Successful completion of objective 2 would require (1) correct entry of classification information for all patients on each eight-hour work shift, (2) an ongoing unit-based program of evaluating staff members' use of the tool, (3) a functional computer program for collecting, processing, and reporting individual and cumulative tool output, and (4) completion of developmental work on baseline information and formatting used in management reports.

The Illini tool was intended to be completed using the hospital computerized information system. Cumulative tool output for each patient (with total actual and total predicted nursing care given separately) is to be collected along with nursing work schedule information through a software package. This information constitutes a piece of data in a cumulative data bank to be applied in decision making by unit-based managers and centralized staffing personnel. Adaptation of the tool on all units remains in process.

Completing the Workload Estimate

Completing the workload estimate entailed four steps: (1) collection of work-sampling data, (2) review of results by administrative staff, (3) application of a workload estimate to a staffing methodology, and (4) formatting of management reports. This work is still in process.

Forms and techniques tested during the second phase of the project for collecting work-sampling data were modified to accommodate departmental uses. To balance the benefit of a good sample with the high cost of work-sampling personnel, the length of data collection was reduced from seven to two unconsecutive days. In addition, data could be collected on a "composite day" consisting of three workshifts that might not have occurred in the same calendar day. When a composite of two or three separate days of data collection was used, an effort was made to control for staff composition, patient census, and demand for direct nursing services (as documented on the patient classification tool), and any major variations were taken into account during the initial review of data.

The data were initially analyzed according to personnel classification (staff nurse I, staff nurse II, and so forth) and type of activity (direct, indirect, and personnel fatigue and downtime). Further analysis was done by work shift and by each of the composite 24-hour days. This format was used for two reasons: to facilitate the unit manager's evaluation of current work patterns and to assist in speculation about new work patterns, such as 10- or 12-hour shifts.

After review by unit and departmental managers, the data were further analyzed to meet their individual needs. At no time were the data analyzed for the purpose of generating a departmental standard of work activity. This remains the responsibility of the unit manager, and information from one clinical area is not comparable with that from another.

An Operative System

For a patient classification system to be considered fully operative, four elements must be in place. Two elements involve the tool itself; that is, a tool must be designed for clinical nursing areas where direct nursing services are offered, and the tool must be put into use. Of course, the tool and its use will be modified in response to changes in professional practice and technology. The other two elements relate to the processing of information generated by the patient classification system. A report format must be developed to provide accurate and timely information for the most effective management of human and material resources by the department of nursing. And finally, a fully operative patient classification system will provide a basis for exploring extended clinical, educational, and research uses of the system. This will occur through planned evaluation activities.

Table 1
Fit Between Patient Classification Project Objectives
and Departmental Goals

Overall Project Objectives	Research-Based Departmental Applications
1. A method of categorizing and organizing information in a retrievable manner.	Quality assurance, research, and departmental utilization review activities.
2. A method of documenting 98 percent of direct care.	Documentation of actual nursing services delivered.
3. A method of documenting direct care projected for the next work shift.	Establishing or updating a timely plan of care; predicting staffing resources for each shift based on nursing assessment.
4. A method to measure a unit of service.	Measurement of activity used in construction of models for:
	a. Estimating costs of nursing service for budgeting, planning, and reimbursement schemes.
	b. Profiles of services delivered to clients by individual clinicians, types of specialized units to determine necessary skill mix, and orientation and continuing educational needs as dictated by changes in professional practice and client population.

Unlike the diagnostic and developmental evaluation activities associated with the first and second phases of the project, respectively, evaluation in the third phase of the University of Illinois Hospital's patient classification project has a variety of purposes. The first is to measure planned and unplanned effects of project activities against the Department of Nursing's goals, the project's plan of action (prospective), and the annual report (retrospective). The second purpose of evaluation is to monitor activities at the user and delivery system levels. Third, since the patient classification project is a relatively new program, evaluation will provide information for subsequent decision making about the program itself. A systematic evaluation framework has been designed to provide assessment of activities associated with program planning, program monitoring, program impact, and economic feasibility.

APPLICATIONS

The overall objectives of the patient classification project were based on departmental goals. Thus, the design for information retrieval reflects both these departmental objectives and the specific aims of the project. An illustration of the fit between project objectives and departmental operations are displayed in Table 1. Thus, the information format design provides a language with which we can talk about our work.

Using the Warp Concept of Graphics in Patient Classification

Jonelle E. Wright

Given the competitive circumstances in which financially constrained, technologically top-heavy health care providers must function today, health care personnel are having to make difficult decisions about allocation of resources based on available data about consumers and providers. To effectively match the resources of health care providers to the needs and eligibility status of consumers is most difficult in and of itself, but to answer demands for efficacy of services in the process creates an almost insurmountable challenge using present-day data management techniques.

The purpose of this paper is to examine current case-mix and patient classification instruments in light of health care management needs and to propose a model for data management that would better organize consumer, provider, financial, resource, and biopsychosocial data to inform policy decisions on allocations and appropriations.

CASE MIX CLASSIFICATION METHODS

Table 1 highlights characteristics of selected case-mix models that relate directly to the purposes of this paper (for an in-depth review of current case-mix classification methods, see Horn, 1981).

The author wishes to acknowledge the contribution of Robert R. Widdowson in the conceptualizing of the model presented.

51

All the patient classification models presented in the table use a combination of requisite tools to give the patient an overall score, usually the sum of z-scores of the tools. As always, when we collapse these data, we lose sensitivity and information. For example, if a patient's total score decreases from one measurement to the next, there is no indication of the area in which the patient changed, or in what direction. Perhaps the patient's physiological functions score is zero; the patient is dead. What happens to the patient's scores on measures representing family, legal, or cost factors? Of course, we can always examine the raw scores for the individual tools, but then we can't progress past this raw data. Thus, the total score is not very helpful.

THE WARP CONCEPT

There is another way to represent at least three factors in a model in summary form—graphics. Consider the cube. Any point inside a cube can be represented by values for the three axes of the cube, x, y, and z (see Fig. 1), and these three coordinates can give the location of any point in the cube. If the three factors we wish to examine are represented by these axes, we can watch the patient—represented by the point (x,y,z)—"float" around the cube—that is, change on the three factors— as we measure him or her periodically.

In other words, patients are characterized differently according to different dimensions—in this instance, three. For example, the three dimensions might represent the patient's physiological functioning, nursing care intensity, and community service support. In actuality, the number of these dimensions is unlimited, depending on the different ways in which we want to characterize the patient. The cube, then, represents an area that will accommodate (multidimensionally) all the dimensions of a patient being characterized. Thus, a patient can be characterized without collapsing data in many different areas. The cube might represent the field in the computer where patient data are stored.

One can also define specific regions within a space. In the cube, for example, we might define a spherical region (see Fig. 2). These regions, known as *warps*, are defined by coordinates of x, y, and z, just as the points (patients) are. A region might represent, for example, level IV of a nursing intensity classification system. Unlike total scores, regions allow us to create boundaries (limits) for the factors as well as combinations of factors.

We can now define regions in the patient's "progress" space. If the patient passes into the intensive care unit region of care, for example, we could switch to a new cube with different factors or different weights for the same factors, depending on the philosophical tendency of the

Table 1
Characteristics of Selected Case-Mix Models

Features	Model and Date of Origination						
	Commission on Professional Hospital Activities[a] (1975)	International Classification of Diseases[b] (1978)	Staging[c] (1978)	Generalized Patient Management Paths[d] (1979)	Diagnosis Related Groups[e] (1980)	Iso-Cost[f] (1981)	Severity of Illness[g] (1981)
Number of classification groups	6,940	1,000 or 10,000	1,600	Incomplete	467	Incomplete	Incomplete
Data base	Discharge summary	Discharge summary	Discharge summary or chart	Discharge summary or chart	Discharge summary	Discharge summary	Patient chart
Defining variables	Principal diagnosis Secondary diagnosis Surgery Age bracket	Principal diagnosis	Physiological severity of principal diagnosis Diagnostic testing	Admitting signs and symptoms Diagnostic and therapeutic interventions	Length of stay, which accounts for age, presence of secondary diagnosis, and therapy	Charge	Seven factors, relating to therapy, dependency, condition, and burden of illness
Objective of system	Considers principal diagnosis plus other patient variables and groups them likewise	Places same patient diagnoses together	Produces clinically homogeneous principal diagnosis groups	Produces homogeneous intervention groups	Produces groups homogeneous for length of stay	Produces groups homogeneous for charge	Differentiates total patient burden of illness

Table 1
(cont.)

	Model and Date of Origination						
Features	Commission on Professional Hospital Activities[a] (1975)	International Classification of Diseases[b] (1978)	Staging[c] (1978)	Generalized Patient Management Paths[d] (1979)	Diagnosis Related Groups[e] (1980)	Iso-Cost[f] (1981)	Severity of Illness[g] (1981)
Comments	Considers more patient features	Considers only principal diagnosis	Clinically based principal diagnosis grouping	Considers reason for admission and intervention	Uses empirical data to produce homogeneous groups	Uses empirical data to produce homogeneous groups	Conceptually based homogeneous patient severity groups
Advantages	Accessibility Simplicity of data Data source More sensitive than ICDA	Accessibility Simplicity Little time required to gather data Same diagnosis grouping	Sensitive to patient complications Simplicity of required data Medically meaningful	Clinically usable Produces homogeneous resource utilization groups	Accessibility Simple data source Simple applicability	Accessibility Considers interventions Charge is dependent variable Medically meaningful Simplicity of data	Conceptually based Clinically usable Considers severity of illness Considers patient response Not disease specific

Disadvantages						
Hard to manage Inaccurate measure of actual burden of treatment Potential for diagnosis inflation Loss of sensitivity in abstract	Hard to manage Unstable estimates (low N in groups) Heterogeneity within groups Potential for diagnosis inflation Loss of sensitivity in abstract	Hard to manage Insensitive to any but primary diagnosis Does not consider patient response Subjective rating	Hard to gather data Ratings inflated in teaching hospitals Large number of paths (diagnoses) Influenced by individual differences in physician practices No indication of burden of illness	Used as measure of resource consumption Potential for diagnosis inflation Insensitive to individual patient burden Loss of sensitivity in abstract	Uses mortality rates as indicators of burden of illness Loss of sensitivity in abstract Potential for diagnosis inflation	Subjective rating Increased time required for data collection Influenced by individual physician practice

[a] *Hospital Mortality, PAS Hospitals, U.S. 1972–73* (Ann Arbor, MI: Commission on Professional and Hospital Activities, 1975).

[b] V. M. Slee, "The International Classification of Diseases: 9th Revision (ICD-9)," *Annals of Internal Medicine, 88* (March 1978): 424–426.

[c] M. L. Garg, D. Z. Louis, W. A. Gliebe, C. S. Spirka, J. K. Skipper, and R. Parekh. "Evaluating Inpatient Costs: The Staging Mechanism," *Medical Care,* 16 (March 1978): 191–201.

[d] W. W. Young, "Measuring the Cost of Care Using Generalized Patient Measurement Paths," Year 1 Final Report (Pittsburgh, PA: Blue Cross of Western Pennsylvania, November 1979).

[e] D. Simborg, "DRG Creep, A New Hospital Acquired Disease," *New England Journal of Medicine,* June 25, 1981, 1602–1604; R. B. Fetter, Y. Shin, J. L. Freeman, R. F. Averill, and J. D. Thompson, "Case Mix Definitions by Diagnosis-Related Groups," *Medical Care, 18* (February 1980): 1–53.

[f] D. A. Bertram, D. N. Schumacher, S. D. Horn, C. J. Clopton, J. G. Lord, and C. Chan, "Hospital Care Mix Groupings: Concepts and Generic Algorithms" (Baltimore, MD: Center for Hospital Finance and Management, Johns Hopkins University, October 1981).

[g] S. D. Horn, D. N. Shumacher, D. Bertram, and P. D. Sharkey, "Measuring Severity of Illness: Homogeneous Case Mix Groups" (Baltimore, MD: Center for Hospital Finance and Management, Johns Hopkins University, November 1981).

Figure 1

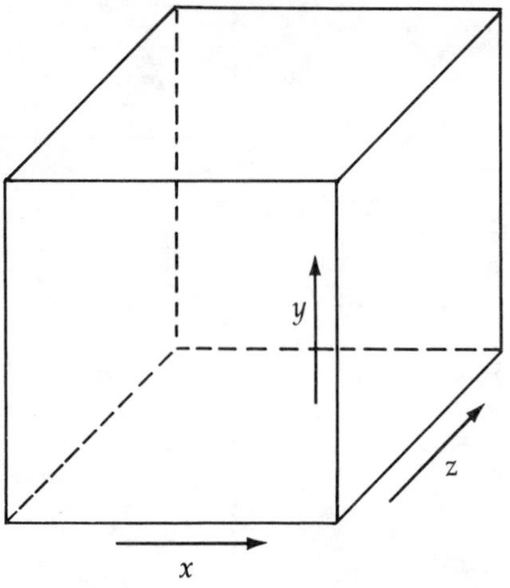

policy body—in other words, we would have a cascade of patient spaces, each with regions leading in and out. One could also telescope the regions, or connect them together in other ways. The lesson is to work from a visual model in three dimensions.

Imagine, for example, a moldable structure—in this case made up of cubes connected by tubular tunnels to one another. Let this structure visually represent the warp model and its definitions. The mathematics describing this structure represent technical descriptions and tools for intervention as patients progress through the health care system. As an example, when we switch to a new cube, the decision of whether to use different factors to describe patient coordinates or to use the same factors with different weights is, as just noted, a theoretical one. Does a patient's state of health depend on pressures common to all environments, albeit in varying proportions? Or do different environments "create" new factors that influence a patient's progress? In the former case, the cubes could nest inside one another like Chinese boxes—what I have described as telescoping. In the case where new factors arise, a new space (cube) must be defined. We then define warps (that is, describe tunnels) to connect this space to the rest of the structure. For example, we might add the dimension of day care to the previously defined dimensions of physiological functioning, nursing care intensity, and community service support. The final step is to define the borders of the structure and the regions of warp in mathematical statements. The computer can monitor passage from space to space quite easily.

One can also work backwards. The patient's coordinates place him or her at point A. The computer can search for warps—tunnels to other places—and ask:

Figure 2

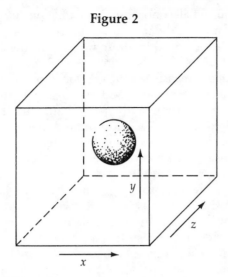

1. What combinations of changes in factors will move a patient from A to any given region?
2. Given a region defined elsewhere in the structure, what is the best way to get the patient there?

I've represented space as three-dimensional because of our conceptual limitations, but no mathematical difficulties arise with increasing the number of dimensions, so we can use as many factors as necessary. These equations are solved with matrix operations, so the formulas are all generalized to n dimensions—otherwise known as *hyperspace*—where n is a position integer. The use of computers with artificial intelligence capabilities accommodates this method of classification.

Thus, we can have an x axis, a y axis, a z axis, an aa axis, and so forth, which would accommodate quantification and qualification of several patient characteristics (such as physiological status, financial resources, and psychosocial status) simultaneously. Even more important, we would not be losing sensitivity from our data because we no longer use an amalgamation of numbers, but warps in hyperspace from a graphic positional perspective.

CONTINUUM OF CARE

Having established the concept of warping, let us now consider which dimensions—patient characteristics—it would be helpful to have information about for patient and resource management. It is generally accepted that such factors as diagnosis, severity of illness, age, charge, and nursing hours required all contribute to the total picture of patient care. Now we can look at all of them simultaneously.

Concerns have been voiced by those working in the area defined by the relationship of diagnosis related groups (DRGs), nursing costs, and nursing intensity about measuring the relationship of these factors. This warp contains data concerning medical diagnosis, length of stay (DRG), cost of nursing care provision, and type and amount of personnel and procedures required to provide appropriate patient care. A primary concern in this area is the relationship of the intensity of nursing service to nursing diagnosis and practice. The routine per diem method of charging for nursing care is just not accurate across or within DRGs. To my knowledge, no system acknowledges the difference between nursing care given in intensive care units and care given in routine patient care areas. Intensive care alone accounts for a significant portion of Medicare expenditures reported in the past. In addition to the type of care given, the length of care provided has also been inadequately represented in the areas of budgeting, forecasting, cost containment, and variance analyses of costs within and among DRGs. These two primary concerns must be answered.

The Continuum of Care Model presented in Figure 3 addresses these problems. Patients are provided care along a continuum of health status and intervention. A patient progresses (or regresses) along this line. Because we view the patient in light of a given system—the health care or medical system—the patient's progress must be plotted according to the system's points (stages) and boundaries, as depicted in Figure 3. Plotting each patient on this continuum according to provider characteristics and facility, as well as type of care emphasized at a particular stage in the care, pinpoints for management the patient's goals for progress, utilization of services, rate of progress, and utilization of different types of personnel during different stages of care and allows predictions about where on the continuum the patient will move next.

With this model, the patient is not lost in the system between services and facilities. In-house services are coordinated with outpatient services, and individual patients' progress from a low level of health to a high level of health (or vice versa) can be charted. A mechanism for a central data bank is thus put into effect. All facility and provider data can be organized according to the model to provide systemwide data collection, storage, and retrieval. Even though different facilities, providers, and services provide care at different times, the patient is still kept track of. The patient's rate of progress is also followed. Since emphasis is placed on different types and degrees of service during the various stages of care on the continuum, the model also allows for budget planning and forecasting the needs for service or facilities for policy and reimburse-

Figure 3
Continuum of Care Model

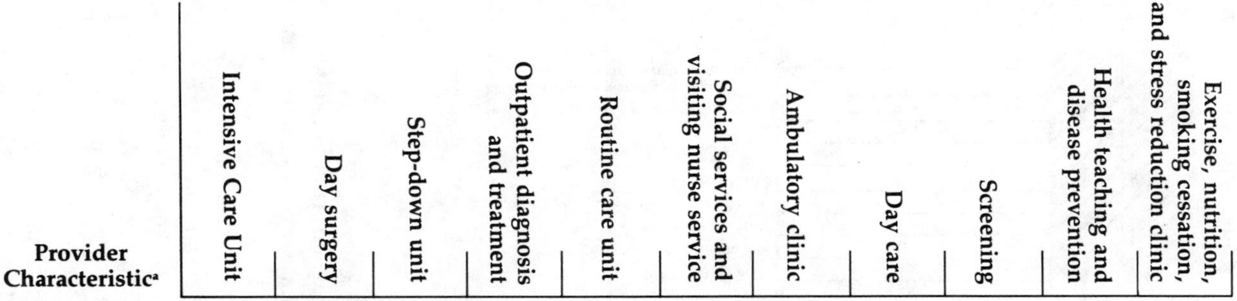

Exercise, nutrition,
smoking cessation,
and stress reduction clinic

Health teaching and
disease prevention

Screening

Day care

Ambulatory clinic

Social services and
visiting nurse service

Routine care unit

Outpatient diagnosis
and treatment

Step-down unit

Day surgery

Intensive Care Unit

**Provider
Characteristic**[a]

[a]Provider characteristic is defined by provider type (RN, LVN, social worker, etc.), level of care needed (critical, skilled, unskilled, sitter, etc.), and hours per day of service needed.

Figure 4
Warp Model with Continuum of Care

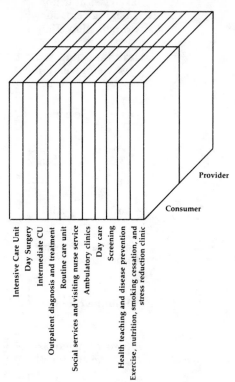

ment decisions. From the information generated by the use of this model, we can easily learn what services are emphasized during which stage of the patient's care.

To integrate this model with the warp model, the Continuum of Care Model becomes the *x* axis of the cube. A map of services and provider characteristics is then graphed along another point on the *z* axis but parallel to the *x* axis (see Fig. 4). When the two are compared, discrepancies between available provider personnel, facilities, and funding and consumer needs quickly become evident. The gaps, overlaps, and inadequacies of staffing, facilities, and funding for services in each stage of care can be realized and documented for future problem solving and policy decisions. Measures of psychosocial, physiological, financial, and other factors can be placed along the *y*, *aa*, and other axes, as discussed previously.

APPLICATION OF THE WARP MODEL

Although these models are roughly sketched, they offer a new perspective on the way classification techniques are usually conceptualized. The different kinds of patient information this model makes available for planning and evaluation have the potential to expand the idea of patient acuity and consequently to:

1. Broaden the range of resources in health care data sets.
2. Allow tracking of patient trends.
3. Evaluate individual practices for competitive positioning and marketing.
4. Evaluate the appropriateness of substitution of services.
5. Evaluate the match between provider and consumer.
6. Negotiate for services.
7. Facilitate health planning.
8. Control overlap in the system.
9. Control internal pricing and volume expenditures of diagnostic testing and possible unnecessary procedures using the supply and demand theory.
10. Manage payment as
    a. a unit of account to develop prospective institutional budgets by adjusting hospital budgets to reflect changes in case mix other than those expected,
    b. a unit of payment to assure adequate cash flow during the fiscal year, and
    c. a command and control regulatory system in accounting to create hospital budgets, set limits to reimbursement in Medicare, and restrict eligibility of patients to certain providers or settings on an individual rather than group (population) basis.
11. Assess the impact of new programs.
12. Assess efficacy of services by analyzing services provided in particular cases rather than using aggregate data.
13. Assess efficiency of services for hospital management, insurance carriers, and federal and state administrators of services.

In conclusion, use of such a model on the policy level would facilitate effective characterization of the mix of patients in all systems in light of resource utilization. Moreover, the information obtained through this model has innumerable uses for research, management, and administration of services.

REFERENCES

Horn, Susan D. (1981). *The Role of Severity-Adjusted Case Mix in Hospital Management.* Unpublished paper. Center for Hospital Finance and Management, Johns Hopkins University, Baltimore, MD.

Patient Management Categories and the Costs of Nursing Services

Wanda W. Young, Marlene S. Carson, and Susan A. Lander

The implementation of Medicare's prospective payment system has precipitated a number of investigations, both large-scale demonstrations and individual hospital studies, aimed at determining the costs of hospital services. Few attempts have been made, however, to associate nursing costs with disease-specific patient categories based on the type or intensity of nursing care required. Instead, in those studies that have been conducted, the allocation of nursing costs is based on either an undifferentiated day of care or a relative value system that reflects nursing time actually spent with particular patients (as opposed to nursing time required to care for certain patient types).

There are a number of reasons why nursing costs have not been linked effectively to patient types. First, present hospital cost-accounting systems make it difficult to determine actual costs accurately. More important, however, is the fact that most studies are based on patient classifications that are not linked to well-defined patient management processes. That is, neither nursing services nor other hospital services that are required in patient management have been associated with the disease-specific patient classifications used in most analyses. Thus, even when the cost of nursing care has been identified for a patient category, that information is not necessarily a useful basis for making hospital management

This paper previously appeared in F. A. Shaffer (Ed.), *Costing Out Nursing: Pricing Our Product* (New York: National League for Nursing, 1985), 209–223.

decisions unless the category means something in terms of the clinical requirements of the patients assigned to that category.

The need to associate the costs of nursing care with clinically specific patient types has become particularly acute in light of recent federal initiatives in the area of hospital reimbursement (Medicare's prospective payment system). Faced with the potential of reduced hospital payment and thus reduced departmental budgets, most hospital departments, including nursing, are actively seeking ways to maintain their current share of the payment received for each patient. Within such a case-mix payment environment, it is critical that the patient categories that are the basis of hospital payment not only predict hospital resource use on average but also reflect the nursing services required, as well as the hospital services used by physicians, to diagnose and treat particular patient types. These linkages, however, cannot be made effectively unless the patient categories that are the basis for payment are recognized by physicians and nurses as homogeneous clinical entities. Only in this way will hospitals be able to identify inefficiencies and assess the utilization of nursing services.

The patient classification that is currently the basis of Medicare's prospective payment system is diagnosis related groups (DRGs). Although this classification system may predict hospital resources used on average (e.g., average length of stay, or average charges or costs of services), it does not define patient types that are clinically specific. Medical professionals have difficulty relating to the DRG classification because it is not consistent with their clinical frame of reference. Because of the clinical heterogeneity within DRGs, it is unlikely that meaningful service profiles can be specified for DRGs, using either data or professional judgment.

Without the ability to link payment to hospital resource use, hospitals will be unable to manage effectively. Translation of payment incentives into acceptable measures of performance and productivity in a particular hospital will be possible only if the basis of payment is consistent with the medical care process. Similarly, only with a clinically based system will cost-effective changes in technology and practice patterns be identified and incorporated in the system over time.

The object of this paper is to describe a patient classification and cost-weighting system that is consistent with the medical care process and to demonstrate its applicability and usefulness in addressing the problems associated with measuring nursing costs and productivity. This case-mix system, developed under a grant from the Health Care Financing Administration by the Health Care Research Division of Blue Cross of Western Pennsylvania, has the following distinct parts:

- *Patient management categories (PMCs)*—computerized patient classification developed with extensive clinical input from physician panels.

- *Patient management paths*—physician-specified clinical management strategies, each of which consists of diagnostic and treatment services for a patient type.

- *Relative cost weights*—a set of relative weights (one for each patient management category) that reflect the cost of physician-specified services.

Some of the ways in which this case-mix system can be used to measure relative nursing costs will be discussed after a general description of the system.

PATIENT MANAGEMENT CATEGORIES

Patient management categories were designed to represent clinically specific patient types, each requiring a distinct diagnostic and treatment strategy for effective care. Within clinically defined disease or disorder groups, patient types were initially identified in clinical terms by expert panels of physicians, independent of patient data. Approximately 50 disease-specific panels were formed to define patient categories. Each panel consisted of four to six physicians (both generalists and specialists) who treat patients with the disease in question. More than 100 physicians from southwest Pennsylvania participated in identifying 800 patient management categories.

Only after patient types were defined by physicians were International Classification of Disease codes (ICD-9-CM) mapped to the resulting categories in order to computerize the classification. That is, physicians identified patient types on their own terms based on their clinical knowledge base; then diagnosis and procedure codes and other patient data were used to computerize the assignment of patients to categories. The actual operational definitions of patient management categories use combinations of diagnoses and, when necessary, specific procedures to capture the clinical specificity of the patient types identified by physicians. Age and sex are also used to assign patients to categories in the few instances where these variables are pertinent.

In addition to defining clinically distinct patient types that should be managed differently, physician panels were asked to specify explicitly the types and quantities of services required for the effective management of a typical patient in each category (Young, 1985b). Each physician-specified management strategy consists of diagnostic and treatment services (for example, specific X-ray examinations, scans, laboratory studies, and operative procedures required, if any) as well as expected lengths of stay in special-care units and in total. An example of the way in which this information was specified by physicians is shown in Figure 1. This format was used to accommodate the way physicians think about the process of patient care. That is, for each patient type within a disease area (in this case, burns), physicians stated the possible reasons for admission, the services or components of care required for diagnosis, the specific diagnoses, and the components of care required for treatment.

In the example shown in Figure 1, there are two patient management categories: smoke inhalation with inhalation injury, and smoke inhalation without inhalation injury. These categories are defined based on the disease characteristics and the severity of the illness, not on the components of care or the typical treatment of that illness as specified by physicians. That is, the existence of the inhalation injury distinguishes a more severely ill patient type that is identified using combinations of diagnosis codes. The hospital services associated with diagnosing and treating a patient type were identified in order to provide a basis for the detailed cost finding that was done in a small but diverse sample of western Pennsylvania hospitals. The result, however, is a management strategy for each patient category that links the patient type to needed hospital services.

Assignment of a patient to a patient management category is done by computer using currently available discharge abstract data. The classification software can be applied to any data base that is compatible with the Uniform Hospital Discharge Data Set (UHDDS) and is thus readily transportable. It is the way in which diagnosis and procedure codes are aggregated, however, and the use of combinations of codes, that is critical to the accurate definition of patient categories. Most important in this regard is the fact that the sequence of diagnoses listed on the patient's abstract (principal versus secondary) does not affect patient assignment to a patient management category. This feature of the classification software minimizes the potential for manipulation of patient categorization (which is especially important within a reimbursement context).

In the example shown in Figure 1, each of the two patient management categories (smoke inhalation with inhalation injury and smoke inhalation without inhalation injury) has a different set of components of care or services, representing physicians' opinions of an effective management strategy for the typical patient in each category. These components of care are not used in the assignment of a patient to a category. Rather, they were specified by physicians to provide a basis for the derivation of a set of cost weights (one for each patient management category)

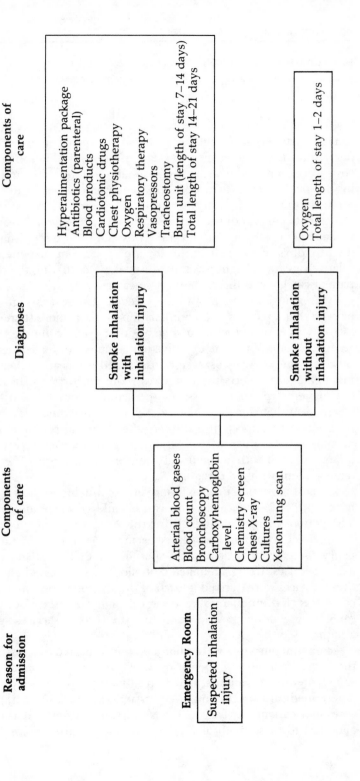

Figure 1
Patient Management Path

reflecting the relative cost of services required (as opposed to services provided) to treat a typical patient in each category.

COST WEIGHTS

The relative cost weight for each patient management category was derived using actual hospital cost data in a sample of hospitals. Standard costs were identified in six study hospitals (both teaching and nonteaching hospitals with 175 to 625 beds) and then allocated to the patient services provided in each institution. These service costs (rather than charges or charges adjusted to reflect costs) were assigned to each patient management category based on the hospital service requirements specified by physician panels in the form of patient management paths. A relative category weight was then derived by comparing the cost of each patient category to the cost of a base category.

By applying this method to the categories shown in Figure 1, it can be seen that a patient with an inhalation injury is more than eight times as costly as a patient without such an injury, reflecting the more costly resources required in the effective management of that patient type. In this way, the relative cost weight associated with each patient management category reflects the resources required for the effective care of that patient type, not necessarily the actual resources used by patients assigned to that category (Young, 1985a). This approach enables comparison of the expected resource use with actual resource use. It also permits estimation of a relative cost weight for each case type that is independent of both hospital inefficiencies and diversity of actual clinical management within a category.

The cost-allocation process as it relates to nursing services is illustrated here for PMC 0305, acute myocardial infarction: pulmonary edema. The patient management path for this category is shown in Figure 2. There are 13 components of care specified on this path, including emergency room services, acute- and special-care unit days, and specific ancillary services. Using a detailed cost-allocation process, the unit costs of these services were derived in each of the six study hospitals. An average cost for each component of care was calculated and the cost for a patient category was derived by accumulating the costs of services specified on a path.

Actual nursing costs were identified and allocated as a distinct part of the cost of particular patient care units (for example, medical-surgical units, intensive care units, newborn nursery, and coronary care units). These medical-surgical units were assumed to produce components of care on a patient-day basis. That is, nursing costs as well as other costs allocated to these medical-surgical units were differentiated for acute

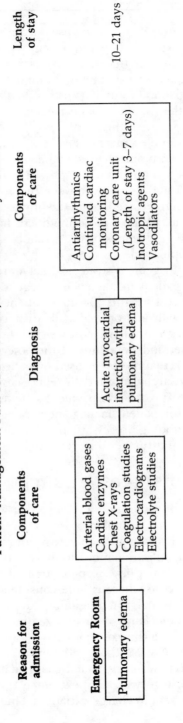

Figure 2

Patient Management Path for PMC 0305, AMI: Pulmonary Edema

Reason for admission	Components of care	Diagnosis	Components of care	Length of stay
Emergency Room	Arterial blood gases	Acute myocardial infarction with pulmonary edema	Antiarrhythmics	10–21 days
Pulmonary edema	Cardiac enzymes		Continued cardiac monitoring	
	Chest X-rays		Coronary care unit	
	Coagulation studies		(Length of stay 3–7 days)	
	Electrocardiograms		Inotropic agents	
	Electrolyte studies		Vasodilators	

care (general or nursery) and intensive care, but within each type of unit, service costs were assigned to patient types on a patient-day basis. The assumption here is that the services and staff on each unit are available to all patients treated on that unit on an equal basis. Although further differentiation of nursing costs is possible based on the specific patient types or the specific patients treated on a unit, such distinctions were beyond the scope of this study.

Thus, in the example shown in Figure 2, nursing costs were assigned to PMC 0305, AMI: pulmonary edema, based on a 5-day stay in a coronary-care unit (the midpoint of the physician-specified range) and 8.94 acute-care days (the difference between the geometric mean length of stay for patients in this category and the physician-specified special-care-unit days). This allocation can be modified, however, to reflect other physician-specified guidelines or the actual hospital utilization of a different patient population.

The clinical management strategies that were specified by physician panels for each patient management category served as the basis for deriving relative cost weights. Because patient management categories are both conceptually and operationally distinct from the clinical management strategies and relative cost weights, however, each part of the system can be used independently of the others. For example, weights can be based on actual resources used by patients assigned to each category. Average charges adjusted to reflect costs for each category (as used in Medicare's prospective payment system) can also be the basis of relative weights for patient management categories. Similarly, certain parts of the cost-finding process, such as the allocation of nursing costs, could be refined and further differentiated.

ISSUES IN COST-WEIGHT DERIVATION

In the process of associating a relative cost weight with each patient management category, a number of issues have been addressed that are important in the determination of relative nursing costs. First, in order to reflect resource utilization more accurately, costs, as opposed to billed charges, were used. Because hospitals typically set charges without an analysis of actual costs, there is little consistency in charge structures, not only among hospitals but also among departments within the same institution. Based on charge data analyzed in this study, it appears that both intra- and interfacility cost comparisons are distorted when charges are used to reflect costs. Although the overall impact of this distortion is unknown at this time, using patient-charge data to identify the relative cost of a patient category makes it extremely difficult to isolate real cost differences from built-in charge variation. Thus, hospital charges for a day of nursing care (within room and board charges) are likely to be quite different from the hospital's cost for a day of nursing care.

The second important issue addressed in this method of cost finding involves the variation in services provided for the same patient type. The question is, to what extent should the set of relative cost weights that is the basis of hospital payment reflect the cost of required hospital services versus the cost of services actually provided? Optimally, it is desirable to implement a hospital payment program that pays for needed services; realistically, this goal cannot be achieved at this time. Because of current data and measurement limitations, it is necessary to use weights based on the costs or charges of services provided or based on some combination of actual and expected utilization.

In most disease-costing studies, all relevant hospital costs or charges (including nursing costs) are identified and allocated to particular patients by one method or another. The resultant cost or charge associated with a patient category is the average cost or average charge of the patients who are grouped together. This is a reasonable strategy for estimating the cost of actual care provided at a particular institution, but it does not necessarily reflect required services or a reasonable relative cost structure on which to base payment. The cost of services actually used by patients assigned to each category may not yield an appropriate cost weight, since all of the services provided may not have been required; conversely, needed services may not have been provided. Although patient data can be analyzed to determine the variability in services and associated costs within and across institutions, the differential use of nurses within patient categories should not affect the development of a relative value index used to allocate nursing costs.

It should be noted that for any particular patient type, multiple management strategies are both possible and appropriate. The particular diagnostic and treatment strategy selected depends on the differential availability of resources across hospitals and nurse staffing patterns as well as the physician's discretion in the selection and substitution of alternative components of care for a particular patient. These management differences, however, should not necessarily be incorporated into the derivation of relative levels of payment for patient care. The differential use of services by patients in the same category (or by the same patient treated by two different physicians at two hospitals that have different levels of technological sophistication and nurse staffing) should not influence the derivation of cost weights.

In the research we conducted, actual patient-related costs at each of six western Pennsylvania hospitals were allocated to each patient management category, holding the clinical management strategy constant. This is emphasized because it represents a significant departure from previous work in this area, which has generally used actual patient data to associate costs or charges with a patient type. Both of the two major studies in the measurement of nursing intensity and nursing costs—the development of relative intensity measures (the New Jersey State Department of Health completed its first study in 1980 and its second in 1981; see New Jersey Department of Health, 1979) and the Stanford University Hospital study to examine nursing costs within DRGs (Mitchell, Miller, Welches, & Walker, 1984)—used a time-based approach to identify the actual services (in nursing time) rendered to particular patients.

In these studies RNs, LPNs, and nurses' aides recorded the exact time spent performing direct and indirect care. This approach, however, has a number of disadvantages. Potential problems related to the use of this method include the following:

- Actual time used to perform a task may be distorted by factors such as demanding patients or nurses who lack proficiency in performing certain nursing skills.
- The number of patients in each category is frequently inadequate for determining averages based on nursing times.
- Inaccurate time estimates may result when staff members either fail to record the time of nursing care directly after it was given or intentionally falsify the times recorded.

These studies have demonstrated the importance of using a clinically specific patient classification in determining the cost of nursing care. They have also identified the need to have specific nursing services linked to the patient categories that are used. The issue that they have not addressed is whether to measure actual nursing services that patients receive during their hospital stay or to estimate relative costs based on nursing services typically required.

MEASURING NURSING COSTS AND PRODUCTIVITY

The usefulness of patient management categories to measuring nursing costs and productivity is based on two unique characteristics of this case-mix system. First, each patient category was defined to be clinically specific enough to enable physicians to infer similar clinical management for the patients who are assigned to that category. Consequently, severity-of-illness distinctions among patient types were incorporated in the design of the patient classification where physicians expected those distinctions to reflect differences in patient management and hospital resource requirements. Second, for each patient management category, physicians specified types and quantities of services required for the effective management of a typical patient. This management strategy provides the link between patient types and the resources that are required for effective care. This link is necessary to allow for both financial analysis and effective quality assessment within a hospital environment.

This system can be translated and used to measure the relative costs of nursing services in a number of ways. Given that patient management categories represent clinically specific patient types, nurses should be able to specify nursing care requirements in the same way that physicians specified the diagnostic and therapeutic services required for the typical patient in a category. Nursing costs can then be associated with services required or rendered for specific patient types.

The determination of the approach to be used in costing out nursing care is influenced by the decision to link patient types with either (1) the intensity and types of nursing services that are actually being rendered by hospital nursing staffs or (2) the intensity and types of nursing services considered by experts to be necessary for the effective care of a patient type during a particular episode of care. The first approach can be used with any patient classification, since it is empirically based. The results, however, will be useful in hospital management only if the patient categories are clinically specific enough to be interpretable by nurses. The second approach may be possible only with a clinically specific patient classification. That is, nurses and physicians will not be able to specify even a general management profile to use in cost finding if the patient categories are not consistent with their clinical frame of reference.

Both of these general methods of identifying the unit costs of nursing care can be used with patient management categories. Nursing costs can be associated with clinically specific patient types by averaging the nursing costs of all patients assigned to each PMC. This method has been used in most other studies to date. In addition to this type of investigation, however, patient management categories can be used to estimate the relative differences in needed care for various patient types. Because of the clinical basis of patient management categories and the detailed information used in the specification of clinical management strategies, this system provides the framework necessary for specifying the nursing services required for each patient type.

This can be accomplished in a number of ways, depending on the level of detailed nursing service and cost information available. The relative cost weights associated with patient management categories already include nursing costs for acute (general and nursery) versus special care. Daily special-care-unit costs were generally three times greater than daily acute-care costs. A hospital payment based on this level of service specification reflects the availability of different levels of service intensity from acute and special care, but it assumes that all acute-care patient units and all special-care units have the same overall case complexity. If it is found, however, that certain acute-care units or special-care units vary significantly from the average nursing intensity and costs, more detailed costing and further differentiation of nursing services will be necessary.

Because patient management categories are clinically specific, this system provides the flexible framework needed for such investigations. For example, the nursing services required on an acute-care medical unit may be quite different from those required on an acute-care orthopedic surgery unit. Patient management categories can be aggregated into these service units and linked with the associated nursing costs to determine differences in unit costs.

The use of patient management categories with current per diem costing methods will also yield more specificity because of the clinical and severity distinctions that are incorporated in the category definitions and the classification software. For example, patients in DRG 141 (syncope and collapse, age greater than 69, and/or complications and comorbidities) discharged in 1983 from western Pennsylvania hospitals were assigned to the PMCs listed in Table 1. Assuming a nursing cost of $25 per day for these patients (Grimaldi & Micheletti, 1982), the average DRG nursing cost for each of these patients is $132.00. Using the same costing method with PMCs would yield much more diverse payment levels, as shown in Table 1—from $97.75 per case for PMC 3920 to $282.25 per case for PMC 4603.

All of the applications discussed thus far are based on the actual utilization of services by patients assigned to a particular patient category. Patient management categories, however, go beyond other patient classifications and provide the basic structure necessary to link needed nursing services with patient types. This linkage is essential in determining the costs of nursing services that are required for effective patient management.

Nursing costs can be associated with services by specifying general levels of nursing intensity for each patient management category or, more specifically, by specifying the nursing tasks required for each component of care listed on the patient management path. The process of identifying nursing tasks is illustrated using the clinical management strategy for PMC 3801, GI disorders: bleeding varices with operation (Figure 3). As noted, this patient type requires the availability of emergency room facilities. One or more emergency room nurses might be needed to help the physician control this bleeding episode while maintaining or restoring the patient to a stable enough condition to permit transfer to an intensive care unit or directly to the operating room for definitive surgery.

Table 1
Patient Management Categories (N ≥ 10) Included in DRG 141

Patient Management Category		N	Average Length of Stay (days)	DRG Nursing Cost per Case	PMC Nursing Cost per Case
0000	Nonspecific/ambulatory diagnoses	251	4.44	$132.00	$111.00
3903	Cardiac: stable angina w/o operation	171	5.23	132.00	130.75
3917	Cardiac: tachyrhythmia	134	6.06	132.00	151.50
3915	Cardiac: bradyrhythmia/ heart block w/o operation	70	5.24	132.00	131.00
3920	Cardiac: valvular/congenital disease w/o operation	53	3.91	132.00	97.75
0401	COPD: chronic bronchitis/ asthma	50	5.00	132.00	125.00
4609	Neurologic disorder: other seizures/epilepsy	42	4.19	132.00	104.75
4511	Psychiatric: organic mental disorder	31	6.73	132.00	168.25
3925	Cardiac: cardiomyopathy/ hypertensive disease w/o operation	29	6.77	132.00	169.25
3501	Head injury: linear skull fracture/scalp laceration	26	4.30	132.00	107.50
4715	Supplementary category: nonspecific urinary infections	24	4.78	132.00	119.50
3606	Bone and joint: other arthritis w/o operation	21	5.12	132.00	128.00
4515	Psychiatric: alcoholism	16	4.67	132.00	116.75
1704	Cerebrovascular: transient ischemia w/o operation	15	5.20	132.00	130.00
3620	Bone and joint: back pain, disk w/o operation	15	6.15	132.00	153.75
4102	Vascular disorder: Peripheral w/o operation	15	6.84	132.00	171.00
3903	Cardiac: Stable angina w/o operation }	14	5.10	132.00	127.50
0401	COPD: chronic bronchitis/ asthma				
3917	Cardiac: tachyrhythmia }	14	5.10	132.00	127.50
0401	COPD: chronic bronchitis/ asthma				
4102	Vascular disorder: peripheral w/o operation }	13	8.58	132.00	214.50
3903	Cardiac: stable angina w/o operation				

Table 1
(cont.)

Patient Management Category		N	Average Length of Stay (days)	DRG Nursing Cost per Case	PMC Nursing Cost per Case
1702	Cerebrovascular: embolus/ intracerebral bleed w/o operation	12	8.15	132.00	203.75
4503	Psychiatric: neurotic/reactive depression	11	5.35	132.00	133.75
4603	Neurologic disorder: movement disorder w/o operation	10	11.29	132.00	282.25
3917	Cardiac: tachyrhythmia	10	9.29	132.00	232.25
1704	Cerebrovascular: transient ischemia w/o operation				
3903	Cardiac: stable angina w/o operation	10	6.27	132.00	156.75
3606	Bone and joint: other arthritis w/o operation				
Total		1,057	5.28		

The nursing tasks during this critical period may include drawing blood for laboratory studies (blood urea nitrogen, coagulation studies, creatinine, liver function studies, blood counts, type and crossmatch); initiating intravenous lines for the administration of medications (cardiovascular drugs), fluids, and blood products; assisting in the insertion of esophagogastric tubes for treatment involving balloon tamponading or ice lavaging; preparing the patient for panendoscopy or angiography; and frequent monitoring of vital signs. Operating room nurses will be involved in the surgical intervention and recovery room care. Once the patient has had surgery and is no longer in an intensive care unit, the level of nursing care can be determined for the number of acute-care days that remain. Major nursing functions at this time involve general daily care (feeding, bathing, ambulation, and so forth); dressing changes; tube care; medication and fluid administration; observation, assessment, and recording; and patient education and discharge planning.

The process of specifying nursing services will require review of the management strategy associated with each patient management category by panels of nurses. The purpose of these panels is to determine direct nursing care requirements for the patient types defined by patient management categories. Although this is a major investment of time, it is

Figure 3
**Patient Management Path for PMC 3801, GI Disorder:
Bleeding Varices with Operation**

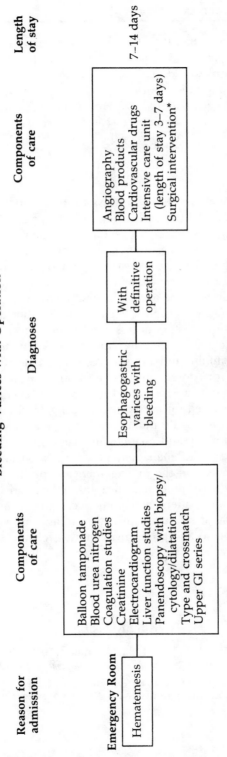

Reason for admission	Components of care	Diagnoses	Components of care	Length of stay
Emergency Room Hematemesis	Balloon tamponade Blood urea nitrogen Coagulation studies Creatinine Electrocardiogram Liver function studies Panendoscopy with biopsy/ cytology/dilatation Type and crossmatch Upper GI series	Esophagogastric varices with bleeding → With definitive operation	Angiography Blood products Cardiovascular drugs Intensive care unit (length of stay 3–7 days) Surgical intervention*	7–14 days

*Surgical intervention includes one or a combination of the following procedures: portal systemic shunt, transesophageal ligation, gastrectomy, esophageal transection, bowel interposition, esophagogastrectomy.

much less intensive than the original identification of patient types and specification of patient management paths. In this application, patient management paths would be a starting point to be used by nurses as a guide in specifying typical nursing services and the intensity of nursing care required by each patient type. Hospital costs related to direct nursing care could then be assigned to each service based on nursing time spent in completing the function or the level of nursing intensity involved.

SUMMARY

The search for more equitable ways to differentiate nursing service costs requires a clinically specific categorization of patients. Without this clinical specificity, the linkage between patient types and nursing services cannot be made effectively. Patient management categories and the management strategies that are associated with them provide the clinical foundation necessary to undertake more systematic and theoretically sound investigations in the areas of nursing costs and productivity.

For management purposes, it is clear that further differentiation of nursing services and costs is necessary. Further, given the dynamic nature of medical knowledge and the clinical practice of medicine, whatever method of determining nursing service costs that is developed must be flexible enough for subsequent modification. The clinical specificity of patient management categories and the level of detail of the physician-specified services listed for each category provide this flexibility. Patient management paths can be updated on a regular basis to account for changes in technology and changes in diagnostic and treatment regimens. With these clinical management strategies available, the impact of technological change on the management of specific patient types can be assessed and the resultant modification to the relative cost of care can be made. In this way, patient management categories and their associated clinical management strategies provide the analytic tools necessary to measure nursing costs and productivity more effectively than past efforts.

REFERENCES

Grimaldi, P. L. & Micheletti, J. A. (1982, December). DRG reimbursement: RIMS and the cost of nursing care. *Nursing Management, 13* (12), 12–20.

Mitchell, M., Miller, J., Welches, L., & Walker, D. (1984, April). Determining cost of direct nursing care by DRGs. *Nursing Management, 15,* 29–32.

New Jersey Department of Health (1979, September). *A prospective reimbursement system based on patient case mix for New Jersey hospitals, 1976–1983 case mix performance study, instruction manual.* Trenton: State of New Jersey Department of Health.

Young, W. W. (1985a). *Measuring the Cost of Care Using Patient Management Categories, Final Report, Vol. II: Patient Management Category Relative Cost Weights.* Baltimore, MD: Health Care Financing Administration.

Young, W. W. (1985b). *Measuring the Cost of Care Using Patient Management Categories, Final Report, Vol. III: Patient Management Paths.* Baltimore, MD: Health Care Financing Administration.

Part 2
Patient Classification, DRGs, and Nursing Costs

Correlating Patient Classification and DRGs

Elizabeth A. Buck

The cost of health care in the United States has been increasing faster than the general rate of inflation. President Reagan signed P.L. 98–21, the Social Security Amendment of 1983, in an effort to contain these spiraling costs. Title VI of this law provides for payment for hospital inpatient services through Medicare under a prospective payment system, in which a hospital is reimbursed at a predetermined rate based on a list of diagnosis related groups (DRGs). The previous retrospective method of payment was based on the costs incurred by a hospital, which did not provide any incentive to decrease costs of health care. The new system became effective at the beginning of the hospital's fiscal year after October 1, 1983. At present, the prospective payment system applies only to Medicare patients; however, most experts agree that all third-party payers will adopt this method of reimbursing hospitals.

The new legislation has had far-reaching implications for the entire medical community, including nursing. Tomsky (1983) states that hospitals usually concentrate their cost-containment and cost-cutting measures on departments of nursing, because nursing costs have traditionally been the largest part of the operating budget. Consequently, as Curtin (1983) notes, there is considerable evidence that nursing departments will be required to justify costs for nursing services according to patient acuity, which must correlate with the patient's DRG.

PATIENT CLASSIFICATION SYSTEMS

One of the initial steps for nursing administrators to take in preparing for the implementation of DRGs is to make their patient classification systems parallel with DRGs (National League for Nursing, 1983). That is, patients' classification on the basis of nursing resources consumed should be related to the DRG into which the patient's condition falls.

Curtin (1983) has developed a model to develop a system for determining the cost of nursing services based on the DRG system. The patient should be classified, using a patient classification system, according to the number and complexity of his or her nursing care needs. When the patient is assigned to a final DRG at discharge, the patient's classification should then be correlated with that specific DRG.

The use of patient classification systems has been mandated by the Joint Commission on Accreditation of Hospitals (1984). Its Nursing Service Standard III states: "Nursing department/service assignments in the provision of nursing care shall be commensurate with the qualifications of nursing personnel and shall be designed to meet the nursing care needs of patients" (p. 113). The interpretation of this standard directs that "the nursing department/service shall define, implement and maintain a system for determining patient requirements for nursing care on the basis of demonstrated patient needs, appropriate nursing intervention, and priority for care" (p. 114).

Nursing administrators use patient classification systems "to monitor productivity levels, to predict and justify staffing needs, and to assist in the budgeting process for their divisions (Alward, 1983, p. 14). Although patient classification systems are used primarily for staffing decisions, they are also a useful tool for measuring the amount of nursing resources used per patient, enabling an institution to respond to variable needs for nursing care.

A patient classification system was implemented at Stanford University Hospital in October 1980 in order to charge patients for levels of nursing care received, as opposed to a flat daily room rate, and to document nursing care hours for reimbursement from third-party payers (Ames & Madsen, 1981). Using this patient classification scheme, which indicates all components of the nursing process, researchers at Stanford University Hospital's Department of Nursing conducted a study relating nursing resources consumed (defined as hours of nursing care), costs, and DRGs (Mitchell, Miller, Welches & Walker, 1984). Patients whose condition fell into several DRGs were identified on admission, and the number of hours of nursing care received were obtained from the patient classification tool. One finding was that nursing resource use for different DRGs varied considerably. The researchers also determined the range of resource use within a specific DRG and found that there was a considerable span of hours used, depending upon where the patient fell on a severity of illness continuum. Their ultimate conclusion was that a patient classification system can be used to determine the use of nursing resources.

Another study utilizing patient classification in determining patient charges for nursing care was done at St. Luke's Hospital Medical Center in Phoenix, Arizona (Cisarik, 1983). An analysis of the data collected indicated a definite positive relationship between a patient's acuity and the amount of nursing care provided. As the patient acuity increased, more professional nursing care was required, and a higher rate was charged.

The cost of nursing care has traditionally been included in the room charge, putting nursing into a non-revenue-producing cost center. Because attempts to decrease hospitals' operating costs have been aimed at cutting the nursing department budget, it has become necessary to justify the nursing budget by determining the portion of a patient's hospital bill that is attributable to nursing care. However, a considerable amount of information is needed about nursing hours for patient care before such costing can be attempted.

CORRELATING PATIENT CLASSIFICATIONS AND DRGs

The first step in justifying the nursing portion of a hospital's budget was taken through a descriptive study that attempted to identify the amount of nursing care given per DRG. Nursing care hours were identified through patient classification type for a selected group of DRGs. Five DRGs that were common in the two hospitals studied were selected. The patient classifications of those patients whose diagnoses fell into these DRGs were tabulated over their length of stay and were correlated between the two hospitals.

The following objectives were explored for each of five designated DRGs:

1. To determine the extent to which patients' classifications within a given DRG were homogeneous at each of three time points: (1) the day of admission, (2) the midpoint in the hospital stay, and (3) the day prior to discharge.

2. To determine whether the two hospitals differed in their respective distributions of patient classifications for patients in a given DRG. Again, this comparison was done at three time points.

3. To determine the extent to which the patients' lengths of stay were homogeneous for a given DRG.

4. To compare length of stay between the two hospitals for each of the five DRGs.

5. To determine the extent to which the total number of hours of nursing care were homogeneous for a given DRG.

The subjects for this study were drawn from two hospitals in a large midwestern city: a large university-affiliated teaching hospital and a 200-bed religious-affiliated community hospital. Both hospitals use a similar patient classification tool. The university-affiliated hospital uses the Medicus System, a commercially produced computerized system. The religious-affiliated hospital uses a modification of the Medicus System using the same critical indicators, only calculated manually.

For the Medicus System used by Hospital 1, the patient classification types, point ranges, and the corresponding hours of nursing care given in a 24-hour period are as follows:

Patient Type	Point Range	Hours of Care per 24 Hours
1	0–24	0–2
2	25–48	2–5
3	49–120	5–10
4	121–180	10–16
5	180 +	16 +

For the modified Medicus system used by Hospital 2, the patient classification types, point ranges, and hours of care are the following:

Patient Type	Point Range	Hours of Care per 24 Hours
I	0–11	0–2.2
II	12–27	2.2–5.4
III	28–40	5.4–8.0
IV	41 +	8.0 +

Each point is equal to four minutes of direct nursing care per shift.

Although the Medicus system tool has five classifications and the modified Medicus system tool has four, the range of nursing hours per classification was similar. None of the patients in the sample from Hospital 1 fell into classification V. The classifications are defined as follows:

Classification I: A patient who requires only a minimal amount of nursing care.

Classification II: A patient who requires an average amount of nursing care.

Classification III: A patient who requires above average nursing care.

Classification IV: A patient who requires maximum nursing care.

The sample for the study included all patients falling into each of the five selected DRG categories from May 11, 1984, through September 9, 1984, at each hospital. The five DRGs were selected based on the frequency of their occurrences at the smaller hospital in order to obtain a sufficient number of subjects within each DRG category. The five DRGs were DRG 88, chronic obstructive pulmonary disease; DRG 89, simple pneumonia and pleurisy, age greater than 69 years; DRG 127, heart failure and shock; DRG 138, cardiac arrhythmia and conduction disorders, age greater than 69 years; and DRG 296, nutritional and miscellaneous metabolic disorders, age greater than 69 years.

METHOD OF DATA COLLECTION

Because the classification of patients into DRGs was mandatory only since January 1984 for each of the hospitals studied, there was no common standardized method for assigning DRGs in each hospital. Therefore, the method of data collection was slightly different in the two hospitals.

Hospital 1

At Hospital 1, the university-affiliated teaching hospital, the researcher identified those patients whose diagnoses might fall into one of the five DRG categories from a computer list of all Medicare admissions compiled by the Medical Records Department. The patient classification data on these individuals were collected from the Medicus Scantron printouts located in the nursing office. The patient classification points were calculated only once in a 24-hour period, during the early day shift, and these were tabulated along with the patient classification type over each patient's length of stay.

This hospital had a direct computer linkup with the Medicare intermediary, and within seven days of a patient's discharge the final DRG was assigned and entered in the hospital's computer. The researcher then looked up the DRG corresponding to each patient, chosen on the basis of his or her admitting diagnosis. The original sample of patients whose patient classifications and points were tabulated over their lengths of stay numbered 233. However, only 88 of these patients actually had diagnoses that fell into the five selected DRGs and were included in the study.

Hospital 2

At the religious-affiliated community hospital, Hospital 2, patients who were assigned to each DRG were identified by the DRG coordinator. Each Medicare patient was assigned a tentative DRG based on the history and physical examination data collected within 24 to 48 hours following admission. The patient classification tool used by this hospital was obtained from the nursing office.

At this hospital the patient classification points were tallied on each shift, and a separate classification was recorded. However, to allow a more reliable comparison with the other hospital, which only makes one classification determination early in the day shift, only the points recorded on the day shift and the corresponding classification type were recorded over each patient's length of stay.

Because the Medicare intermediary had reviewed the coordinator's DRG assignments in July 1984 and found a high percentage of agreement and minimal disallowances, all 82 patients whose diagnoses fell into one of the five DRGs to be studied were included in the sample.

RESULTS

The first research objective involved determining the homogeneity of patient classifications for a given DRG within each hospital. In fact, for all DRGs in both hospitals at each of the three time points, more than 65 percent of the patient classifications were distributed within one or two consecutive classifications. This finding substantiates the homogeneity of DRGs with respect to the use of nursing resources. According to a study by Giovannetti (1984), one of the purposes of categorizing patients according to DRGs is to identify patient groups that are similar in their consumption of hospital resources, part of which is hours of nursing care. Since the patient classification to which each patient is assigned is a representation of the number of nursing care hours needed by each patient, it follows that if the frequency distribution indicates a consistency in the patient classifications assigned for a particular DRG, the number of hours of nursing care required for patients within that DRG will also be homogeneous.

There were two exceptions to this homogeneous distribution: (1) for Hospital 1 in DRG 89, only 62.5 percent of the patient classifications were grouped within two consecutive classifications on the day prior to discharge (see Table 1); and (2) for Hospital 1 in DRG 296, at the midpoint in the hospital stay, the classifications were evenly distributed (see Table 2). A possible explanation for the first exception is found in the fact that 31.3 percent of the sample in that DRG were in classification

Table 1
Frequency Distribution of Patient Classifications for DRG 89

Time of Classification	Patient Classification							
	I		II		III		IV	
	Number	Percentage	Number	Percentage	Number	Percentage	Number	Percentage
Day after admission[a]								
Hospital 1	4	25.0	4	25.0	8	50.0	0	0
Hospital 2	0	0	7	63.6	4	36.4	0	0
Midpoint of stay[b]								
Hospital 1	1	6.3	6	37.5	9	56.3	0	0
Hospital 2	1	9.1	5	45.5	5	45.5	0	0
Day before discharge[c]								
Hospital 1	8	50.0	2	12.5	5	31.3	1	6.3
Hospital 2	1	9.1	9	81.8	1	9.1	0	0

[a]Chi-square = 5.41, df = 2 (not significant at .05 level).
[b]Chi-square = 0.32, df = 2 (not significant at .05 level).
[c]Chi-square = 13.09, df = 3, $p < .01$.

Table 2
Frequency Distribution of Patient Classifications for DRG 296

	Patient Classification							
	I		II		III		IV	
Time of Classification	Number	Percentage	Number	Percentage	Number	Percentage	Number	Percentage
Day after admission[a]								
Hospital 1	3	60.0	1	20.0	1	20.0	0	0
Hospital 2	7	53.8	6	46.2	0	0	0	0
Midpoint of stay[b]								
Hospital 1	1	20.0	1	20.0	2	40.0	1	20.0
Hospital 2	1	7.7	5	38.5	6	46.2	1	7.7
Day before discharge[c]								
Hospital 1	1	20.0	2	40.0	2	40.0	0	0
Hospital 2	0	0	10	76.9	2	15.4	1	7.7

[a]Chi-square = 3.26, df = 2 (not significant at .05 level).
[b]Chi-square = 1.38, df = 3 (not significant at .05 level).
[c]Chi-square = 4.71, df = 3 (not significant at .05 level).

III, which may indicate some patients were discharged to skilled nursing facilities or had expired. No conclusion can be drawn about the second exception, because of the small size of that sample.

The second research objective, concerning homogeneity of patient classifications between hospitals, was tested using qualitative and quantitative comparisons with a series of chi-square and t-tests respectively. In only two instances were there statistically significant differences between the two hospitals in frequency distributions, both on the day prior to discharge. For DRG 89 at Hospital 1, 50 percent of the sample were in classification I, while at Hospital 2, 81.8 percent were in classification II (see Table 1). For DRG 127, Hospital 1 had 61.3 percent of the sample in classification I, while 71.4 percent of the sample at Hospital 2 were in classification II (see Table 3).

Both of these exceptions show a larger percentage of patients in classification I at Hospital 1 on the day prior to discharge, while at Hospital 2 a larger percentage of predischarge patients were in classification II. This may relate to the fact that Hospital 2 had greater control over the discharge of patients then Hospital 1, because the DRG coordinator was also the leader of the discharge planning committee. The mean length of stay at Hospital 2 was also shorter than at Hospital 1, which indicates that patients were being discharged sooner and might, therefore, be sicker, hence rating a higher classification. Another possible explanation is that because Hospital 2 is smaller, there is greater pressure to decrease costs. One way to do this is to decrease length of stay, meaning again, that some patients will have a higher patient classification on discharge. However, the data from the quantitative analysis using the t-test showed no significant difference between the hospitals on the basis of patient classification, once again pointing to the homogeneity of resource use in the five DRGs studied.

The next two research objectives referred to the homogeneity of lengths of stay within hospitals and between hospitals. No significant difference was found between the lengths of stay, except in DRG 89, where the mean for Hospital 1 was significantly higher than the mean for Hospital 2. This could be explained by the fact that as a large university-affiliated teaching hospital, Hospital 1 had a higher level of technology, resulting in the patients' receiving more testing than in Hospital 2. Also, 31.5 percent of patients in DRG 89 discharged from Hospital 1 were in classification II, compared to only 9.1 percent in Hospital 2, showing that the discharged patients generally required more nursing care in Hospital 1. For each hospital, the mean length of stay exceeded the national mean of 7.5 days with Hospital 2 being the closer. A recent study by McClain and Selhat (1984) also found length of stay exceeding national norms. According to Health Systems Agency statistics, the metropolis studied

Table 3
Frequency Distribution of Patient Classifications for DRG 127

	Patient Classification							
	I		II		III		IV	
Time of Classification	Number	Percentage	Number	Percentage	Number	Percentage	Number	Percentage
Day after admission[a]								
Hospital 1	8	25.8	12	38.7	10	32.3	1	3.2
Hospital 2	3	27.3	20	71.4	5	17.9	0	0
Midpoint of stay[b]								
Hospital 1	14	45.2	11	35.5	5	16.1	1	3.2
Hospital 2	5	17.9	15	53.6	8	28.6	0	0
Day before discharge[c]								
Hospital 1	19	61.3	9	29.0	1	3.2	2	6.5
Hospital 2	7	25.0	20	71.4	1	3.6	0	0

[a]Chi-square = 6.8, df = 3 (not significant at .05 level).
[b]Chi-square = 6.4, df = 3 (not significant at .05 level).
[c]Chi-square = 11.59, df = 3, $p < .01$.

has one of the higher mean lengths of stay in the nation, probably because of the large number of hospital beds per capita, so these findings are not surprising.

Results pertaining to the final research objective, concerning the homogeneity of the hours of nursing care for each DRG are displayed in Figures 1 and 2. For Hospital 1, in four out of five DRGs (88, 89, 127, and 138) the distribution of total points followed a similar pattern. The distribution was negatively skewed; that is, the bulk of the patients had low classification scores. For DRG 296 the graph appeared to be bimodal (see Figure 1), but it is hard to draw any conclusions from this because the sample only included five subjects. Hospital 2 displayed no clear pattern across DRGs. The distribution for DRG 296 appeared to be negatively skewed (see Figure 2), but otherwise the frequencies of patient classifications seemed to be more uniformly distributed than for Hospital 1.

The total number of hours of nursing care was represented by the total number of patient classification points assigned to each patient falling into each DRG. The ranges of these points are quite variable for all DRGs, a finding consistent with that of several previous studies (Giovanetti, 1984; McClain & Selhat, 1984; Mitchell, Miller, Welches & Walker, 1984). Mitchell et al. (1984) state that "the greater the variety of diagnoses within given DRGs, the greater the possibility of a wider range of resource use" (p. 31). The wide range and large standard deviation they found indicate that similar nursing resources are not used within the DRGs studied. This inconsistency between the findings of homogeneous patient classification and the wide range of total nursing care hours within each DRG could be a result of the range of hours of nursing care within each classification. It appears that use of a classification consisting of only four or five separate classes should be limited to staffing purposes. The actual number of patient classification points, which more precisely relates to the number of hours of nursing care, should be used in the cost analysis.

LIMITATIONS

This study had several limitations. The sample size for three of the DRGs was less than 20; a larger sample size would have made a stronger study.

Using only two hospitals was another limitation, although because of their diversity, the homogeneity statistics are more meaningful than if two similar hospitals were used. Despite the similarities in the patient classification systems of the two hospitals in critical indicators and the definitions of the classifications, the point systems used were different,

Figure 1
Distribution of Patient Classification Points During Hospital Stay: Hospital 1

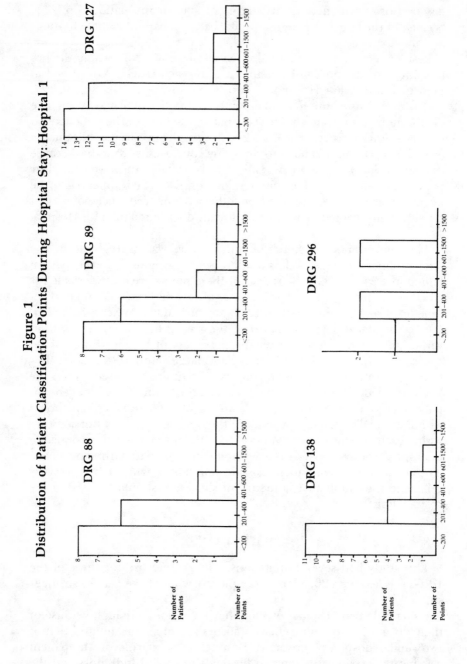

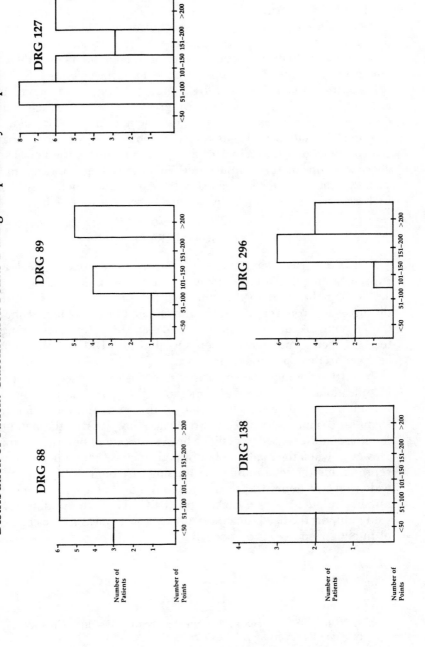

Figure 2
Distribution of Patient Classification Points During Hospital Stay: Hospital 2

which prohibited a statistical comparison of the total number of points for hospital stays between the two hospitals. However, when the total number of hours of nursing care were calculated, the ranges were similar, despite the difference in the ranges of the actual points.

Other studies have used the number of nursing hours over the entire length of stay instead of choosing only three time points (McClain & Selhat, 1984; Mitchell et al., 1984). The use of only three points limits the results of this study because wider variations of frequency distributions may have been seen if the entire length of stay was used.

A final limitation is the unknown reliability of each of the patient classification tools used. In Hospital 1, an ongoing periodic reliability check was done on the computerized Medicus System. However, in Hospital 2, although internal reliability testing of the patient classification tool was carried out initially, it was not done on a routine basis.

SUMMARY

The DRG system was devised as a means for decreasing health care costs, including the cost of nursing care. Because nursing administrators are feeling the need to determine costs of nursing care in order to distinguish it from room charges, initial data must be obtained showing the amount of nursing resources used per DRG. By determining the total number of nursing care hours used in each DRG, a price can then be given to that specific nursing care.

From the findings shown in this study, it can be seen that patient classifications are not a reliable method of determining the amount of nursing resources used. The results of this study showed a statistically significant similarity between two diverse hospitals in the amount of nursing resources used per DRG when classifications only are compared. However, when the total number of patient classification points, directly representing the total number of nursing care hours were compared, a wide range of hours was seen. This indicates that a similar amount of nursing resources was not used per DRG. Thus, the findings of this study support the need for a more precise tool to measure exact amounts of nursing resources used per DRG.

REFERENCES

Alward, R. R. (1983, February). Patient classification systems: The ideal vs. reality. *Journal of Nursing Administration, 13*(2), 14–19.

Ames, D. L., & Madsen, N. L. (1981). Developing a patient classification system. *Nursing Administration Quarterly, 5*(2), 17–21.

Cisarik, I. M. (1983). A unique approach for salient classification, resource allocation, variable charges. In *Nurse staffing based on patient classification: An examination of case studies* (pp. 1–9). Kansas City, MO: American Nurses' Association.

Curtin, L. (1983, April). Determining costs of nursing services per DRG. *Nursing Management, 14*(4), 16–20.

Giovannetti, P. (1984, October). *DRG-based patient classification systems.* Paper presented at the meeting of the National Association of Nursing Service Administrators, Chicago, IL.

Joint Commission on Accreditation of Hospitals (1984). *Accreditation manual for hospitals.* Chicago, IL: Joint Commission of Accreditation of Hospitals.

McClain, T. R., & Selhat, M. S. (1984, October). Twenty cases: What nursing costs per day. *Nursing Management, 15*(10), 26–34.

Mitchell, M., Miller, J., Welches, L., & Walker, D. D. (1984, April). Determining cost of direct nursing care by DRGs. *Nursing Management, 15*(4), 29–32.

National League for Nursing (1983). *The world according to DRGs.* Public Policy Bulletin, II(2).

Tomsky, C. N. (1983, October). Acuity based staffing controls cost. *Nursing Management, 14*, 16–20.

Relationships among Nursing Care Requirements, Nursing Resources, and Charges

Jan R. Atwood, Ada Sue Hinshaw, and Helen C. Chance

Since "financial constraints imposed by cost reimbursement intensified with the introduction of prospective pricing" (Joel, 1985, p. 10), and with the accompanying DRG system, corporate creativity has responded to identify the health product delivered relative to consumption and generation of resources. Nurses are part of that corporate creativity in their effort to relate DRGs to patient care needs.

Identifying the relationship of DRGs to nursing care requirements is vital for management of nursing resources. Curtin (1983), Grimaldi and Micheletti (1982), Hamilton (1984), and others since them have highlighted the importance of monitoring and predicting nursing resources in a definitive manner in order to provide high-quality care that is managed well.

The Institute of Medicine (1983) report on nursing clearly documented that "lack of precise information about current costs and utilization of nursing service personnel makes it difficult for nursing service administrators and hospital managers to make the most of appropriate and cost effective decisions about assignment of nurses" (recommendation 17). The report called for studies to identify the fiscal implications for nursing care. This paper presents one such study. Its purpose is to identify the links among the complexity of patients' nursing care re-

The authors wish to acknowledge the contributions of Roberta Hagaman, MA, statistical consultant, who managed the operational data sets.

quirements, costs of patient care, and charges under DRGs. In the current study, DRGs are related to nursing care requirements based on the University Medical Center (UMC), Tucson, Arizona, patient classification system (PCS). (Hinshaw & Atwood, 1981a; Hinshaw, Verran, & Chance, 1977). Patient stays in medical-surgical, general and intensive care units (ICUs) are primarily considered.

NURSING RESOURCE MODEL

The primary resource question of the current study was whether patients' nursing care needs are the basis for determining the nursing resources needed and, subsequently, the nursing resources used and replaced. A model of nursing resources based on the nursing care requirements of the patient or client was created to explain patterns of nursing care requirements (as measured by PCS scores), nursing resources needed (nursing time and costs), and the rate of resource replacement (charges to patients) within DRGs.

The study was designed to address questions related to the degree to which the delivery of nursing care is determined by a meaningful match among patients' needs for nursing care, concomitant nursing resources (both predicted and actual), and resource replacement rate, rather than being defined by an arbitrary standard used by some organizations nationally in response to the tremendous economic pressures, such as DRGs.

The Nursing Resource Model consists of four stages (see Fig. 1). These stages and the concepts they encompass illustrate the causal or predictive relationships assumed to guide traditional staffing methodology (Adyedottle, 1973). In addition, the model incorporates the concept of charging for patient care based on requirements for nursing care incorporated (see, for example, Grimaldi & Micheletti, 1982; Van Slyck, 1985). The relationships in the model can also be studied conjointly with DRG categories, as was done in this study.

Stage I of the model consists of the patient's nursing care requirements as measured by the patient's score on the patient classification system. The complexity of such requirements—that is the amount of professional knowledge and skill needed to handle the nursing care—guides not only the number but also the type of nursing staff needed, such as registered nurse, practical nurse, or nursing assistant (NA). The patient classification system considers patients' nursing care requirements on several dimensions: entry, exit, and transfer activity; activities of daily living (hygiene, feeding, and mobility); medications; vital signs; behavioral demands; treatments and medical orders; impaired conditions; and independent nursing actions, such as planning and referral, counseling and support, teaching and updating, assessment and observation, and

Figure 1
Nursing Resource Model Based on Patient Care Requirements

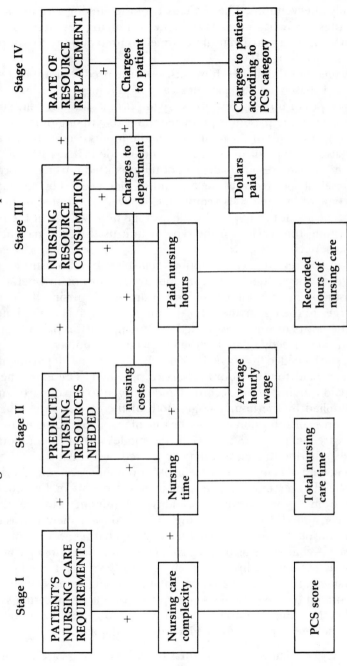

family interventions. The complexity of the nursing care needed to handle these activities predicts the type of nursing resources necessary to provide nursing care in terms of time required and the cost of providing the service (stage II).

Stage II of the model thus consists of the predicted nursing resources needed, based on the patient's care requirement (Giovannetti, 1979). Two types of nursing resources are important: nursing time and cost of the services the patient is predicted to need. Nursing time is considered not only in terms of the total hours and minutes needed for patient care, but also the type of nursing personnel needed: RN, LPN, or NA. The second nursing resource, the cost of the predicted nursing services, clearly is closely associated with the amount of time needed by patients and by the type of nursing staff required. Costs were computed by multiplying the time spent per patient by the average hourly wage of the personnel providing the service on the type of unit used by the patient (general unit or ICU).

Nursing resource consumption (Feldstein, 1983) constitutes the third stage of the model. Two concepts are important in operationalizing consumption of nursing resources: number of nursing hours used and charges to the department for the nursing hours. Nursing hours refers to the hours of service provided by nursing staff in patient care. These hours are directly related to the prediction of number and type of nursing staff needed in stage II. The charges to the department are the dollars paid for the hours of service provided. These are the number of paid nursing hours recorded and charged to the department budget multiplied by the hourly wage. Both of the concepts defining nursing resource consumption predict the rate of resource replacement for nursing care (stage IV). Stage III of the model was not operationalized in this study due to a lack of data organized by patient stay.

The rate of resource replacement for nursing care, stage IV, is defined as the charges made to the patient based on his or her nursing care requirements and the number and type of nursing resources the patient has consumed. In this study, the charges to the patient consisted of the total hospital charges. A subset of these charges was examined more closely—charges reflecting the room rate, of which nursing charges were a part. Ideally, in this model, charges to the patient would reflect the nursing care charges based on patient nursing care requirements and computed by the patient's score on the patient classification system.

The Nursing Resource Model was used to generate the following six specific research questions, which guided the study:

1. To what degree do DRGs describe nursing care requirements?
2. How much variability exists in nursing care requirements within DRGs?

3. For DRGs with a high degree of variability in 'nursing care requirements, to what degree is a meaningful pattern of variability formed by viewing clusters of DRGs for general units and ICUs?

4. To what degree is a pattern of variability in prediction of nursing resource needs (time and cost) noted in general units and ICUs?

5. What is the relationship between nursing care requirements and rate of revenue replacement (charges to patients)?

6. What are the patterns in resource replacement rate within DRGs?

DATA COLLECTION

The research design for this study was correlational and descriptive. The unit of analysis was inpatient stay. Two data sets were used from the hospital's operational data base for the 1982–83 fiscal year. The patient classification data indexed patients' nursing care requirements and the financial data set indexed patient charges.

The financial data set which contained a population of 12,522 inpatient stays, including stays in both general and intensive care units on all clinical services. The patient classification data set contained the patient classification scores for 5,788 stays on general and intensive care units for medical-surgical patients only, a subset of the population in the financial data set. The actual sample used for various analyses was determined by the degree to which the two data sets (financial and patient classification system) had to be merged. For example, when both patient classification and financial information were needed, the maximum sample size was just under 6,000 inpatient stays. Guided by the financial data set, the study included only those stays from which the patient was discharged by the end of the data-collection period and for which complete billing information was therefore available.

DRGs were determined for all inpatient stays in both the patient classification system and financial data sets. The study examined primarily those DRGs that were highly prevalent at the hospital—those with at least 50 patient stays during the study year. The DRGs with a high volume of patient stays were more likely to show typical and replicable patterns.

The UMC Department of Nursing patient classification system was used to index patient care requirements (stage I of the Nursing Research Model) (Hinshaw & Atwood, 1981a; Hinshaw & Atwood, 1983; Hinshaw, Verran, & Chance, 1977). In this system, complexity of patient care is defined as the amount of professional knowledge and skill needed to handle the nursing care requirements or factors. In practice, the scores range from 11 to approximately 45, with higher scores indicating greater complexity of nursing care requirements. The patient classification instrument is updated every four to five years to maintain its clinical credibility and validity. Construct validity has been estimated to be moderate to strong, using predictive modeling (Hinshaw & Atwood, 1981b). To estimate the completeness of the instrument, factor scores on the UMC PCS were compared with scores from a second subjective form of the same instrument using regression analysis, with a 75.8 percent explained variance (R^2) (Hinshaw, 1984). Factor analyses have shown a correspondence in nine out of ten factors. Results of criterion validity tests with the Johns Hopkins instrument (Connor, 1961) and the Saskatchewan, Canada, instrument (Giovannetti, 1978) ranged from $r = .74$ to $r = .77$. The reliability of the UMC instrument has been estimated as moderate, with test-retest correlations of $r = .80$ and higher. Staff reliability using the PCS instrument is moderate to strong, with agreement figures ranging from 65 percent to 99 percent, depending on the factor, and gamma coefficients of .70 and higher.

The two nursing resources whose need was predicted, time and cost, were indexed in accordance with stage II of the Nursing Resource Model. To compute nursing time in hours, the time coefficients from a validation study of the patient classification system (Hinshaw & Atwood, 1981b) were multiplied by each patient's PCS score from the operational PCS data set. To compute the costs of nursing time, the average hourly wage for staff on general units and on intensive care units was multiplied by the computed nursing time.

The rate of resource replacement (stage IV) was indexed by the dollars charged to each patient, obtained from the operational financial data set. To compute the total charges, the various types of charges to the patient were summed, including charges for room, pharmacy and supply, occupational and physical therapy, respiratory therapy, diagnostic labs and X-ray, therapeutic X-ray, special services, emergency and operating room, and special medical services. At the time of the study, charges to the client for nursing services were included in the room charge and were based on a daily rate for the type of room the patient occupied. Therefore, the charges for nursing care were represented in the room rate.

DATA ANALYSIS

Secondary data analysis was used to address each of the six research questions generated by the Nursing Resource Model. The methods of analysis included frequency and percentage distributions, means and standard deviations for description of central tendency and dispersion, bivariate correlations, and eta squared for description of relationships and coefficients of variation for description of differences within a DRG category (Polit and Hungler, 1978). The coefficient of variation (the mean divided by the standard deviation of the PCS scores in a given DRG) was used to identify DRGs with a great deal of variation in nursing care requirements.

The research questions will be considered individually in turn.

1. To what degree do DRGs describe patients' nursing care requirements?

The first question addresses the identification of nursing care requirements according to stage I of the Nursing Resource Model. Since the UMC patient classification system had been validated previously as a solid estimate of nursing care needs, the focus was on the degree to which DRGs index those needs.

Little relationship was found between patients' DRG and their nursing care requirements or resource demand. The eta squared between patients' PCS scores and their DRG was .23 for general unit stays, .47 for intensive care unit stays, and .38 for total stays, indicating that only 23 percent, 47 percent, and 38 percent, respectively, of the patients' nursing care requirements were indexed by their DRG.

DRGs alone are obviously not adequate to index nursing care requirements, so nursing care resources cannot be meaningfully allocated on the basis of DRGs, nor can nursing services be charged on that basis. When adopted as national policy for the prospective payment, DRGs were based on medical care but not nursing care parameters (Fetter, Shin, Freeman, Averill, & Thompson, 1980). Several systems are being tested to address the problem of the insensitivity of DRGs to nursing care parameters, including the Severity of Illness Index (Horn 1983) and APACHE (Jones, 1984). Patient classification systems, such as that used at UMC, have also been devised to index nursing care requirements, some predating DRGs by several years (Hinshaw, Verran, & Chance, 1977).

2. How much variability exists in nursing care requirements within DRGs?

Patients' nursing care requirements (stage I of the model) vary little within some DRGs but a lot in others. Average PCS scores ranged widely from 23.1 for DRGs 372 and 383 to 28.5 for DRG 91. Tables 1, 2, and 3 show the PCS scores and their degree of variation in nursing care requirements within DRGs for patients' general unit, ICU, and total stays. Variability is considered high when the coefficient of variation approaches or exceeds the .10 (Giovannetti, Edwardson, & Busch, 1984).

Table 1
Nursing Care Requirements (PCS Scores) by DRG
for General Unit Stays

DRG	Number of Stays	Mean	SD	Coefficient of Variation
12	52	25.6	3.23	.13
14	50	25.9	2.54	.10
39	55	24.3	1.07	.05
60	65	25.4	1.92	.07
82	103	25.9	2.07	.08
88	74	25.8	2.27	.09
89	68	26.3	2.09	.08
91	54	28.5	2.30	.08
98	71	26.9	2.84	.10
105	62	24.5	2.02	.08
107	88	24.6	1.34	.05
122	53	24.5	1.14	.04
125	133	25.6	2.24	.09
127	53	26.1	2.29	.09
138	77	25.6	1.87	.07
140	46	24.4	1.50	.06
143	71	24.7	1.71	.07
182	85	25.5	1.82	.07
184	63	26.9	2.62	.10
209	94	25.7	1.31	.05
222	63	25.2	1.33	.05
243	78	24.1	1.90	.08
295	50	24.6	1.68	.07
296	59	25.1	2.72	.11
298	65	26.5	3.14	.12
355	64	24.0	1.13	.05
370	74	23.3	1.05	.05
371	117	23.4	1.10	.05
372	219	23.1	0.97	.04
373	1,047	23.2	1.00	.04
374	83	23.5	1.18	.05
383	90	23.1	1.18	.05
389	140	26.2	3.72	.14
390	617	25.6	3.69	.14
391	633	24.7	3.35	.14
403	86	25.9	1.93	.07
408	69	25.1	1.40	.06
409	50	24.7	1.75	.07
410	248	24.6	1.98	.08
426	58	25.8	2.09	.08
430	201	26.3	1.66	.06
467	62	24.9	2.74	.08
468	202	25.4	2.07	.08
470	60	25.3	2.34	.09

Table 2
Nursing Care Requirements (PCS Scores) by DRG for Intensive Care
Unit Stays

DRG	Number of Stays	Mean	SD	Coefficient of Variation
105	59	34.1	1.74	.05
107	89	34.1	1.57	.05
122	52	29.3	1.29	.04
138	54	29.4	2.09	.07
143	80	29.5	1.51	.05
386	74	36.1	2.69	.07
389	93	36.0	2.70	.08
390	72	35.4	4.37	.12
468	74	32.3	2.92	.09

For general units, of the 44 DRGs with 50 or more stays and complete PCS data, 9 (21 percent) showed a high degree of variation in the mean PCS score for the patients' entire stay (see Table 1). For ICU stays, among the 9 DRGs with at least 50 stays, only one (11 percent) showed high variability (see Table 2). This finding indicates that the average complexity of nursing care needed by patients varies less within most DRGs during stays in the ICU than in general units.

Taking general units and ICUs together, among the 48 DRGs with at least 50 stays and complete PCS data 18 (38 percent) show at least the criterion amount of variation in the average PCS score for patients' entire stay (see Table 3). This finding indicates that for nearly half of the high-volume DRGs, even the average complexity of nursing care is highly variable.

In sum, average (mean) nursing care complexity for entire patient stays is least variable for stays with ICU days and most variable when stays are not distinguished by ICU or general units stays. (These findings apply only to the average complexity of patient care per DRG; PCS scores of individual patients vary considerably more in some DRGs.) Over 10 percent of the stays in ICUs that are classified in high-volume DRGs vary considerably in nursing care requirements; general unit stays vary considerably for 21 percent of the stays; and, without considering the type of unit, 38 percent of the stays vary notably. The high variability in general unit stays is important because more patients are on general units than ICUs. There is less range in the ICUs, but the PCS scores are higher (ranging from 29.3 to 36.0), as would be expected. These findings have profound cost implications for the higher-cost care at higher levels of complexity. For example, estimates of nursing care complexity and, therefore, staffing, must have greater accuracy than that afforded by

Table 3
Nursing Care Requirements (PCS Scores) by DRG for Total Stays

DRG	Number of Stays	Mean	SD	Coefficient of Variation
12	53	25.9	3.51	.14
14	52	26.6	3.07	.12
39	55	24.3	1.06	.05
60	65	25.4	1.92	.07
82	107	26.1	2.32	.09
88	74	26.0	2.26	.09
89	68	26.6	2.52	.09
91	55	26.1	2.73	.10
98	71	27.1	3.04	.11
105	63	29.1	2.82	.10
107	92	29.4	2.25	.08
122	58	26.5	1.58	.06
125	134	25.9	2.39	.09
127	55	26.9	2.66	.10
138	83	26.9	2.09	.08
140	50	26.2	1.95	.08
143	94	27.1	2.18	.08
182	87	25.8	1.91	.07
184	63	27.0	2.65	.10
209	94	25.8	1.41	.05
222	63	25.1	1.33	.05
243	79	24.2	2.08	.09
295	50	25.2	1.98	.08
296	60	25.2	2.89	.12
298	65	26.5	3.21	.12
355	64	24.1	1.14	.05
370	74	23.3	1.11	.05
371	117	23.4	1.10	.05
372	219	23.1	0.97	.04
373	1,047	23.2	1.00	.04
374	83	23.5	1.18	.05
383	90	23.2	1.32	.06
385	54	35.5	4.93	.14
386	77	33.5	3.62	.11
389	188	29.7	4.99	.17
390	634	26.5	4.01	.15
391	636	24.9	3.52	.14
403	87	26.2	2.34	.09
408	69	25.1	1.42	.06
409	50	24.7	1.75	.07
410	248	24.6	1.99	.08
426	58	25.8	2.09	.08
430	201	26.3	1.66	.06
442	50	26.5	2.06	.08
449	52	28.2	3.33	.12
467	62	25.0	2.74	.11
468	211	26.4	3.11	.12
470	63	26.2	3.36	.13

DRGs so that prediction of staffing needs is feasible and use of expensive overtime and registry nurses, resulting in budget excesses, is avoided. Variability of nursing care requirements within DRGs is explored further in the next research question.

3. **For the DRGs identified as having a high degree of variability in nursing care requirements, to what degree is a meaningful pattern of variability formed by viewing clusters of DRGs for general and intensive care units?**

Based on coefficients of variation in nursing care requirements for individual DRGs (stage I of the model), four clusters of DRGs were considered: DRGs 12 to 15, which contain nervous system and cerebrovascular disorders; 182 to 184, dealing with the digestive system; 296 to 298, concerning nutrition and metabolic disorders across the age span; and 385 to 391, regarding newborns (see Table 4). The clusters were formed by grouping the DRGs in the original sample that were highly variant with other similar DRGs that formed meaningful anatomical units.

In the first cluster of DRGs, nervous system disorders, only DRGs 12 and 14 had 50 or more stays and were therefore examined in the original screening. The sample size for the entire cluster ranged from 10 to 52 patient stays. The coefficients of variation in nursing care requirements ranged from .07 to .13. The criterion of .10 was used for identifying high variation in individual DRGs, and viewing the pattern in the clusters of DRGs suggests that a criterion of .08 to .10 is a meaningful one for clusters. Using the latter criterion, the cluster of DRGs 12 to 15 would be viewed on the average as highly variant in average nursing care requirements.

In the second cluster, DRGs related to digestive disorders, only DRG 183 was not found in the original screening of high variation in nursing care requirements. (DRG 183 had only 33 patient stays.) The coefficients of variance for this cluster ranged from .07 to .10, again indicating that the cluster was to be relatively variant in average requirements for nursing care.

In the third cluster, concerning nutrition and metabolic diseases, only DRG 297, with 15 patient stays, was not in the original screening. Consistent with the two previous clusters, the coefficient of variance range of .08 to .12 indicated that patients in this cluster were highly variable in average requirements for nursing care.

In the fourth cluster of DRGs dealing with neonates, DRGs 389, 390, and 391 had at least 50 stays and therefore were included in the original screening. The range of stays for the cluster was 19 to 633. All of the coefficients of variation for the general unit stays were at least .10 and

Table 4
Clusters of DRGs with High Variance in Nursing Care
Requirements (PCS Scores)

Cluster and DRG	Number of Stays		Coefficient of Variation	
	General Unit	ICU	General Unit	ICU
Nervous system				
12 Degenerative nervous system disorder	52	—	.13	—
13 Multiple sclerosis and cerebellar ataxia	10	—	.12	—
14 Specific cerebrovascular disease (expect TIA)	50	—	.10	—
15 Transient ischemic attacks	28	—	.07	—
Esophagitis, gastroenteritis, misc. digestive disorders				
182 Age greater than 69 and/or CC.	85	—	.07	—
183 Age 18–69 without CC.	33	—	.10	—
184 Age 0–17	63	—	.10	—
Nutritional and miscellaneous metabolic diseases				
296 Age greater than 69 and/or CC.	59	—	.11	—
297 Age 18–69 without CC.	15	—	.08	—
298 Age 0–17	65	—	.12	—
Neonates				
385 Neonate died or transferred	19	48	.13	.08
386 Extreme immaturity of neonate	46	74	.10	.07
387 Prematurity with major problems	28	34	.13	.06
388 Prematurity without major problems	25	27	.13	.07
389 Full-term neonate without major problems	140	93	.14	.08
390 Full-term neonate with major problems	617	72	.14	.12
391 Normal newborn	633	23	.14	.14

ranged up to .14. In addition, some of the stays in the DRGs in this cluster were in the ICU. Consistent with earlier findings, nursing care requirements varied less during ICU stays, with coefficients of variation ranging from .06 to .14, and all but three above .08.

The high-prevalence DRGs can serve as indicators to identify clusters of DRGs that form a pattern with other anatomically similar DRGs. In this case, the clusters grouped around individual DRGs that were highly variant in their nursing care requirements also manifested relatively high variance. These clusters of DRGs are meaningful units to use when planning and evaluating nursing care.

4. To what degree is a pattern of variability in prediction of nursing resource needs (time and cost) formed by viewing clusters of DRGs in general units and ICUs?

The patterns in prediction of the need for nursing resources (stage II of the Nursing Resource Model) may be seen by examining nursing care time and dollar costs. As may be expected from the variability in the PCS scores examined in research question 3, nursing care hours per patient stay range broadly for all kinds of medical-surgical patient stays without considering DRGs (see Table 5). The median hours of care required are lowest for general unit stays (43.8 hours) and highest for ICU patient stays (73.6 hours), as would be expected, and average 52.5 hours for all stays. However, the standard deviations are at least as large as the means, validating the need to further refine classification of patients' nursing care requirements beyond the categories of general unit, ICU, or total hospital stays. For some time, nursing managers have been convinced of the variability in patients' nursing care requirements and the difficulty in predicting the need for nursing resources. The data here document the magnitude of variability in patients' nursing care requirements. Even patients in ICUs varied several hundred percent in their requirements.

Consistent with these findings, when hours of care are used as a base for computing the dollar cost of nursing time, the median cost is noticeably higher for ICU than for general unit stays (see Table 5). The dollar costs also vary phenomenally by patient stay for each type of unit when DRGs are not considered.

5. What is the relationship between nursing care requirements and rates of revenue replacement (charges to patients)?

Charges by patient stay are shown in Table 6 according to type of charges, not considering DRGs. It is interesting to recall that the Nursing

Table 5
Nursing Resources Needed Predicted by PCS for Medical-Surgical Patients

Type of Unit	N	Hours of Nursing Care Time per Stay[a]			Cost of Nursing Care Time		
		Range	Mean (SD)	Median	Range	Mean (SD)	Median
Total stays	5,788	8.51–1,690.00	95.93 (130.33)	52.50	$77.16–15,294.50	$868.55 (1,179.49)	$475.13
General unit portion of stay	5,551	8.51–935.55	63.53 (63.29)	43.75	$74.77–8,214.13	$557.82 (555.68)	$384.12
ICU portion of stay	1,569	16.80–1,663.20	129.12 (157.90)	73.63	$160.14–15,850.29	$1,230.54 (1,504.85)	$701.71

[a]Accounts for 100 percent of nursing time (direct and indirect time).

[b]Dollar costs computed on the basis of $8.78 per hour for general unit, $9.53 per hour for ICU, and $9.05 per hour for total stays.

Table 6
Description of Charges by Patient Stay

		Charge per Patient Stay		
Type of Charge	Number of Patient Stays	Mean Amount (SD)	Median Amount	Mean Percentage of Bill (SD)
Room[a]	12,516	$1,341.97 (2,403.26)	$628.00	42.4 (21.0)
Pharmacy and supply	12,522	884.62 (2,505.67)	265.80	17.8 (11.7)
Occupational therapy, physical therapy, etc.	1,165	227.89 (342.66)	108.00	2.8 (3.1)
Respiratory therapy	5,388	650.52 (2,317.29)	157.00	7.7 (7.9)
Lab and X-ray	12,270	850.71 (1,981.31)	307.28	19.6 (15.3)
X-ray	182	398.35 (280.75)	363.60	13.1 (10.3)
Special services	237	2,155.37 (3,666.31)	848.00	12.5 (8.7)
Emergency room	2,665	182.97 (177.74)	145.00	8.2 (7.3)
Operating room	5,283	1,077.05 (1,286.40)	683.40	31.8 (14.6)
Special medical services	5,240	122.72 (179.85)	36.50	3.4 (4.7)
Total charges	12,522	$1,769.79	[b]	$3,951.93 (8,114.71)

[a]Nutrition included in room charge.
[b]Adds up to more than 100 percent because some very high charges in some charge types elevated the averages.

Resource Model predicts that resources—nursing care time and costs (stage II)—are related directly to resources consumed and indirectly to the rate of resource replacement (patient charges) (stage IV). The correlation between flat-rate room charges, which include nursing care, and hours of nursing time is the highest of that for any type of charge for general unit stays ($r = .75$; $r^2 = .57$); the correlation of nursing time with room charges for ICU stays ($r = .78$; $r^2 = .61$) is second only to that with total charges ($r = .80$; $r^2 = .64$) (see Table 7). Few nursing departments today could survive with the ability to accurately predict only 57 or 61 percent of the need for nursing resources. The recom-

Table 7
Relationship Between Patient Charges and Nursing Time, Based on PCS Patient Complexity[a]

Type of Charge	General Units			Intensive Care Units		
	Number of Patient Stays	Correlation[b]		Number of Patient Stays	Correlation[c]	
		r	r^2		r	r^2
Room	5,551	.75	.57	1,569	.78	.61
Pharmacy and supply	5,551	.50	.25	1,569	.72	.53
Occupational therapy, physical therapy, etc.	920	.59	.35	274	.24	.06
Respiratory therapy	3,242	.36	.13	1,393	.72	.51
Lab and X-ray (Dx)	5,440	.49	.24	1,567	.76	.58
X-ray (Rx)	155	.22	.05	15	−.46[d]	.21
Special services	74	.54	.30	45	.28[e]	.08
Emergency room	1,562	.11	.01	778	.12	.01
Operating room	2,461	.21	.05	747	.19	.03
Special medical services	3,932	.17	.03	1,394	.35	.12
Total charges	5,551	.61	.37	1,569	.80	.64

[a]PCS coefficients adjusted to equal 100 percent of nursing time.

[b]$p \leq .005$.

[c]$p \leq .001$.

[d]$p = .08$.

[e]$p = .057$.

mendation of the Institute of Medicine's (1983) report to refine nursing resource management systems is well supported by these data.

6. What are the patterns in resource replacement rate within DRGs?

The next research question dealt with patterns of charges for selected DRGs (stage IV of the Nursing Resource Model). Table 8 illustrates the patterns of charges for DRG 14, specific cerebrovascular disease, and DRG 209, major joint procedures. DRG 14 is one of the DRGs with high variability in nursing care requirements. The charges are also highly variant, with wide ranges in both individual and total charges. On the average, room charges, which include nursing care charges, amount to about half of the charges for this DRG. In contrast, the room charges are a little under 25 percent of the charges for DRG 209, which was not a highly variable DRG. The nature of the diagnosis is reflected in the pattern of charges. Neither DRG had charges for treatment X-ray or special services. DRG 14 had no operating room charges, but DRG 209, which deals specifically with a major joint procedure, had notable operating room charges.

Interpretation of these data in terms of the rate of replacement of nursing resources is limited, because the data for the study year were not a precise indicator of nursing charges. The room charges, which contain nursing care revenue, are a function of the number of days of stay in a particular type of room (ICU, private, double, or triple), providing a rough categorization of the complexity of nursing care into four levels, rather than the more desirable factor-type patient classification index of nursing care requirements. Sovie, Tarencale, VanPutte and Stunden (1985) estimated that, based on the most prevalent medical DRGs, the room charges by DRG reflect 15.8 to 23.6 percent of the nursing costs, supporting their contention that nursing costs should be specified rather than part of the room charges.

IMPLICATIONS

DRGs alone do not provide a firm basis for managing nursing resources. Based on the research findings described here, patients' nursing care requirements can readily be used in conjunction with DRGs not only to predict needed nursing care resources but also to target groups of DRGs for which flexible resources will be needed.

Three primary implications are apparent from this study. The first relates to DRGs as a predictor of nursing care requirements. That DRGs are not consistently sensitive predictors is known. The new finding here is that DRGs predict the average patient's nursing care requirements

Table 8
Patient Charges for DRG 14 and DRG 209

Type of Charge	DRG 14 (N = 47)			DRG 209 (N = 94)		
	Range	Mean (SD)	Median	Range	Mean (SD)	Median
Room	$169–6,495	$2,110 (1,594)	$1,763	$954–6,727	$2,614 (952)	$2,366
Pharmacy and supply	24–3,242	689 (843)	292	639–119,251	2,820 (12,232)	1,221
Occupational therapy, physical therapy, etc.	24–1,442	421 (351)	378	18–853	318 (188)	296
Respiratory therapy	42–4,714	681 (1,013)	341	38–2,035	234 (340)	126
Lab and X-ray (Dx)	150–4,108	1,298 (870)	1,247	220–6,803	795 (845)	552
X-ray (Rx)	0	0	0	0	0	0
Special services	0	0	0	0	0	0
Emergency room	58–688	191 (110)	145	93–230	159 (40)	145
Operating room	0	0	0	878–6,595	3,301 (1,706)	2,843
Special medical services	36–893	208 (217)	73	36–365	55 (54)	36
Total	$919–18,789	$5,063 (3,755)	$3,881	$4,373–139,917	$10,122 (13,950)	$8,148

reasonably well for ICU stays, but in the general units, where most of the patient days are spent, they do not even predict the average patient's requirements. In the ICU, patients' care is much more homogeneous than in the general units, where a patient with a given diagnosis may be hospitalized for diagnostic tests, for specific treatment, because of exacerbation of symptoms, or for all these reasons. Thus, DRGs predict nursing care requirements least well on the general units, where nurse staffing must be sensitive to patients' heterogeneous needs in order to provide cost-effective, safe, satisfying care.

The second implication is that DRGs with high variability in complexity of requirements for nursing care cluster into groups of similar diagnoses. Thus, identifying such clusters is a significant management strategy for predicting the kinds of patients whose needs for nursing care resources are likely to fluctuate widely in a short time.

The third implication relates to the fact that charging for nursing services as part of the room rate is not sensitive to the variation in nursing care requirements. As documented in this study, it would be equally insensitive to charge a flat rate for nursing care by DRG, especially for those categories that vary greatly in the cost of patients' care requirements. Just knowing a patient's DRG does not solve the problem of being able to predict the complexity of nursing care needed, the amount of staffing needed or the amount to charge the patient.

Costs can vary for two reasons. The first is heterogeneity in nursing care requirements, as in certain clusters of DRGs. This phenomenon affects more patients in general units than in ICUs. The second reason for variation in costs is the exponential increment in nursing care requirements with slight increases in the PCS score. That is, for every increment in complexity of care at the upper end of the PCS continuum, representing patients with great care needs, nursing care time and therefore costs rise rapidly, as they do in ICUs. In contrast, the increase is very gradual at the lower end of the continuum (Hinshaw & Atwood, 1981b). More variation in nursing care requirements can be tolerated for patients with less complexity without greatly affecting staffing and budgeting. Thus, it is essential to use patients' requirements for nursing care as a basis for charging patients.

A careful look needs to be taken at the complexity of nursing care and the specific resources needed and charged. If patients' nursing care needs are the basis for determining nursing resources needed as well as the nursing resources used and replaced, nurse managers need effective, efficient mechanisms for identifying the need for nursing resources. The UMC patient classification system is a valid and reliable system to measure complexity of nursing care. It has been documented to show sensitivity to variations in nursing care requirements both within DRGs and independent of DRGs. Such a system is vital to the effective management of nursing resources.

REFERENCES

Aydelotte, M. K. (1973). *Nursing staffing methodology: A review and critique of selected literature* (DHEW Publication No. NIH 73–433). Washington, D.C.: U.S. Government Printing Office.

Connor, R. J. (1961, May). Effective use of nursing resources: A research report. *Hospitals, 35,* 30–39.

Curtin, L. (1983). Determining costs of nursing services per DRG. *Nursing Management, 14*(4), 16–20.

Feldstein, P. J. (1983). *Health care economics* (2d ed.). New York: Wiley.

Fetter, R. B., Shin, Y., Freeman, J. L., Averill, R. F., and Thompson, J. D. (1980). Case mix definition by diagnoses related groups. *Medical Care, 18*(2 suppl.), iii, 1–53.

Giovannetti, P. (1978). *Patient classification systems and their uses: A description and analysis* (DHEW Publication No. HRA 78–22). Springfield, VA: National Technical Information Service.

Giovannetti, P. (1979). Understanding patient classification systems. *Journal of Nursing Administration. 9,* 4–9.

Giovannetti, P., Edwardson, S., & Busch, W. (1984). *Relationship between DRG and patient classification data for nursing costs and allocations.* Paper presented at a meeting of the American Society for Nursing Service Administrators of the American Hospital Association, Chicago, IL.

Grimaldi, P. L., & Micheletti, J. A. (1982). DRG reimbursement: RIMs and the cost of nursing care. *Nursing Management, 13*(12), 12–22.

Hamilton, J. M. (1984). Nursing and DRGs: Proactive Responses to Prospective Reimbursement. In F. A. Shaffer (Ed.), *DRGs: Changes and challenges* (pp. 99–107). New York: National League for Nursing.

Hinshaw, A. S. (1984). *Shaping patient classification systems for reimbursement.* Paper presented at University of Pittsburgh Sigma Theta Tau Research Conference, Pittsburgh, PA.

Hinshaw, A. S., & Atwood, J. R. (1981a). Factors impacting on the delivery of quality nursing care. *Nursing Research, 31*(2), 120–121.

Hinshaw, A. S., & Atwood, J. R.(1981b). Time distribution among nursing care activities. *Western Journal of Nursing Research, 3*(3), 39–40.

Hinshaw, A. S., & Atwood, J. R. (1983). Independent nursing action: An integral part of patient classification. In J. Verran (Moderator), Patient classification research: New directions (Symposium). *Western Journal of Nursing Research, 5*(3), 91–93.

Hinshaw, A. S., Verran, J., & Chance, H. C. (1977). A description of nursing care requirements in six hospitals. *Communicating Nursing Research* (Western Interstate Commission for Higher Education, Boulder, CO), *9,* 261–283.

Horn, S. (1983). Measuring severity of illness: Comparisons across institutions. *American Journal of Public Health, 73*, 25–31.

Institute of Medicine (1983). *Nursing and nursing education: Public policies and private action.* Washington, DC: National Academic Press.

Joel, L. A. (1985). "The economics of health care: Trends and problems." In *The economics of health care and nursing.* Kansas City, MO: American Academy of Nursing.

Jones, K. R. (1984). Severity of illness measures: Issues and options. *Nursing Economics, 2*(5), 312–317.

Polit, D., & Hungler, B. (1978). *Nursing research: Principles and methods.* Philadelphia: J. B. Lippincott.

Sovie, M. D., Tarcinale, M. A., VanPutte, A., and Stunden, A. (1985). Amalgam of nursing acuity, DRGs, and costs. *Nursing Management, 16*(3), 22–42. Reprinted in this volume, pp. 121–148.

Van Slyck, A. (1985). Costing nursing care with the GRASP system. In F. A. Shaffer (ed.), *Costing out nursing: Pricing our product* (pp. 39–53). New York: National League for Nursing.

Amalgam of Nursing Acuity, DRGs, and Costs

Margaret D. Sovie, Michael A. Tarcinale,
Alison VanPutte, and Ann Stunden

The effective management of patient care resources under prospective payment systems requires new knowledge and a comprehensive and integrated patient care and financial information system. One data element that is essential to both components of such a management information system is the identification of the nursing care hours associated with the diagnosis related groups (DRGs) that constitute a hospital's case mix.

In order to study, predict, control, and assign hospital costs to specific hospital outputs or products—that is, patient care—the DRG patient classification system has been adopted as the basis of case-mix management and pricing in the Medicare prospective payment system.

The current DRGs constitute a revised medical classification schema that has 23 major diagnostic categories (MDCs), organized by organ system and disease etiology, and 468 DRGs. The individual DRG is assigned on the basis of the patient's principal diagnosis, secondary diagnosis, surgical procedures, and age. To have a complete picture of hospital resource utilization, it is necessary to correlate DRGs (a medical

An earlier version of this paper appeared in *Nursing Management*, *16* (March 1985): 22–42, and it is reprinted by permission of the author and publisher. This study was supported in part by a grant from the Rochester Area Hospital Corporation (Hospital Experimental Payments Program Contingency Fund) and in part by Strong Memorial Hospital of the University of Rochester Medical Center.

classification system), with a nursing patient classification system that indicates the nursing care hours required to meet the patient's care needs. To accomplish this objective, a correlation study of nursing patient classification, DRGs, other significant patient variables and total costs of patient care was designed and conducted. The purposes of the study were to identify the nursing classification of patients associated with the various DRGs; to determine the average nursing care hours requirements per category of patient classification by unit, service, and DRG; and to develop, implement, and evaluate a nursing budgetary system that combines DRGs and nursing classification of patients as the predictors of nursing resource utilization.

The objectives of the study were:

1. To design and develop a computer program to capture and retain daily classification of each patient with all other patient-specific data.

2. To determine the required nursing care hours per patient day per category, per unit, and service, according to the nursing patient classification system.

3. To identify and analyze the relationship of a nursing patient classification schema to DRGs with their required nursing care hours per category and direct costs.

4. To develop a program budgeting system for nursing practice that uses patient volume projections according to DRGs and their associated nursing patient classification system categories for determining budgetary requirements for designated cost centers.

5. To evaluate the resulting program budgeting system design for nursing practice and determine the effectiveness and efficiency of the amalgamation of DRGs and the nursing patient classification system in budgetary planning, monitoring, and control.

This study was conducted at the University of Rochester's Strong Memorial Hospital (SMH). This 741-bed teaching hospital is the primary educational facility for the School of Nursing and the School of Medicine and Dentistry. The nursing practice organization of the hospital is the responsibility of the School of Nursing and the hospital under the "unification model." The nursing staff mix at SMH during the study period was 92 percent registered nurses and 8 percent licensed practical nurses, nursing assistants, and technicians. Primary nursing is practiced throughout the inpatient settings.

Data were studied from a total of 24,879 patients. Collectively, these patients represented 218,182 patient days, which accounted for 92.8 percent of the hospital's total patient days during the data-collection period of July 1, 1982 to June 30, 1983. Daily nursing patient classification data were collected on patients in 34 patient care units constituting eight clinical departments (medicine, surgery, obstetrics/gynecology, pediatrics, psychiatry, neurology, orthopedics, and rehabilitation). Data on nursing care hours were collected in these same 34 units during selected weeks of this time period and again for 21 consecutive days in June 1984.

NURSING PATIENT CLASSIFICATION

The SMH nursing patient classification system measures the relative nursing effort required in the care and management of specific types of patients and groups patients into four categories of nursing acuity. In this study, nursing acuity is defined as the relative amount of nursing care required by a patient, as determined by the sum of the patient classification indicator weights and represented by the assigned category of acuity, 1 through 4.

The nursing patient classification system used for data collection has been in use in the hospital since 1977. Two instruments comprise the system: one for medical, neurological, rehabilitation, orthopedic, pediatric, obstetrics/gynecology, and surgical patients (hereafter referred to as the general instrument); and a second instrument for psychiatric patients.

Instruments

The general instrument consists of 35 indicators that are descriptive of a patient's potential nursing needs. The psychiatric instrument has 40 indicators describing the potential nursing needs of this group of patients. Each day, primary nurses classified each of their assigned patients by selecting the indicators that are most descriptive of the patient's nursing needs. These indicators are descriptive cue words or phrases that represent conditions or needs that, when present in a patient, require a nursing response. These cue words or phrases are defined and illustrated with examples in a nursing patient classification manual available on each unit. Although not displayed on the form, each indicator has an assigned weight (see Figs. 1 and 2).

The patient classification instrument, with its marked indicators, is optically scanned, and the weights for the selected indicators are summed. Using the sum of weights, a category of nursing acuity is assigned to each patient for that particular day. The process is completed with a computer program.

Figure 1
Nursing Patient Classification
Medicine, Surgery, Obstetrics/Gynecology, Pediatrics

Assigned Weight	Indicators
	Assessment Observation Needs
3	Admission/transfer in
3	Discharge/transfer out
8	Confused/retarded/disoriented
2	Specimen collecting/testing
8	Respirator
8	Physiologic instability/major trauma/psychological instability
2	Intake and output
5	IV and site care
8	Monitor
6	Frequent vital signs
	Nursing Intervention Needs
4	Sensory/communication impairment
5	Elimination
6	Extensive wound/skin care
2	Simple wound/skin care
6	Tube care
4	Pulmonary treatment
2	Discharge planning
4	Patient/family teaching
4	Emotional needs greater than usual
	Functional Needs
4/6	Age (0–2 yrs. old = 4 pts; 3–4 yrs. old = 6 pts)
3	Partial immobility
6	Complete immobility
2	Bath with assistance
6	Complete/total bath
0	Up ad lib
2	Up with assistance
4	Bed rest
4	Difficult transfer/turn
2	Assist with oral/tube feeding
6	Total oral/tube feeding
2	Assist with exercise
	Special Needs
6	Isolation/isolette
4	Prepared for test/procedures
6	Assist patient off unit
151	24-hour attendance

Category I	0–15	Category III	27–49
Category II	16–26	Category IV	50 +

Figure 2
Nursing Patient Classification
Psychiatry

Assigned Weight	Indicators
20	Admission/transfer in
10	Discharge/transfer out
5	Out on pass
30	Confused/disoriented
5	Delusional
30	Withdrawn—high
20	Withdrawn—low
30	Hyperactivity
20	Aggressive
30	Complete immobility
15	Partial immobility
121	One-to-one restriction
80	Close observation
80	Monitor q 15 minutes
40	Monitor q 30 minutes
20	Incontinent bowel or bladder
10	Sensory deficits
30	Bed rest
10	Bath—total
5	Bath with assistance
20	Oral/tube feeding—total
5	Oral/tube feeding—with assistance
0	Oral feeding—no assistance
10	Intake and output
10	Tube care
30	Extensive wound/skin care
10	Simple wound/skin care
20	Vital signs q 2 hours/more often
20	Monitor IVs
10	Activity supervision
25	Room restriction
20	Restraint application
10	Additional teaching needs
10	Special family emotional needs
20	Patient/family conference
5	Room search
10	Room change
10	Accompany off unit
10	Test and/or procedures
5	Specimen collection

Category II	0–48 points	Category IV	121 + points
Category III	49–120 points		

The psychiatric patients have only three categories of nursing acuity: 2, 3, and 4. There are no category 1 inpatients in psychiatry since patients with this degree of nursing acuity are treated in the ambulatory units.

The general instrument was designed by SMH nurses who used the Rush Medical Center nursing patient classification instrument as a model. In a validity study of the SMH general instrument, Jezek (1978) compared a sample of 127 patients representing the various services. These patients were rated by two specially trained raters, each using a different set of indicators. The overall rate of agreement between the two forms was reported to be 66 percent, and Jezek concluded that although there were some differences in the category assignments, there was no significant difference between the instruments for assigning patients to categories of nursing acuity. The psychiatric instrument was adopted with only minor changes from the Rush Medical Center psychiatric instrument. Since the Rush form had been developed with several intensive studies to support its validity (Jezek, 1978), the degree of agreement in the categorization of patients using the SMH and Rush forms was accepted as congruent validity for the SMH forms (Fox, 1969).

An interrater reliability study was conducted using two different raters for each patient, each using the general instrument. The findings in this study reported that the staff nurses and special raters agreed 88 percent of the time (Jones, Kunz, Hanna, & Downey, 1981).

Automating Patient Classification

A major objective of the study was to design and develop a system to automate the process of patient classification and to capture and retain daily patient classification data in computer files along with all other captured patient-specific data. The components of the automated system are as follows:

- A patient-specific, computer-generated classification instrument. Preprinted continuous forms are used for the classification instrument, and a form is printed each day for each patient in the hospital. The primary or associate nurse classifies each patient once during each 24-hour period, at the end of the day shift.
- Blank back-up forms for new admissions and transfers.
- A master list of patients on each patient care unit.
- Computer weighting of indicators selected by the nurse, calculation of the sum of weights, and assignment of patient classification category.

- A computer-generated daily summary report of the classification of each patient on each unit.
- A data base of all data collected.

The automated system was initiated on June 22, 1982, and all study data were collected with the automated system. In March 1983, a mark-sense-reader (optical scanner) was introduced, and the format of the patient classification instrument was changed to permit optical scanning. The major benefits resulting from the addition of the scanner were reduction in the cost of data entry from $3,800 a month to $400 a month; seven-day scanning of patient classification data; and redesigned patient classification forms that were easier for staff to read and use.

TIME STUDY

In order to assign nursing care hours to categories of nursing acuity, a detailed study of nursing time spent in patient care and unit-related activities was required. Two time studies were conducted. Time Study II data were accepted as valid and reliable. Time Study II procedures included:

- A process to ensure that each nurse reported all hours worked on each shift in the data-collection period.
- Clarification of definitions to ensure that all patient-assignable time was reported, as well as all other paid time.
- Simplification of the time study self-report forms.
- Securing the support of the nursing unit leadership for the time study.
- Availability of study staff on all shifts to answer staff's questions as the time study was initiated.
- Appointment of unit leadership person on each shift to assure proper data collection.
- Standardization of the placement of time study data-collection instruments on the patient care units.
- Simultaneous collection of 21 days of time study data on each unit in the hospital.
- Provision of electronic calculators for nurses on each unit to use to verify totals of time distributed in various categories of time.

Definitions of Categories of Time

Direct time (patient-assignable time) was defined as all patient-centered activity carried out directly with the patient and/or family or significant other. Direct time included all patient group activity that involved nursing supervision or direction. Time spent for group supervision or direction was assigned to the individual patients by dividing the total time spent with the group by the number of patients in the group. Examples of direct time are all hands-on care, admission history and assessment, patient or family teaching, medication administration, dressing change, specimen collection, group therapy, group pre- or postoperative teaching, and health teaching to a group of new mothers.

Other time (patient-assignable time) was defined as all time spent in activity away from a specific patient, family, or significant other, but in preparation for completion of direct care for that patient. Examples include development or documentation of comprehensive care plan, family-team conference, extensive progress notes, and preparation of medications.

Unit-related time was defined as time related to the entire unit and its patient population or group. Unit-related time cannot reasonably be divided among patients to be individually assigned. Unit-related time also included all productive activity in support of the unit that was not directly related to the patients. Examples include inservice education, committee work, emergency cart check, administrative activity (charge nurse or clinician), personnel policy–related activity (evaluation, time scheduling), and narcotic count.

Personal time was defined as paid time spent on breaks, personal hygiene, or personal errands.

Unit constant time was defined as the time derived for each unit by adding the average personal hours per patient day to the average unit-related hours per patient day. Each patient, independent of acuity, received an equal assignment of unit constant time.

Total time was defined as the total nursing care time assigned to each category of nursing acuity on each patient care unit. Total time is the sum of the average direct time, the average other patient-assignable time, and the unit constant time assigned to the respective unit.

Staff reported the time spent in minutes in each defined category on two color-coded forms. Once every 24 hours, a new patient time study form was printed for patient identification and placed at the respective patient's bedside or on the patient's room door. This form was used by nurses to record all patient-assignable direct time immediately after a direct patient care activity was completed. A nurse's time study form was completed by each nurse on each shift during the data collection period.

On this form the nurses recorded all patient-assignable direct and other time, as well as unit-related and personal time expended during the shift. In addition, a shift summary of total time spent in each category of time was recorded. To ensure that all time worked had been reported, the nurse totaled all time in each category to reach a grand total time, in minutes, and then compared this grand total against actual minutes worked.

During the time study, nurses continued classifying their assigned patients once every 24 hours at the end of the day shift. To facilitate correlation of each patient's direct and other time with the patient's nursing classification, a "time box" was added to the patient classification form. In the time box nurses entered a summary report of 3 shifts (24 hours) of patient-assignable time, taken from each patient's patient time form, after completing the classification of each respective patient.

Validation and Processing of Time Study

Once daily, at the end of the day shift, the unit leadership nurse, who was responsible for assuring the accuracy of the time study data, checked each patient classification form to ensure that the time box for reporting shift totals of direct and other care time was complete. These forms were then sent to the study office, along with all completed time study forms for the previous 24-hour period. Following a second check for completeness and accuracy, the patient classification forms were forwarded to the computing center for data entry and processing. Daily, the time study staff totaled all unit-related and personal time reported for each of the 34 units. These data were recorded on a separate summary sheet that was also forwarded to the computing center for data entry.

Since time study data were not collected on randomly chosen days, but rather were collected during a block of 21 consecutive days in one month, it was possible that the constant time on each unit was atypical. Through discussion with clinicians, the investigators determined that some units had experienced unusually high numbers of new staff being oriented, atypical amounts of administrative activity, and very high demands for time spent in staff educational activities while the Time Study II data collection was going on. To correct for this error, clinicians reported to the investigators the usual number of staff class days, orientations, and administrative work days that would occur during a three-week interval. Obviously atypical amounts of unit constant time were then adjusted to make the unit constant data more representative of a normal calendar year.

The validity of average hours of care assigned to patients was assured through the daily accuracy check on the patient care units and by study staff. In addition, preliminary results from the study were carefully scrutinized by study staff to identify units where results appeared extremely unusual. A computer program was created to identify patients included in these results, and their data was double checked. This included rechecking the sum of weights and time (in minutes) that had been key punched to detect obvious human error and reviewing the patient's record and patient classification sheet to determine if the classification was accurate. The exclusion of erroneous or incomplete data at this point resulted in a loss of 34 records, or 0.24 percent of the total of 13,863 records, leaving 13,829 time records for analysis. The major error source in these 34 records was inaccurate classification of patients. For example, all normal newborn infants require a certain minimal amount of nursing care. When the patient classification instrument is correctly used for these infants, the sum of weights always is great enough to place them in category 2. Therefore, the classification of any infant on an obstetrics/gynecology unit into category 1 was reviewed via a chart audit. If the audit revealed that nursing care was given that allowed reclassification of the infant into category 2 or higher, the classification was corrected. If such documentation was lacking, the case was dropped. A similar process was applied to the review of other selected cases.

Validity of self-reported time was determined by comparing hours reported for the purposes of the time study with hours reported as worked taken from payroll sheets. The total time reported was 85,517 hours, while the total time worked was 84,749 hours. This constituted an overreporting of 768 hours in the time study, or 100.9 percent reporting of the payroll hours worked. When records were searched and documents rechecked, explanations for the overreporting of hours were found and were attributed to data-entry errors or to the existence of overtime hours reported for the purposes of the time study but unreported to payroll. The final results of Time Study II were considered satisfactory by the investigators and these data were used to assign average nursing care hours to categories of patient acuity on each of the patient care units.

Assigning Nursing Care Hours to Categories of Nursing Acuity

The time study was designed to assign nursing care hours to each category of acuity for specific patient care units. This is an essential step, since units have particular constellations of patients with varying nursing care requirements.

To achieve this objective, patient classification data collected during the time study were merged with time study data. The resulting data base included a daily record for each patient, by unit, showing both the time required to deliver nursing care and the patient's classification category for that day. A computer program was created to calculate from these data the average patient-assignable direct and other care hours required by patients in each acuity category for each of the 34 units involved in the study. Unit-specific hours of unit-related and personal time were calculated by dividing the daily reported totals of unit-related and personal time by the daily patient census. The daily totals were then averaged to yield average unit-related and personal time by unit, and the averages were summed to yield the unit constant figure for each unit. The unit constant figure was assigned equally to each category of acuity and added with the average direct and other hours for the total hours assigned per category.

DATA ANALYSIS

All study data were entered or optically scanned and fed to a computer for tape file generation. This resulted in multiple computer files. The first two separate computer files were named CLASS (for the classification data) and CARE (for the time study data). All data were analyzed using the SAS (Statistical Analysis System) software. SAS was chosen to process the study data for its ease of data modification, file handling, information storage and retrieval, and report writing. Two additional data files were supplied to the study, one from the hospital's patient data base, called PDB, and the other from patient accounting, called FINANCE.

In order to conduct the analysis, a merge of the data sets was necessary. Data sets were merged such that observations in CLASS were matched with PDB using the variable Patient-ID. This identification is assigned to an individual upon admission to the hospital and is unique to that patient for that admission.

The first merge, CLASS + PDB, depicted in Figure 3, resulted in a large cumulative file of 218,182 patient days for 24,879 patients and the file was retitled CLASSDRG. To assign costs, another file, FINANCE, was passed against the CLASSDRG file using the Medicare step-down methodology described in the section which follows.

The second merge, CARE + CLASS, resulted in a file of 13,829 patient records containing nursing classification and time study data. This data base, called CARECLASS, was created in June 1984 using patient classification data from the same period and was used to determine nursing care hours assignments per category of acuity per unit.

To create the final data base, called CLASSCAREDRG, the "total care" average nursing care hours per patient classification category, per unit,

Figure 3
Creation of Final Data Base

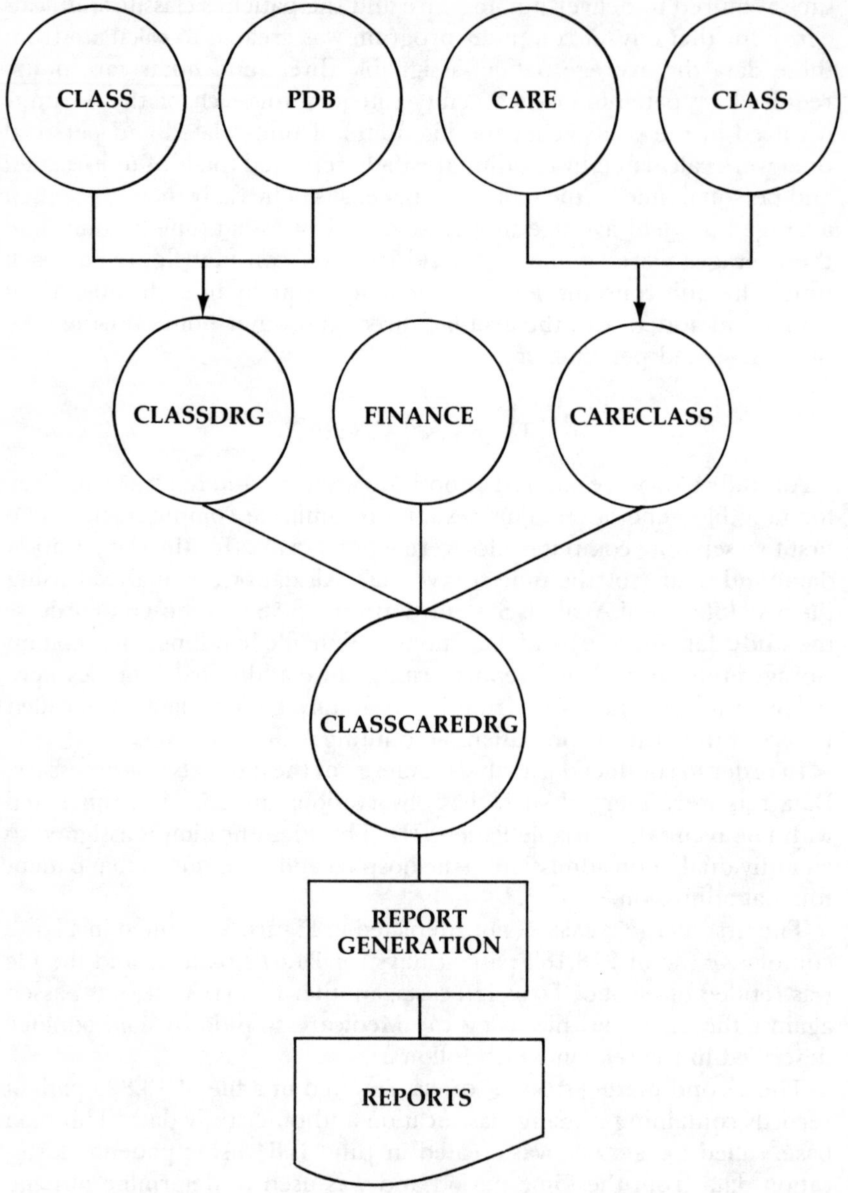

from the CARECLASS file were assigned to each patient day on the CLASSDRG file. Thus the final data base, CLASSCAREDRG included a figure for nursing care hours per patient day for every patient, for each day of the patient's stay, that reflected both the nursing acuity of the patient and the unit where the nursing care was delivered.

Costs of Ancillary and Room Services: Medicare Step-Down Methodology

To compute the cost of services for our study, the single-apportionment Medicare step-down methodology was used to generate a ratio of costs to charges for patients discharged in 1982.[1] The result of the Medicare step-down methodology was that the costs of all non-revenue-producing centers were allocated to revenue-producing centers. The Medicare step-down methodology first identifies all non-revenue-producing centers in the institution. These are not only departments, but centers such as building depreciation and capital equipment. Using a set of statistics for each department such as square feet, hours worked, and so forth, the costs of the non-revenue-producing centers were allocated to other non-revenue-producing centers and to the revenue-producing centers. Medicare provides guidelines as to the sequence of the allocation, with building depreciation being the first center allocated, and administrative and general costs being the last center allocated. This sequence of allocation is what is referred to as the "step down." An example of an allocation might be a housekeeping department, where the costs are allocated to patient care units, clinics, labs, and the like, as well as to the other non-revenue-producing centers such as dietary and administration. Housekeeping costs would be allocated to all departments based on the total square footage in each department. In addition to the allocation of housekeeping costs to administration, administrative and general costs were allocated to housekeeping.

After the first step down (or allocation) of all non-revenue-producing centers to all centers, the costs (which were now the result of the step down) of the non-revenue-producing centers were allocated to revenue-producing centers only. Again, the sequence for allocation is prescribed in the Medicare guidelines. Once this is complete, no costs reside in non-revenue-producing centers. All costs, both direct, and indirect (allocated), reside in revenue-producing centers, that is, centers where charges are generated.

---

[1] Specific information on the Medicare single-apportionment step-down methodology is available in Medicare and Medicaid guide-books or from a hospital financial officer.

At this point, ratios of costs to charges were computed for each revenue-producing center. These ratios were computed by dividing the total costs for a center (as determined using the methodology just described) by the total charges generated by the center. (A charge was generated when it was posted to a patient's account as the result of a service provided or a supply or drug dispensed). Once this was done, a cost-to-charge ratio was available for each department.

To compute the costs of ancillary services for each DRG, the appropriate cost-to-charge ratio was applied to each charge for each patient. The resulting "cost" was aggregated for the ancillary areas within each DRG, and then those ancillary costs were added together for the DRG and divided by the number of patients in the DRG to develop an average cost of ancillary services for each DRG. The same procedure was repeated to develop the average room costs for each DRG.

As the hospital's Medicare step-down analysis for 1983 had not been completed when the study data were being processed, the ratios developed for 1982 were applied for 1983 data. The costs that were computed were adjusted upward by a factor of 7 percent, which was the difference in the hospital's cost base for those two years.

Average Cost of a Nursing Care Hour

To compute the average cost per nursing care hour for the period from July 1, 1982 to June 30, 1983, actual salaries and benefits were adjusted to remove all costs for nursing administration above the level of head nurse and all unit secretarial costs. The adjusted actual salaries and benefits totaled $19,532,279.

Using the hospital's Manpower Utilization Control Report, the number of full-time equivalent (FTE) staff was adjusted for each patient care unit to remove all nursing administration staff above the level of head nurse and the unit secretarial personnel. The adjusted total number of FTE staff was 869.72. Each FTE staff member has 2,080 paid hours per year. The total number of paid hours in this study year was 1,809,017.6.

The adjusted annual salaries and benefits, divided by the annual adjusted hours, determined the direct average hourly rate, including benefits. The direct average cost per nursing care hour was calculated to be $10.80.

Nursing Hours and Direct Nursing Costs per Patient and per DRG

The average direct nursing costs per patient and per DRG were derived by using the daily nursing patient classification, its assigned hours, and multiplying by the average hourly rate. The following sequence was used:

- Each patient was classified daily, using the nursing patient classification instrument. This resulted in a sum of weights, from which an assignment was made to a nursing acuity category of 1 to 4.

- Each unit, through a time study, had assigned nursing care hours for each of the four categories of acuity. This time was assigned to each patient depending on the patient's category of acuity and the patient care unit.

- The patient's total nursing requirements, by hours of nursing care required on each day of hospitalization, were summed.

- To obtain costs, the totaled hours were multiplied by the cost of an average hour of nursing care. This resulted in the assigned direct nursing costs for each patient's hospitalization.

- To calculate the hospital's average direct nursing costs for each DRG, all patients' direct nursing costs in each DRG were summed, and then divided by the number of patients in the particular DRG.

CONCLUSIONS AND IMPLICATIONS

The study results validated an approach that integrates nursing patient classification data with other important patient care information using information-processing technologies. The merged data provide the basic information required to move from the traditional assignment of average nursing care hours per patient day to a patient classification–centered assignment of nursing hours based on a daily assessment of each patient's nursing needs. The daily patient classification data, coupled with the results of the time study and the other hospital data on each patient, have produced a DRG composite of the patients treated at SMH that includes essential information on nursing acuity for each DRG and the associated average hours of nursing required to care for these patients.

Need for Consensus

When the investigators attempted to compare results from this study with similar findings from other reported studies, the comparisons were limited. Selected findings from only four studies could be compared because of differences in definitions and methodologies. This limitation creates a sense of urgency in regard to developing some national consensus among nursing leaders and researchers on definitions of key

terms, and the inclusion of some common components in the methodological approaches. For example, what nursing staff members on a
patient care unit should be included in the calculations and assignment
of nursing care hours? In this study, all nursing staff members up to
and including the head nurse were included for the calculation of nursing hours. Also, the decision was made to exclude clinical nurse specialists
and all other nursing administrative staff. These two groups are considered part of the indirect costs, which were not assigned in this study.
The secretarial costs were excluded and remain in the room costs as part
of the unit support services. Caution must be exercised by all investigators to ensure that the concepts of costs and charges are kept as discrete
entities. Methodologies for moving from charges to costs must be similar
if dollar results are to be compared. Furthermore, whenever costs are
compared, allowances must be made for known regional differences.
Consequently, the investigators have concluded that it is more meaningful to compare average nursing hours per DRG, and report the statistics that describe the variances in the sample (for an example, see
Table 1), than to report average direct nursing costs per DRG. An important demographic variable that should be included consistently, to
enable meaningful comparisons, is a description of the mix of nursing
staff that is included in the average nursing care hours assigned to the
DRGs. In addition, comparisons across institutions of distributions of
nursing acuity within DRGs would be facilitated if there was agreement
on the number of categories or classes necessary to reflect the nursing
acuity level of patients. Based on this study, the investigators concluded
that unit-specific assignment of nursing care hours to a four-category
system of nursing acuity can adequately account for the variations in
nursing care requirements for all patients in the hospital.

Unbundling Nursing Costs

The ability to determine the nursing care hours that are spent in caring
for individual patients enables the identification of direct nursing costs
assignable to specific patients. This is the first step in the process required
to unbundle nursing costs from room costs and to make nursing care a
discrete, identified service provided to patients in varying amounts, depending on need. Other steps in the unbundling process include determining the indirect costs that must be added to the direct costs and
calculating the total nursing costs to be assigned to the patient for each
day of hospitalization. Unbundling of nursing costs from the room costs
enhances the accountability of nurses in patient care. Experiences in this
study with both daily patient classification and the time studies have
impressed upon the investigators the importance of a well-informed staff
who understand and support the system's requirements.

Table 1
Nursing Hours for a Sample of DRGs

MDC	DRG	Number of Patients	Mean Nursing Hours	SD	Coefficient of Variation	Minimum Nursing Hours	Maximum Nursing Hours
1	1 Craniotomy, age 17 or over, except for trauma	127	171.6	250.3	145.9	1.9	365.5
	12 Degenerative nervous system disorders	107	69.2	98.7	142.6	7.9	818.6
2	42 Intraocular procedures, except iris, lens, retina	81	17.6	11.6	65.7	2.7	65.5
	44 Acute major eye infections	33	24.1	12.8	52.9	6.7	62.8
3	55 Misc. ear, nose, and throat procedures	138	12.9	11.7	90.4	2.5	127.2
	73 Other ear, nose, and throat diagnoses, age 17 or older	32	30.1	37.5	124.7	5.7	161.4
4	75 Major chest procedures	74	138.1	287.8	208.4	4.2	2,484.4
	82 Respiratory neoplasms	153	48.9	48.7	99.6	4.2	308.7
5	107 Coronary bypass w/o cardiac cath.	307	106.5	100.2	94.1	4.2	1,594.6
	122 AMI w/o CV compl., discharged alive,	211	56.6	37.4	66.1	2.9	307.8
6	148 Major small and large bowel procedures, age ≥ 70 or CC	111	110.4	103.6	93.8	18.5	786.4
	174 GI bleeding, age ≥ 70 or CC	67	52.9	135.4	256.0	7.3	1,109.3
7	198 Cholecystectomy w/o CDE, age < 70	101	31.9	8.7	27.3	18.0	68.3
	203 Hepatobiliary or pancreas malignancy	43	40.0	32.5	81.2	6.5	171.3
8	209 Major joint procedures	232	93.9	57.2	60.9	3.8	451.2
	243 Medical back problems	247	18.0	21.1	116.9	3.0	154.1
9	258 Total mastectomy for malignancy, age < 70	35	26.0	7.1	27.5	12.9	40.6
	278 Cellulitis, age 18–69	43	24.3	19.2	79.1	3.7	102.8
10	290 Thyroid procedures	47	19.4	7.5	38.7	6.9	45.2
	295 Diabetes, age 0–35	80	24.2	17.5	72.2	3.5	81.5

If nursing costs are unbundled from room costs by the use of a daily patient classification system, it is imperative that all patients are classified each day. In addition, the classification data must be valid and reliable. Variables selected as indicators of patient acuity must be reflected in documented observations and nursing interventions in the patient's record. Such an accountability and audit trail is a basic requirement for a discrete, chargeable service provided to patients. Furthermore, data from periodic interrater reliability studies will be expected to support the reliability of the patient classification categories assigned daily. Finally, the unit-specific assignment of nursing hours to categories of patient acuity will have to be reviewed at least annually; and revisions made as necessary to reflect advances in technology, new procedures, and treatment modalities that may be in use and that affect nursing care hours.

The findings in this study related to the percentage of direct nursing costs that are included in the room costs of patients in the DRGs are instructive. When the extremes are removed (DRGs with limited numbers of patients), the most common percentage of average direct nursing costs in the average room costs fall within the range of 18 to 24 percent (see Table 2). These data surprise many individuals involved directly in hospital health care, including practicing nurses and physicians as well as observers of the hospital health scene, who have assumed that nursing accounts for a much larger share of the room costs. Moreover, this percentage of direct costs for nursing care at SMH is for a predominantly professional nursing staff, represented by a mix that includes 92 percent registered nurses and 8 percent licensed practical nurses, nursing assistants, and technicians. The data challenge the notion of the "high expense" of RN staff. The methodology demonstrated in this study, if repeated across multiple institutions, should provide evidence of the cost efficiency of a predominantly RN staff.

Variability of Acuity within DRGs

The nursing needs of the individual patients within the DRGs are extremely variable, as reflected in Table 1 by the large standard deviations reported for the average nursing hours associated with the DRGs, the broad range indicated by the minimum and maximum nursing hours, and the high coefficient of variation for these average nursing hours. Early in the study, the investigators had speculated that there might be a predictable pattern of nursing acuity for patients assigned to the same DRG. In fact, the investigators searched for such a pattern within each DRG, and this was not the case. The DRGs, as a case-mix profile, do not predict individual patients' needs. DRGs are not homogeneous from a nursing acuity perspective. Nevertheless, DRGs coupled with nursing patient classification data can be used as predictors of the relative needs of the grouping, as demonstrated by the comparison of estimated budget projections and actual budget expenditures. Nursing patient classification data coupled with DRGs allowed a budget prediction that reflected 87 percent of the actual adjusted expenditures.

Information Systems

Nursing and hospital management need the assistance of information systems technology to develop and track DRG or product data and costs. The comprehensive information provided through this study about the hospital's DRGs and nursing hours and costs would have been impossible without the ability to automate the daily nursing acuity data-collection and reporting process, and the development of a computerized data base. The accelerating demands for management information warrant information systems support. Data on length of stay by DRGs indicate that intervention strategies are warranted to seek potential reductions in length of stay. Comprehensive information systems will facilitate tracking of such data and permit the analysis and evaluation of the effectiveness of clinical and management strategies over time.

Potential for Nursing Management

The findings of this study will contribute to the nursing management objectives of quality care at controlled costs. These contributions are in the areas of budgeting, planning, operations, and control, including productivity monitoring. The uses of the findings in predicting nursing manpower budgets have already been addressed.

DRG data are valuable in succinctly describing patient volume and mix, a finding that is especially useful in program planning. The fact that 80 percent of the hospital's annual admissions can be described by 148 DRGs is useful. In addition, service and unit data are even of more value for patient care and program planning. An example will illustrate the potential that DRG data have for nursing management. Over two-thirds of the annual patient volume on the cardiothoracic unit is described by seven DRGs, as shown in Table 3. These data include all patients treated during the study period, including outliers. Four hundred fifty patients, utilizing 3,249 patient days are included in three DRGs: 107, 105, and 106. These DRGs account for 41 percent of the annual patient volume on the cardiothoracic unit. Assuming that a primary nurse spends a minimum of one to two hours in formulating the nursing care plan for each of these 450 patients, this is equivalent to 450 to 900 nursing hours, or up to one-half of an FTE staff person devoted solely to nursing care planning for 41 percent of the patients on one patient care unit. Given the DRG data of the unit, the nursing staff can plan

Table 2
Hospital Summary Costs for Top 22 DRGs on a Medical Unit

DRG		N	Mean Length of Stay	Average Nursing Care Hours	Average Ancillary Costs	Average Room Costs[a]	Average Direct Nursing Costs	Nursing Costs as Percentage of Average
14	Specific cerebrovascular disorders except TIA	224	25.7	113.4	$2,395	$ 5,544	$1,150	20.7
127	Heart failure and shock	206	13.0	57.0	1,408	3,189	578	18.0
468	Unrelated OR procedure in MDC	365	19.0	98.0	3,806	4,642	996	21.5
122	AMI w/o CV complication, discharged alive	211	11.4	56.6	1,414	3,636	574	15.8
125	Other circulatory disorder w/ cardiac cath.	505	3.4	16.6	1,343	845	169	20.0
89	Pneumonia and pleurisy, age ≥ 70 and/or CC	128	9.6	45.6	1,684	2,396	462	19.3
88	Chronic obstructive pulmonary disease	125	10.2	47.9	1,579	2,775	486	17.5
182	Gastroesophagitis, miscellaneous digestive disorders, age ≥ 70 and/or CC	120	8.1	31.4	1,111	1,841	319	17.3
403	Lymphoma, leukemia, age ≥ 70 and/or CC	71	14.0	62.4	4,570	3,303	633	19.2

415	OR procedure for infectious and parasitic disease	35.1	178.9	4,750	7,699	1,814	23.6
82	Respiratory neoplasms	12.7	48.9	1,762	2,830	496	17.5
79	Respiratory infections and inflammations, age ≥ 70 and/or CC	21.7	113.2	3,477	5,756	1,148	19.9
416	Septicemia, age ≥ 18	14.8	69.0	3,250	3,460	699	20.2
121	AMI w/CV compl., discharged alive	13.3	69.6	1,864	4,481	706	15.8
296	Nutritional and miscellaneous metabolic disorders, age ≥ 70 and/or CC	12.0	53.2	1,403	2,827	539	19.1
18	Cranial and peripheral nerve disorders, age ≥ 70 and/or CC	24.7	100.9	2,237	5,267	1,023	19.4
140	Angina pectoris	7.1	33.1	815	2,027	336	16.6
395	Red blood cell disorders, age ≥ 18	8.2	29.4	1,268	1,857	298	16.0
96	Bronchitis, asthma, age ≥ 70 and/or CC	8.3	38.5	1,555	2,390	390	16.3
174	GI bleeding, age ≥ 70 and/or CC	11.0	52.9	1,896	2,666	537	20.1
129	Cardiac arrest	43.8	234.5	5,886	13,019	2,378	18.3
310	Transurethral procedures, age ≥ 70 and/or CC	11.2	63.3	2,116	3,437	642	18.7

[a]Average room costs include total nursing costs.

Table 3
Seven DRGs Representing 61.7 Percent of Patient Days on Cardiothoracic Unit

DRG		Unit Patient Days	Percentage of Unit Total	Percentage of Patient Days in Classification Category				Hospital Admissions (N)	Hospital Average Length of Stay	Hospital Average Hours of Nursing Care
				1	2	3	4			
107	Coronary bypass w/o cardiac cath.	2,176	27.4	19.2	22.6	47.6	10.6	307	12.7	106.5
105	Heart valve procedure w/pump	670	8.4	19.0	20.9	45.2	14.9	91	19.2	149.4
75	Major chest procedures	558	7.0	16.3	30.3	46.6	6.8	74	19.7	138.1
110	Major reconstructive vascular procedure, age ≥ 70 and/or CC	527	6.6	12.9	25.8	50.1	11.2	124	24.5	173.0
106	Coronary bypass w/cardiac cath.	403	5.1	6.7	17.9	61.3	14.1	52	21.2	149.4
5	Extracranial vascular procedures	338	4.3	24.6	31.4	37.0	7.1	178	12.9	70.2
111	Major reconstructive vascular procedure, age < 70	229	2.9	19.2	36.7	38.9	5.2	81	13.1	74.7

and develop generic care plans to accommodate the most frequent admissions. In this example, one generic care plan for patients having open heart surgery was developed and is adapted for use for patients in all three DRGs. The generic care plan is developed and approved by the nursing and medical staff and incorporates the standards of patient care expected by the specialists in both disciplines. At most, the primary nurse spends up to 30 minutes individualizing the generic care plan to the patient's unique needs. If this example is multiplied by the development of generic care plans on each of the patient care units, there is the potential, based on 25,000 admissions, of shifting the equivalent of 12 to 25 full-time nurses from initial patient care planning to other direct patient care activities with no adverse effects on quality standards. DRG data can also be used in designing content for orientation and inservice programs on specific patient populations, formulating action plans for procedure and policy review, and evaluating potential usage of supplies and equipment.

There is even greater potential in the evaluation of the efficacy of routine medical and nursing practices associated with specific DRGs. Further development of a computerized patient information system along with continued research of the DRGs in hospitals will uncover this potential.

A valid and reliable nursing patient classification system can also be used to assign variable staff, based on patient acuity. A variety of systems to provide data for this purpose are in use. In addition, this information plus staffing data serve as the necessary data elements for a nursing productivity monitoring system.

Age and Length of Stay

The study results provided an interesting finding related to age and length of stay. The investigators had hypothesized that there would be a direct positive correlation between increasing age and prolonged length of stay, particularly for patients 70 years of age and older. The hypothesis was rejected, as there was no direct positive correlation with increasing age alone and prolonged length of stay. Of course, the single variable of increasing age may be too isolated to account for length of stay outliers. Prolonged length of stay is more likely associated with multiple variables, including comorbidities and complications (CCs) that occur with increasing age. Review of the DRG nursing data support this conclusion. A higher average number of nursing care hours are consistently associated with DRGs for patients age 70 or greater and/or with comorbidities or complications than are associated with the same DRG relating to patients less than 70 years of age and without comorbidities or complications. These findings are illustrated in Table 4.

Table 4
Comparison of Age and Comorbidities/Complications in DRGs with Length of Stay and Nursing Hours

DRG		Admissions (N)	Mean Length of Stay	Length of Stay SD	Minimum Length of Stay	Maximum Length of Stay	Mean Nursing Hours	Nursing Hours SD
7	Peripheral, cranial, and other nerve procedure, age ≥ 70 and/or CC	23	32.6	68.3	1	285	84.5	150.1
8	Peripheral, cranial, other nerve procedure, age < 70	70	4.2	3.3	1	18	20.3	17.3
24	Seizure, headache age ≥ 70 and/or CC	45	16.9	24.1	1	127	63.0	91.1
25	Seizure, headache, age 18–69	61	9.6	10.2	1	73	35.6	31.7
96	Bronchitis, asthma, age ≥ 70 and/or CC	66	8.3	9.9	2	66	38.5	70.1
97	Bronchitis, asthma, age 18–69	82	5.3	3.1	1	20	21.1	17.7
110	Major reconstructive vascular procedure, age ≥ 70 and/or CC	124	24.5	20.1	1	106	173.0	209.3
111	Major reconstructive vascular procedure, age < 70	81	13.1	5.8	7	39	74.7	39.1
130	Peripheral vascular disease, age ≥ and/or CC	69	9.6	5.8	1	27	44.5	33.0
131	Peripheral vascular disease, age < 70	43	8.7	8.7	1	55	31.8	20.0

DRG	Description							
148	Major small and large bowel procedures, age ≥ 70 and/or CC	111	22.6	19.7	1	138	110.4	103.6
149	Major small and large bowel procedures, age < 70	49	13.6	12.8	3	93	63.1	70.3
174	GI bleeding, age ≥ 70 and/or CC	67	11.0	22.5	2	185	52.9	135.4
175	GI bleeding, age < 70	36	4.5	2.5	1	12	17.5	11.5
197	Cholecystectomy w/o DEC, age ≥ 70 and/or CC	56	12.2	5.9	6	38	51.6	34.1
198	Cholecystectomy w/o DEC, age < 70	101	7.7	2.0	5	17	31.9	8.7
210	Other hip and femur procedures, age ≥ 70 and/or CC	78	32.1	21.9	6	124	143.0	109.1
211	Other hip and femur procedures, age 18–69	37	38.9	19.7	7	81	127.4	84.3
442	Other OR procedures for injury, age ≥ 70 and/or CC	65	23.8	24.7	1	123	123.2	127.1
443	Other OR procedures for injury, age < 70	50	12.7	14.3	1	89	73.8	116.0

Table 5
DRGs with Highest Nursing Intensity

DRG		Total Admissions	Total Patient Days[a]	Percentage of Patient Days in Each Nursing Intensity Category				Percentage of Days in Categories 3 and 4
				1	2	3	4	
77	OR procedures on respiratory system except major chest w/o CC	8	209	5.7	2.4	7.2	84.7	91.9
385	Neonates, died or transferred	146	2,290	—	1.1	17.2	80.9	98.1
386	Neonates, extreme immaturity	59	2,378	—	2.9	31.3	65.6	96.9
2	Craniotomy for trauma, age ≥ 18	35	1,618	2.4	4.5	23.7	69.5	93.2
387	Prematurity w/major problems	125	3,126	—	6.1	42.6	50.6	93.2
457	Extensive burns	7	330	0.6	6.4	36.4	56.7	93.1
123	Acute myocardial infarct, expired	39	315	5.4	5.4	19.1	70.2	89.3
27	Traumatic stupor and coma, > 1 hour	23	277	3.2	7.9	25.6	63.2	88.8
192	Minor pancreas, liver, shunt procedures	5	213	5.2	6.1	32.4	56.3	88.7
173	Digestive system malignancy, age < 70	9	174	5.7	6.9	32.8	54.6	87.4
1	Craniotomy, age ≥ 18 except for trauma	127	3,383	9.5	11.9	32.7	45.9	78.6
91	Pneumonia, pleurisy, age 0–17	82	440	4.1	11.4	39.3	45.2	84.5
156	Stomach, esophageal, duodenal procedure, age 0–17	30	268	3.4	8.6	43.7	44.4	88.1

213	Amputation for muscle and connective tissue disorders	16	493	3.0	11.0	42.0	44.0	86.0
415	OR procedure for infectious and parasitic diseases	33	940	7.4	14.6	35.2	42.8	78.0
3	Craniotomy, age < 18	84	1,133	6.5	17.2	34.4	41.8	76.2
109	Other cardiothoracic procedures w/o pump	39	647	8.8	11.0	39.3	41.0	80.3
64	Ear, nose, and throat malignancy	25	281	4.3	14.6	40.6	40.6	81.2
29	Traumatic stupor and coma, < 1 hour, age 18–69	22	201	15.4	12.9	30.8	40.8	71.6
81	Respiratory infection, inflammation, age 0–17	14	175	3.4	12.0	46.3	38.3	84.6
74	Other ear, nose, and throat diagnosis, age 0–17	14	169	2.4	13.0	47.3	37.3	84.6
28	Traumatic stupor and coma, < 1 hour, age ≥ 70 and/or CC	13	208	7.0	16.7	40.8	35.6	76.4
137	Cardiac congenital and valve disorders, age 0–17	22	205	2.0	12.7	51.7	33.7	85.4
458	Nonextensive burns w/skin graft	34	802	4.6	14.0	48.0	33.4	81.4
405	Lymphoma, leukemia, age 0–17	39	463	5.0	14.0	46.2	34.8	81.0

[a]Subtotal of patient days = 20,738, 9.5 percent of total patient days in sample.

Nursing Research

The final conclusion is that DRGs are a useful classification for nursing research as well as nursing management. To be able to describe an entire hospital inpatient population with 468 groupings is reasonable and facilitates studies. Investigators can elect to study all or part of the DRGs, and further refinements and improvements will result. DRGs have validity for describing nursing workload when coupled with a nursing patient classification system. Review by practicing nurses of the top 74 DRGs listed according to nursing intensity provides consistent agreement between the lists and the nurses' expectations and knowledge about diagnoses and associated nursing acuity. Table 5 illustrates the 25 DRGs with the highest nursing intensity—the highest percentage of patient days classified into categories 3 and 4. However, the lack of homogeneity of nursing acuity within the DRGs, as reflected by the large standard deviations of the average nursing hours and the broad range of hours describing patients' nursing needs within the DRGs, warrants further study immediately. What is the effect of length of stay on the heterogeneity of nursing care hours within DRGs? Are there particular International Classification of Disease (ICD-9-CM) diagnoses within a DRG that are similar in their utilization of nursing resources or of ancillary resources? Those DRGs that are the most costly, including those with the highest average nursing care hours and those with the highest ancillary costs, should be partitioned and analyzed by individual patients within the DRG and by patients grouped by ICD-9-CM codes. The data are available to answer these questions. Continuing study in these important areas should be commissioned and funded immediately.

REFERENCES

Fox, D. J. (1969). *The research process in education*. New York: Holt, Rinehart & Winston.

Jezek, J. (1978, December 13). *Comparison of indicator sets for determining the nursing requirements of hospitalized patients*. Unpublished study report, Strong Memorial Hospital, Rochester, New York.

Jones, L., Kunz, M. E., Hanna, N., & Downey, J. (1981, May). *SMH patient classification system interrater reliability study*. Unpublished study report, Strong Memorial Hospital, Rochester, New York.

Predicting Nursing Care Costs with a Patient Classification System

Joanne S. Harrell

The implementation in 1984 of the prospective payment system using diagnosis related groups (DRGs) has had far-reaching effects on hospitals. There have been many responses to this attempt to reduce the cost of delivering health care, varying from summaries of the problems ("Unit Leaders," 1985), to suggestions for living with DRGs (Feldman & Goldhaber, 1984), to research aimed at determining nursing care costs in specific DRGs (Curtin, 1983). A few studies have examined nursing care costs related to DRGs using a patient classification system (Mitchell, Miller, Welches, & Walker, 1984; Riley & Schaefers, 1983). Much work has been done with relative intensity measures (RIMS) in New Jersey (Caterinicchio, 1983; Caterinicchio & Davies, 1983; Joel, 1984), but the reliability and value of that complicated approach has been criticized (Grimaldi & Micheletti, 1982). There is a continuing need to develop simpler models to analyze nursing care costs in acute-care settings.

This study used one hospital's patient classification system and DRG reporting system to develop a model to analyze and predict the cost of delivering direct nursing care to patients in major medical-surgical DRGs.

NURSING PRODUCTIVITY

The nursing productivity model of Jelinek and Dennis (1976) provided the conceptual framework for the study. Jelinek and Dennis define nursing productivity as the "relationship between the amount of acceptable output produced and the input required to achieve that output" (p. 9).

This is consistent with general definitions of productivity (Edwardson, 1985; Herzog, 1985). The Jelinek and Dennis model uses a systems approach to incorporate a number of input and output variables. Success in determining nursing productivity, however, requires definitions of input and output that are meaningful and acceptable to nurse managers and chief financial officers.

This study used nursing care cost as the *input* variable and developed some simple measures of that input. Nursing care costs were determined using various measures of the number of nursing care hours provided. These hours were determined by patient acuity, as measured by a patient classification system. Patient acuity can be considered a form of severity-of-illness data readily available in most hospitals. The *output* was defined as the total patient charges per DRG, the same output measure used by Riley and Shaffers (1985) and Mitchell et al. (1984). The development of the DRG system provides for the first time a logical way to organize these input and output variables, that is, by case mix.

The productivity for a specific DRG was defined as the cost of providing nursing care to patients in that DRG, divided by the total income received from the patients in the DRG (Graham-Moore & Ross, 1983). Since total patient charges are always more than nursing care costs, the ratio will always be less than one. The most productive DRGs will be those with the smallest ratios, indicating the greatest difference between nursing costs and total patient costs, here operationally defined as total patient charges.

STUDY METHOD

The descriptive and predictive study presented in this paper sought to answer the following questions:

1. What is the ratio of nursing care costs to total patient charges—the productivity—of selected DRGs?

2. Is there a significant difference in productivity ratios between medical-surgical units and intensive care units?

3. Can a measure of nursing care hours be used to predict nursing care costs per DRG?

4. Can the case mix on a nursing unit be used to predict the number of nursing care hours needed?

Setting and Sample

The study was conducted at a 467-bed acute-care, nonprofit, non-teaching private hospital in a large urban area in the Southwest. The hospital is a magnet hospital, with low turnover. The nursing staff is predominantly registered nurses; 78.5 percent are RNs, 17.5 percent are LPNs, and 4.0 percent are nursing assistants. The hospital has 12 medical-surgical units, each with a 32-bed capacity, and 3 adult intensive care units (ICUs). The hospital uses the Freisen system for supply delivery. It has a computerized hospital information system, the HBO system, using Medpro software. The average occupancy of the hospital in 1983 was 86.7 percent, with an average length of stay of 5.9 days.

An important aspect of the setting is the mandated use of a hospital-specific patient classification system for determining patient acuity on each shift. Daily staffing is determined by the total patient acuity on each unit, and any additional needed staff members are provided from an on-call pool. The fact that the nurses are assigned to units based only on the number and acuity of patients made this study possible.

The study population consisted of 3,757 patients who were discharged from the hospital during a six-week period (March 15–April 30, 1984). Only those age 18 or over and classified in one of the 15 DRGs being studied were included in the sample. Of all patients discharged during this period, 53 percent were included in 30 DRGs. Of these, 57 percent were in perinatal DRGs and so were excluded from the study.

Patient Classification Tools

The patient classification tools used in the study hospital were developed internally. The medical-surgical patient classification tool is a four-level prototype system using a checklist format for nursing care activities. Budgeted hours of care range from 2.6 to 7.8 hours per 24 hours. The classification system for patient acuity is as follows:

Patient Acuity Rating		Budgeted Hours per 24 hours
I	Minimal help	2.6
II	Help with basic needs	4.3
III	Activity severely restricted	6.0
IV	Total care	7.8

The various patient classification tools used in the intensive care unit all utilize prototype classifications based on diseases. They also have four levels, but the hours range from 8 to 36 hours of care per 24 hours:

Patient Acuity Rating	Budgeted Hours per 24 hours
ICU I	8
ICU II	12
ICU III	24
ICU IV	36

The content validity of the tools was established by members of the hospital's patient classification committee. Criterion-related validity of the medical-surgical tool—validity in predicting the number of nursing care hours required for each classification level—was determined by self-report time-and-frequency studies conducted on several of the medical and surgical units in 1979 and 1980. On the basis of those studies, weights were assigned to the patient acuity levels to provide the predicted number of nursing care hours required for each patient. These weights have been revised at least twice since the original studies to reflect the actual budgeted positions for the units. Vanderzee and Glusko (1984) recommend using the budget to determine weights or hours for a patient classification tool. Since the system has been used as a basis for daily staffing for several years, it might also be said to have practical validity.

Reliability of the patient classification tools was examined regularly by the patient classification committee in 1982 and 1983, using audits of randomly selected charts, to see if the tools had been used properly and the patients correctly classified. Interrater reliability was established by this investigator during the study period with a sample of 58 patients. Five ratings were compared for each patient—the independent, simultaneous ratings of four nurses (the investigator, the head nurse or supervisor, the charge nurse, and the nurse assigned to the patient), and the acuity number in the computer. The intraclass correlation coefficient, which is an estimate of the typical reliability of a single rater's ratings, was .83. The reliability coefficient, which is an estimate of the reliability of the mean of the ratings, was .96. The tools were thus determined to be reliable.

Procedure

The DRGs to be studied were selected in a manner designed to maximize both the size of the groups and their relevance to other settings. Thus, 7 of the 15 DRGs to be studied were selected ahead of time using the study hospital's previous year's case mix and a report of the nationwide case mix of urban hospitals. The 8 remaining DRGs were chosen after the specific case mix for the study period was determined in order to ensure sufficiently large groups. The final sample contained 11 of the national top 25 DRGs. The 15 DRGs in the sample and the number of patients in each were as follows:

   14 Specific cerebrovascular disorders except TIA ($N = 37$)
   25 Seizure and headache, age 18–69, without complications ($N = 37$)
   39 Lens procedures ($N = 52$)

75 Major chest procedures ($N = 30$)

88 Chronic obstructive pulmonary disease ($N = 26$)

122 Circulatory disorders with AMI, without cardiovascular complications ($N = 31$)

127 Heart failure and shock ($N = 44$)

162 Inguinal and femoral hernia procedures, age 18–69, without complications ($N = 32$)

182 Esophagitis, gastroenteritis, and miscellaneous digestive disorders, over age 69 or with complications ($N = 42$)

183 Esophagitis, gastroenteritis, and miscellaneous digestive disorders, age 18–69, without complications ($N = 67$)

209 Major joint procedures ($N = 38$)

215 Back and neck procedures without complications ($N = 47$)

243 Medical back problems ($N = 59$)

355 Hysterectomy without complications ($N = 48$)

410 Chemotherapy ($N = 65$)

DRG data were obtained from a special report prepared through the hospital's case-mix library. This provided the following information on all study patients: DRG number, length of stay, nursing unit(s), sex, age, and total charges. The information was coded with the patient's billing number. These variables were used directly, without transformation.

Nursing care hours data were generated from the raw patient acuity information, as follows: The patient classification numbers for all medical-surgical and ICU patients were collected over the six-week study period for each patient's entire length of stay. This information was collated by hand. Complete acuity data were obtained for 157 of the 162 shifts during the study period. Acuity data were missing or incomplete for five nonconsecutive shifts. This raw acuity data and the DRG data were merged into one data base.

Next, the major input variables were developed from the raw acuity numbers by computer transformation, using two methods. In the first, the acuity numbers were replaced with the budgeted hours, and the hours for each day were averaged (the sum of the numbers for the three shifts was divided by three). Then the hours for each day were simply summed. This variable, total hours of nursing care delivered, was divided by the adjusted length of stay to produce the variable nursing care hours—that is, the average daily hours of direct nursing care. (Adjusted length of stay was used to compensate for the fact that some patients' hospitalization was longer than the study. It was calculated by dividing the number of shifts for which there was data by three.)

In the second method, the acuity numbers were weighted by dividing the budgeted hours by two. This allowed for the comparison of medical-surgical and intensive care unit patients, as shown in Table 1. Thus, the acuity levels were now 1, 2, 3, 4, 6, 12, and 18, instead of 1–4 for medical surgical units and 1–4 for the ICUs. These new weighted acuity ratings were treated in the same way as the actual budgeted hours. That is, the acuity level for each day was averaged by dividing the total of the three shifts by three. Summing each day's average acuity level produced the patient's total acuity level for the entire stay. The total acuity level was divided by the length of stay to produce the index of nursing care hours, the average daily acuity rating. The purpose of this step was to provide an alternative to using actual or budgeted hours, which may not be readily available in some hospitals. In such settings it may be possible to make an estimate of the hours, and weight the acuity levels in a manner similar to that described.

Finally, nursing care cost was determined by multiplying the total hours of nursing care delivered by the average hourly salary in the department of nursing. Nursing cost was then considered the input variable in the productivity ratio, and total patient charges the output. Thus, nursing productivity was determined by dividing the nursing cost by the total patient charges.

RESULTS

Of the 3,757 patients discharged during the study period, 679 were age 18 or over and were classified in one of the 15 DRGs being studied. Because acuity data were missing for some patients, the final sample consisted of 655 subjects, or 17.4 percent of the original study population. Of these, 55 percent were female and 45 percent were male. The

Table 1
Assigning Weights to Acuity Levels

Patient Acuity Rating	Budgeted Hours per 24	Budgeted Hours Divided by 2	Weight
1	2.6	1.30	1
2	4.3	2.15	2
3	6.0	3.00	3
4	7.8	3.90	4
ICU 1	8.0	4.00	4
ICU 2	12.0	6.00	6
ICU 3	24.0	12.00	12
ICU 4	36.0	18.00	18

Table 2
Number of Subjects in DRGs Studied

DRG	Number of Patients	Percentage
183	67	10.2
410	65	9.9
243	59	9.0
39	52	7.9
355	48	7.3
215	47	7.2
127	44	6.7
182	42	6.4
209	38	7.2
14	37	5.6
25	37	5.6
162	32	4.9
122	31	4.7
75	30	4.6
88	26	4.4

distribution of patients in DRGs for the study period was similar to that of the previous year.

The distribution of subjects in the 15 DRGs studied is shown in Table 2. The groups ranged in size from 26 to 67. Most of the patients (89.9 percent) were in medical-surgical units only. Just four patients (0.6 percent) were in an ICU only, while 9.5 percent of the subjects were in both a medical-surgical unit and an ICU.

Table 3
Mean, Range, and Standard Deviation for Selected Variables

Variable	Mean	Range	SD
Age	55.4	19–98	19.11
Length of stay	6.10	1–66	6.26
Adjusted length of stay	5.63	.33–46	5.34
Charges	$3,1990	$225–45,957	$4,355
Total hours of nursing care delivered	28.73	1.8–343.9	32.5
Index of nursing care hours	4.56	1.3–31.5	2.19
Average daily nursing care hours	5.68	1.7–42.8	2.90
Total acuity level	23.96	1.5–307.6	28.69
Nursing cost	$290	$18–3,469	$320
Productivity	.105	.001–.41	.410

Table 3 displays summary statistics on patients' age, length of stay, total charges, nursing care costs, and productivity. This table also summarizes the various measures of nursing care hours.

Productivity

Nursing care costs, total patient charges, and their ratio—that is, productivity—are presented in order of increasing productivity in Table 4. The DRGs with the highest ratio of nursing care costs to total patient charges, and therefore the lowest productivity, were 183, 25, 182, and 14. The ratio was lowest, and therefore productivity was highest, in DRGs 209, 215, 39, 75, and 88. A one-way analysis of variance indicated that the difference between the productivity ratios for the 15 DRGs was significant ($F = 14.7, p = .00001$).

The four DRGs that produced the highest average total patient charges were 209, 75, 127, and 14, with average charges ranging from $4,956 to $9,425. The same DRGs also produced the highest average nursing care costs, ranging from $594 to $616.

The four DRGs with the lowest average total charges were 25, 183, 162, and 410. The charges for these groups ranged from $1,329 to $1,545. Three of these DRGs, 410, 183, and 162, also showed the lowest

Table 4
Nursing Care Costs, Total Charges, and their Ratio (Productivity) for 15 DRGs[a]

DRG	Nursing Costs	Charges	Ratio of Averages	Average Ratio
183	$148	$1,329	.111	.139
25	154	1,329	.116	.131
182	244	2,001	.122	.128
14	594	4,956	.120	.127
127	616	6,754	.091	.116
243	212	1,933	.111	.112
122	400	3,748	.107	.106
162	141	1,401	.101	.101
410	131	1,545	.085	.100
355	256	2,586	.099	.099
88	302	3,817	.079	.088
75	564	7,397	.076	.082
39	113	1,423	.079	.080
215	245	2,975	.082	.078
209	594	9,425	.063	.065

[a]Costs are reported for March 15–April 30, 1984. Also, since the average of the ratios is not the same as the ratio of the averages, both are reported.

Table 5
Comparison of Productivity of Medical-Surgical Units and Intensive
Care Units

Variable	N	Mean	SD	t	df	p
Nursing cost						
Medical-surgical unit	589	$ 239	221			
Intensive care unit	66	737	642	−6.26	653	.000
Total patient charges						
Medical surgical unit	589	2,693	3,219			
Intensive care unit	66	7,710	8,610	−4.70	653	.000

total direct nursing care costs, ranging from $131 to $148. The average nursing cost for DRG 39 was actually the lowest, at $113 also within the low range. Although DRG 25 was among the four DRGs producing the lowest income, it is not among the four lowest in nursing care costs.

To determine whether there was a difference in productivity ratios for patients who had been cared for in an ICU and those who had been only in medical-surgical units, a t-test on independent groups was used to analyze the productivity ratios for these two groups of patients (see Table 5). There was no significant difference in the productivity ratios ($t = -.76, p = .45$). This was because both total charges and nursing care costs were significantly higher for ICU patients. It is interesting to note that the gap between ICU patients and patients in medical-surgical units was greater for total charges (2.9 percent more) than for nursing care (2.2 percent more).

Index of Nursing Care Hours

To determine whether an index of nursing care hours could be used to predict direct nursing care costs, hierarchical multiple regression analyses were performed, with nursing cost as the dependent variable (see Table 6). Since studies have previously shown that nursing costs are related to length of stay, the first predictor variable was adjusted length of stay. To test the hypothesis that patient acuity is also an important factor in determining nursing care costs, the next predictor variable was the index of nursing care hours—the average daily acuity rating of the patient. The other predictor variables were DRG, coded for effects as suggested by Cohen and Cohen (1983), and age. Adjusted length of stay accounted for 78.5 percent of the variance in nursing care costs, but an

Table 6
Multiple Regression Analysis of Nursing Cost

Variable Entered	R^2	R^2 Change	F	p
Adjusted length of stay	.78513	.78513	2353.2	0
Index of nursing care hours	.88915	.10437	2588.1	0
DRG[a]	.89767	.00010	344.9	0
Age	.89769	.00003	324.1	.000

[a]Coded for effects.

additional 10 percent of the variance was accounted for by the index of nursing care hours (R^2 change = .104). The findings were similar when nursing care hours (average daily hours of care) was substituted for index of nursing care hours. This indicates that although the main predictor of direct nursing care hours is length of stay, either the index of nursing care hours or nursing care hours can significantly increase the ability to predict nursing care costs. Further research is needed to see if the index of nursing care hours adds significantly to the prediction of nursing care costs in other settings and with other DRGs. It is possible that this simple measure, readily obtained from acuity classifications currently assigned by nurses, could be widely useful as a severity-of-illness measure.

Case Mix

It was also of interest to see if case mix could be used to predict the number of nursing care hours needed. An analysis of variance showed that nursing care hours differed significantly depending on the DRG (F = 8.66, p = .0001). The four DRGs with the highest daily average of nursing care hours were 39, 410, 14, and 127, with averages ranging from 6.8 to 7.7 hours out of 24. The lowest average nursing care hours were found in DRGs 243, 209, 182, and 88. In these DRGs the nursing care hours ranged from 4.1 to 4.95 hours out of 24. Hierarchical multiple regression of nursing care hours on the predictor variables (DRG group, age, and adjusted length of stay) indicated that DRG group accounted for only 22 percent of the variance in nursing hours. Thus, although DRG group is certainly related to nursing care hours, it is premature to say that nursing care hours can be predicted by DRG group.

Rankings of DRGs

A simple ranking of DRGs by various variables provided interesting insights. When DRGs were ranked by total nursing care hours delivered—the variable that included both length of stay and acuity—

Table 7
DRGs Ranked in Order of Total Nursing Care Hours

DRG	Mean	SD
127	61.0	60.5
209	58.9	36.4
14	58.9	38.9
75	56.0	73.7
122	39.6	20.8
88	30.0	17.6
355	25.4	6.5
215	24.2	12.5
182	24.2	15.1
243	21.9	19.2
25	15.3	7.9
183	14.6	6.6
162	14.9	3.9
410	12.9	4.6
39	11.2	3.1

the order was quite similar to that obtained when DRGs were ranked by total charges (see Table 7). The average nursing care hours per DRG ranged from 11.2 to 61.0.

When DRGs were ranked according to either mean nursing care hours (NCH), or the average daily acuity (index of nursing care hours), not considering length of stay, the order was quite different (see Table 8).

Table 8
DRGs Ranked in Order of Mean Nursing Care Hours

DRG	Mean	SD
39	7.7	2.9
410	7.3	2.5
14	7.2	5.2
127	6.8	1.2
183	5.7	2.6
122	5.6	1.2
162	5.5	1.2
75	5.5	1.8
25	5.4	2.8
88	4.9	1.5
182	4.9	1.2
355	4.6	0.6
215	4.6	1.4
209	4.4	0.9
243	4.1	1.2

Two DRGs with very short lengths of stay (DRGs 39 and 410) had the highest average nursing care hours. This variable (average daily nursing care hours) has not previously been described in the literature, but has promise as an alternate method for analyzing costs.

Other Findings

There were no significant relationships between patient gender and any of the other variables. The daily average number of hours of nursing care a patient received was inversely related to length of stay and positively related to total charges, total hours of nursing care delivered, index of nursing care hours, and productivity.

Further support for the model was found when differences by DRG group due to age, length of stay, total patient charges, total hours of nursing care delivered, index of nursing care hours, average daily hours of care (nursing care hours), total acuity level, nursing costs, and productivity were analyzed with a one-way analysis of variance. All the differences were significant beyond the .0001 level.

One important serendipitous finding was an interesting relationship between two of the computed variables, total nursing care hours delivered and total acuity level, and total patient charges. Several hierarchical regressions were performed separately on the dependent variable of total charges, using either total nursing care hours or total acuity level as the predictor (see Table 9). Either variable was able to explain 60 percent of the variance in total patient charges. These measures of patient acuity across hospital stay were much more sensitive to total charges than was DRG group, which only explained an additional 6 percent of the variance.

Table 9
Regression Analysis to Predict Patient Charges

Variable Entered	R^2	R^2 Change	F	p
Total hours of nursing care delivered	.597	.597	955.52	.000
DRG[a]	.660	.063	81.66	0
Age	.662	.002	72.43	.00
Sex	.662	.000	72.43	.00
Total acuity level	.600	.600	967.15	0
DRG[a]	.661	.060	81.72	0
Age	.662	.002	77.07	.000
Sex	.663	.000	75.52	.000

[a]Coded for effects.

DISCUSSION

Several companies are marketing programs to analyze nursing care costs, but there must be objective ways of analyzing the approaches used. This study provides data to help nursing administrators evaluate one system of cost analysis based on patient acuity.

In this study, direct nursing care accounted for from 6.5 to 13.9 percent of total patient charges. This is consistent with the 14 to 22 percent found by Riley and Schaefers (1983) in Minnesota and the 4 to 8 percent found by Mitchell et al. (1984) at Stanford University Hospital. What is striking is that nursing care costs are such a small percentage of total patient charges.

Nursing care hours in this study averaged between 11.2 and 66.0 hours per DRG. Mitchell et al. (1984) reported much higher average nursing care hours—from 88 to 109 hours—but the formula they used to determine hours included nonproductive time, while the present study did not. In future analyses it would be advisable to include nonproductive hours.

Close inspection of the productivity ratios found in this study provides some practical information about the nursing productivity of selected high-volume DRGs. This knowledge can help pinpoint areas of potential inefficiency for further study. For instance, DRGs were shown to be least productive at the study hospital were two neurologic DRGs (25 and 14) and two related to gastrointestinal problems (182 and 183). The nursing care given to selected patients in these DRGs could be analyzed to determine if there are ways to reduce costs without lowering the standard of care.

The productivity measure of specific DRGs should be as clear and easy to understand as possible. To analyze the productivity of various DRGs, this study divided nursing costs by total patient charges (input ÷ output). This produced a fraction, complicating the concept of productivity. To clarify and simplify the concept, in future studies charges should be divided by nursing costs (output ÷ input), as suggested by Edwardson (1985).

Once productive DRGs are identified, it may be possible to increase the number of patients in those DRGs by introducing a marketing plan to create a demand for those nursing services. This would further increase the productivity of those DRGs, as suggested by Shaffer (1984).

Two new variables not previously reported in the literature were used in this analysis of nursing cost. The average hours of nursing care delivered per day, and the index of those hours (the average daily patient acuity), produced cost findings strikingly different from other variables that use total per stay, not daily averages. The study found that two

DRGs with very short lengths of stay had the highest average nursing care hours (DRGs 39 and 410). These findings suggest that patients in certain short-stay, high-volume classifications might possibly be cared for more economically on an outpatient basis.

FUTURE RESEARCH

Many other types of analyses are possible using the method described in this study. Once nursing care hours and costs have been identified, it would be possible to analyze costs by nursing unit, controlling for DRG group, or, alternatively, to compare costs by DRG, controlling for nursing unit. It would also be interesting to compare the ranking of a hospital's high-volume DRGs by total charges and nursing care costs with the ranking of those DRGs in order of maximum Medicare reimbursement.

Although the indexes of nursing care hours used in this study were not excellent predictors of nursing care costs, they were surprisingly good predictors of total patient charges. Sixty percent of the variance in total charges was accounted for by the variable total hours of nursing care delivered, which was a combination of length of stay and total hours of nursing care received, as measured by the patient classification tool. Total hours of nursing care delivered, or a similar measure, such as total acuity level, may serve as a readily available severity-of-illness measure for use in many hospitals.

Hospitals could use their patient classification tools to estimate nursing care hours and costs. Acuity scales could be weighted according to the hours budgeted for each classification level. Either total acuity level or total hours of nursing care delivered could be used, since they are highly correlated. If nursing costs by DRG were determined in the same manner for all hospitals in a region, costs could be compared across hospitals.

Further research needs to be undertaken to test the utility of the index of nursing care hours and total acuity level as severity-of-illness measures in general and to test their use in DRG reimbursement. Further research is also needed to find other predictors of nursing care hours. In particular, an in-depth study of selected DRGs with high variance in nursing care hours is needed to see if patterns in the variation could be established. Finally, research should also be undertaken to see if total acuity level can predict total hospital costs per DRG as well as total patient charges.

REFERENCES

Caterinicchio, R. P. (1983). A debate: RIMs and the cost of nursing care. *Nursing Management, 14*(5), 108–122.

Caterinicchio, R. P., & Davies, H. (1983). Developing a client-focused allocation statistic of inpatient nursing resource use: An alternative to the patient day. *Social Science Medicine, 17*(5), 250–272.

Cohen, J., & Cohen, P. (1983). *Applied multiple progression/correlation analysis for the behavioral sciences.* Hillsdale, NJ: Laurence Erlbaum Associates.

Curtin, L. (1983). Determining costs of nursing services per DRG. *Nursing Management, 14*(4), 17–20.

Edwardson, S. R. (1985). Measuring nursing productivity. *Nursing Economics, 3*(1), 9–14.

Feldman, J., & Goldhaber, F. I. (1984). Living with DRGs. *Journal of Nursing Administration, 14*(5), 19–22.

Graham-Moore, B., & Ross, T. L. (1983). *Productivity gainsharing: How employee incentive programs can improve business performance.* Englewood Cliffs, NJ: Prentice-Hall.

Grimaldi, P. L., & Micheletti, J. A. (1982). DRG reimbursement: RIMS and the cost of nursing care. *Nursing Management, 13*(12), 12–22.

Herzog, T. P. (1985). Productivity: Fighting the battle of the budget. *Nursing Management, 16*(1), 30–34.

Jelinek, R. C., & Dennis, L. C. (1976). *A review and evaluation of nursing productivity.* Bethesda, MD: Health Resources Administration.

Joel, L. A. (1984). DRGs and RIMs: Implications for nursing. *Nursing Outlook, 32*(1), 42–49.

Mitchell, M., Miller, M., Welches, L. W., & Walker, D. D. (1984). Determining cost of direct nursing care by DRGs. *Nursing Management, 15*(4), 29–32.

Riley, W., & Schaefers, V. (1983). Costing nursing service. *Nursing Management, 14*(12), 40–43.

Shaffer, F. A. (1984). Nursing power in the DRG world. *Nursing Management, 15*(6), 28–30.

Unit leaders tell where costs cuts hurt (1985). *American Nurse, 17*(1), 1, 4.

Vanderzee, H., & Glusco, G. (1984). DRGs, variable pricing, and budgeting for nursing services. *Journal of Nursing Administration, 14*(5), 11–14.

Determining the Cost of Nursing Care Within DRGs

Gail A. Wolf and Linda K. Lesic

The impact of the prospective payment system on hospitals has aroused unprecidented concern with the cost of delivering patient care. Like it or not, health care providers have had to develop a stronger business orientation. Instead of "patient care" we now hear about "product lines," and "marketing strategy" has replaced "community awareness." Like any other competitive business, hospitals are constantly looking for ways to expand their market base, improve their product, and reduce their costs.

Because nursing is the largest single department in any hospital, it is the first place most institutions look for cost reductions. It is commonly believed that nursing costs represent 30 to 60 percent of a hospital's total costs. The accuracy of this assumption, however, is determined by what are considered nursing costs. In many institutions these include room-and-board charges and the cost of medical-surgical supplies as well as the salary costs of nursing personnel.

To accurately determine whether nursing inefficiencies exist, a mechanism must be developed to separate the pure costs of delivering nursing care from the overhead costs of operating a hospital. This distillation process becomes critical when one realizes that the primary reason a patient is hospitalized is for nursing care. If patients did not require nursing care, they could have all tests and surgical procedures done on an outpatient basis and see their physicians in the office. Thus, nursing care is a primary product of a hospital.

Successful businesses understand that to stay competitive, they must produce a quality product at a reasonable cost. To accomplish this goal in the hospital industry, nursing administrators must initially determine what it costs to deliver their product of quality nursing care. This will allow for the planning and development of accurate nursing budgets and ensure that inappropriate cost reductions are not made that would affect the quality of the product. Additional information can be obtained if the cost of nursing care is further broken down into costs per diagnosis related group (DRG). Strategies for reducing high-cost DRGs can then be explored.

ALTERNATIVE COSTING METHODOLOGIES

The literature identifies three primary methodologies for determining the cost of nursing care: the per diem method, relative intensity measures (RIMs), and the acuity-based method.

Per Diem Method

The per diem method determines average daily nursing costs based on total nursing care costs and the number of inpatient days. The allocation statistic, which is the determining factor of the nursing care costs, is the number of inpatient days at the institution. The average daily nursing care costs are determined by totaling all nursing costs, including salaries and fringe benefits of nursing personnel, and dividing this total by the number of inpatient days. Nursing care costs per patient are then calculated by multiplying the average daily nursing care costs by the number of days in the patient's stay.

The advantage of the per diem method is that it is easy to calculate, and it is the most frequently used method for determining nursing care costs. The disadvantages are greater than the advantages, however. No allowance is made for variation in a patient's diagnosis and condition, and the patient's nursing needs are measured only indirectly by the length of stay. In using this method, one must assume that a patient utilizes the same amount of nursing resources each day of hospitalization. Obviously, this is an erroneous assumption. Curtin (1984) cites two additional disadvantages: (1) costs are identified but not justified, and (2) the methodology provides none of the information necessary for management decision making, such as staff allocation and skill mix. Thus, the nursing administrator who is concerned with maximizing efficiency in order to survive prospective payment will find this method of identifying nursing costs woefully inadequate.

RIMs Method

Relative intensity measures (RIMs) is a second methodology for identifying nursing care costs, which relates patients' consumption of nursing resources to their medical condition (Grimaldi & Micheletti, 1982). The allocation statistic in this model is the average minutes of care the patient receives, which is noted as RIMs. One RIM is equal to one minute of nursing resource use.

The RIMs methodology was designed to predict the total use of nursing resources throughout a patient's stay (Caterinicchio, 1983). To accomplish this, both nursing and non-nursing functions were identified and time-and-motion studies conducted to determine the amount of time spent performing these functions. Through a system of mathematical formulas, a fixed number of minutes of nursing resource time was determined for each of nine nursing resource clusters (NRCs), each of which contains several DRGs. Each patient assigned to an NRC is assigned a designated number of nursing resource minutes. Nursing care costs are determined by the number of minutes assigned to the patient. The cost of one RIM is equal to the total nursing care costs divided by the total minutes of nursing resource time used. This cost per RIM is then multiplied by the total minutes assigned to the patient to determine the nursing care costs.

An advantage of the RIMs method is that it provides patient-specific, aggregate, interval measures of nursing resource consumption (Joel, 1984). A second advantage is that it tends to identify DRGs that are cost intensive for nursing (Caterinicchio, 1983). A major disadvantage, however, is that the RIMs method allocates a certain amount of nursing time for each DRG, but does not measure actual patient need. In addition, as in the per diem method, nursing care costs are identified, but not justified.

Acuity-Based Method

The third costing methodology is an acuity-based system. In this method, nursing care costs are determined using a patient classification system that identifies the amount of nursing care required based on the complexity of patient care needs. The allocation statistic is patient acuity.

With this method, patients are classified on a daily basis according to their nursing care requirements. This information is tracked for the patient's entire length of stay. Upon discharge, the patient's average daily classification is determined by adding the daily classification figures and dividing this total by the length of stay. The average daily nursing costs are also determined for each level of acuity. The appropriate daily cost for the patient's average daily classification is multiplied by the length of stay to arrive at the total nursing care costs for that patient.

Curtin (1984) identifies several advantages of this method. Important information is gathered regarding patient acuity as well as information to justify staffing levels and mix based on acuity. The allocation statistic is patient specific and therefore most accurate in terms of nursing demand. Finally, with an acuity-based system, control of nursing resources stays in nursing's hands. However, this method, too, is not without disadvantages. Developing a valid patient classification system is both time-consuming and expensive. Accordingly, some patient classification systems are in a crude state of development and do not accurately measure patient acuity. Interrater reliability, which assures that different individuals classify patients in the same manner, is critical to an effective system and often difficult to obtain. Finally, on a daily operational basis, the acuity-based costing methodology is more expensive in terms of both time and money than the other methodologies. However, this is the only method that allows identification of the actual resources required by individual patients within DRGs. This information is vital in determining the actual costs of nursing care and in assuring that adequate resources are provided to meet patient needs. Consequently, the acuity-based costing methodology was utilized for the research study to be described here.

STUDY OF NURSING CARE COSTS

This study was conducted to determine the cost of nursing care for high-volume DRGs at Shadyside Hospital in Pittsburgh, Pennsylvania. Three specific objectives were established:

1. To determine the direct nursing care costs, indirect unit-based costs, and nursing overhead costs for specific DRGs.
2. To compare the total nursing care costs to the total hospital costs for selected DRGs.
3. To identify the DRGs that had the highest nursing care costs.

For purposes of this study, the three components of nursing care costs were defined as follows:

Direct care costs: The salary costs for caregivers providing direct patient care, including RNs, LPNs, and nursing assistants. (Even though nursing assistants are not considered nursing caregivers, they provide direct care for patients' non-nursing needs, such as making unoccupied beds, transportation, and so forth).

Indirect unit-based costs: The salary costs for unit nursing personnel who are not responsible for providing direct patient care, including the unit director and unit secretaries.

Indirect overhead costs: The salary costs for all nursing support personnel. This includes nursing administration, the nursing education department, and all clinical specialists, nurse clinicians, and secretarial help within the nursing division.

Methodology

The study was conducted in a 474-bed acute care, community teaching hospital located in a large metropolitan city. At the time of data collection, the hospital was undergoing a transition from team nursing to primary nursing; thus both systems could be found on various units within the hospital. The Nursing Division is decentralized and maintains a minimum proportion of 70 percent registered nurses on all nursing units. All nursing care is delivered by licensed personnel, with nursing assistants functioning in a support role.

Data were collected for a six-month period beginning July 1, 1984. This date marked the implementation of the prospective payment system for Medicare patients for the hospital.

Using a computerized nursing information system (MDAX), the nursing workload for every patient was determined and tracked every day. Thirty-two specific indicators were used to consistently and objectively measure the daily nursing requirements for each patient. These indicators included measurement of the patient's physical needs, such as those resulting from immobility or intravenous therapy, as well as nonphysical needs, such as teaching and emotional support. Each patient's daily assessment was converted by computer into weighted relative index of workload units (RIWs). The daily number of RIWs generated by a patient were tracked throughout the entire period of hospitalization. Upon discharge, each patient was assigned to the appropriate DRG category.

DRG categories that contained data from at least 20 patients were included in the final analysis. This resulted in a total sample of 1,737 patients representing 37 DRGs.

Interrater Reliability

As stated previously, when using a patient classification system it is important to ensure that all patients are being classified according to the same criteria. Extensive inservice educational sessions were held for all registered nurses concerning the classification system. Practice sessions were held until a minimum interrater reliability of .90 was obtained.

To maintain reliability, unit directors are responsible for randomly monitoring patient classification cards on a daily basis. In addition, interrater reliability measurements for each nursing unit are conducted by the Nursing Information Systems Department on a quarterly basis.

Calculation of Costs

Staffing within the Nursing Division was calculated on the basis of 3.6 hours of direct nursing care for each RIW generated. By determining the average hourly wage for all direct caregivers and multiplying by 3.6, the direct nursing care costs for one RIW can be calculated. This cost, multiplied by the number of RIWs generated by each patient, yields the total direct nursing care costs for each patient's hospitalization. The indirect unit-based costs and the indirect overhead costs were determined by averaging salary costs and establishing a flat rate for each RIW generated.

To compare nursing care costs with total hospital costs, the average hospital cost for each of the DRG categories was obtained from the hospital's fiscal department. The various nursing care costs divided by the hospital costs determined the percentage of hospital costs represented by nursing.

RESULTS

Initial analysis of the data indicated a large variation in cost within each of the DRG categories. A coefficient of variation was calculated for each DRG by dividing the standard deviation by the mean cost. This statistic is designed to show how much variation is present. A coefficient of variation of less than 0.10 indicates a relatively similar population with little variability. The DRGs studied had coefficients of variation ranging from 0.31 to 1.31. This indicates that within each DRG there is a wide range of nursing care costs reflecting wide variability in nursing care requirements.

A comparison of direct and indirect nursing care costs showed that 83 percent of the nursing costs were spent in providing direct patient care. Indirect unit-based costs represented 10 percent of the total, and nursing overhead costs constituted 7 percent. When nursing costs were compared to total hospital costs, the direct care costs accounted for 21 percent, indirect unit-based costs 2.5 percent, and nursing overhead 1.7 percent of the total. Overall, nursing costs averaged 15 percent of the total reimbursement received by the hospital for the DRGs studied.

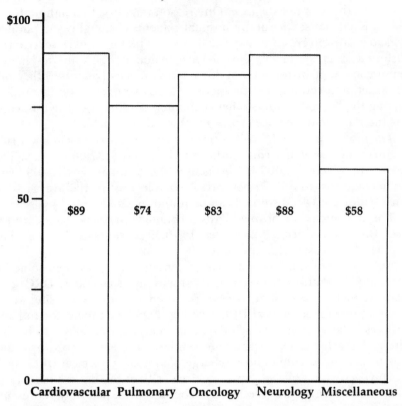

Figure 1
Average Nursing Care Cost per Day,
by Clinical Service

In comparing nursing costs and hospital costs, it is important to bear in mind that a hospital's actual total costs will affect the percentage represented by nursing. For example, suppose the nursing costs per DRG are exactly the same in Hospital A and Hospital B; however, Hospital A has lower total operating costs. The percentage of hospital costs represented by nursing will be greater in Hospital A, even though the actual costs are the same. Therefore, if cost comparisons are done between hospitals, the actual dollar cost is a more accurate statistic than percentages.

To analyze the data by clinical service, the DRGs were classified into five categories representing the main services within the hospital: cardiovascular, neurology, pulmonary, oncology, and miscellaneous. The average DRG nursing care costs by clinical service ranged from $58 to $89 per day (see Fig. 1). As might be expected, the cardiovascular service was the most expensive—largely because of monitoring costs. The oncology DRGs were expected to be among the DRGs with the highest costs because of patients' extensive psychosocial and teaching needs; however, this was not the case. One reason might be that although oncology is a major service at this hospital, patients with highly complicated oncological problems are not usually seen. The pulmonary service is a different story, however. The hospital maintains the only designated pulmonary unit in the city, and, as a result, sees patients with more advanced and complicated problems. The patient acuity on this unit is among the highest in units other than intensive care. Despite this, costs for the pulmonary service can be considered reasonable.

The most expensive DRG in terms of nursing care costs was DRG 106, coronary bypass with cardiac catheters which cost $137.00 per day. The least expensive was DRG 97, bronchitis and asthma, ages 18–69, with an average cost of $40.76 per day. A complete list of the average cost for each of the DRGs studied can be found in Table 1.

The percentage of hospital costs accounted for by nursing care for each DRG ranged from 9.28 percent to 70.59 percent (see Table 2). The average DRG cost was 24 percent.

An analysis of nursing workload by length of stay revealed some interesting differences between medical and surgical DRGs. DRG 294, diabetes mellitus, age 36 or older, is representative of the nursing workload pattern for a medical DRG (see Fig. 2). The demand for nursing services is fairly constant each day, until the patient is about to be discharged. At that time, nursing intervention increases sharply, probably due to patient teaching and discharge planning. A surgical DRG, such as DRG 257, total mastectomy, age greater than 69, has a bimodal demand for nursing care (see Fig. 3). The first peak probably represents the immediate postoperative period. The nursing workload levels off as recovery continues and then peaks again prior to discharge, when the demand for discharge planning and health teaching occurs.

Analysis by nursing workload, especially for high-cost DRGs, can be very helpful in determining ways to reduce costs of care. For example, projection of nursing demand by case mix on a nursing unit can assist in projecting staffing requirements as well as staff mix. Methods for equalizing demand for nursing care can also be proposed, such as beginning discharge planning when the patient is admitted and meeting teaching requirements throughout the period of hospitalization.

RECOMMENDATIONS

In this study, the nursing care salary costs were found to constitute approximately one-quarter of the total hospital costs. Thus, nursing

Table 1
Direct Nursing Care Costs per DRG

Service and DRG		Direct Cost per Day
Cardiovascular		
143	Chest pain	$66.74
138	Arrhythmia and conduction disorder, age > 69 and/or CC	70.09
125	Circulatory disorders except AMI, with cardiac catheter, w/o complex diagnosis	70.53
124	Circulatory disorder except AMI with catheter and CC	75.03
130	Peripheral vascular disorders, age > 69 and/or CC	76.93
127	Heart failure and shock	79.05
140	Angina	80.57
116	Permanent pacemaker w/o AMI or CHE	91.34
108	Cardiothoracic procedures except valve and bypass w/pump	91.97
121	Circulatory disorder w/AMI plus CV comp.—discharged alive	96.39
122	Circulatory disorder w/AMI, discharged alive	98.14
110	Vascular procedure, age > 69 and/or CC	102.97
107	Coronary bypass w/o cardiac catheter	112.41
106	Coronary bypass with catheter	137.53
Pulmonary		
97	Bronchitis and asthma, age 18–69 w/o CC	40.76
88	Chronic obstructive pulmonary disease	56.99
96	Bronchitis and asthma, age > 69 and/or CC	75.07
87	Pulmonary edema and respiratory failure	85.74
82[a]	Respiratory neoplasms	89.26
89	Pneumonia and pleurisy, age > 69 and/or CC	98.12
Oncology		
410	Chemotherapy	64.39
257	Total mastectomy, age > 69 and/or CC	69.44
413	Other myeloprolif disorders, age > 69 and/or CC	75.22
203	Malignancy of hepatobiliary system or pancreas	77.24
82[a]	Respiratory neoplasms	89.26
403	Lymphoma or leukemia, age > 69 and/or CC	98.10
10	Nervous system neoplasms	109.93
Neurology		
15	Transient ischemic attacks	54.03
5	Extracranial vascular procedures	70.75
10[a]	Nervous system neoplasm	109.93
14	Specific cerebrovascular disorder except TIA	117.49
Miscellaneous		
162	Inguinal femoral procedures, age 18–69	41.73
183	Esophagitis, gastroent., age 18–69 w/o CC	42.16
182	Esophagitis, gastroent., age > 69 and/or CC	49.25
243	Medical back problems	53.62
294	Diabetes, age 36 or greater	56.16
39	Lens procedure	59.93
174	GI hemorrhage, age > 69 and/or CC	73.26
296	Nutrition and metabolic disorder, age > 69 and/or CC	91.69

[a]These DRGs appear twice, grouped both by speciality and disease process.

Table 2
Nursing Care Cost as Percentage of Total Hospital Cost per DRG

Service and DRG	Percentage of Hospital Cost
Cardiovascular	
116 Permanent pacemaker w/o AMI or CHF	11.08
107 Coronary bypass w/o cardiac catheter	13.57
106 Coronary bypass with cardiac catheter	14.01
110 Vascular procedures, age > 69 and/or CC	15.53
108 Cardiothoriac procedures except valve and bypass w/pump	17.75
124 Circulatory disorders except AMI, with catheter and CC	18.15
125 Circulatory disorders except AMI, with cardiac catheter, w/o complex diagnosis	19.93
143 Chest pain	24.13
121 Circulatory disorder w/AMI and CV comp., discharged alive	24.98
122 Circulatory disorders w/AMI, discharged alive	27.35
130 Peripheral vascular disorder, age > 69 and/or CC	29.69
140 Angina	30.09
138 Cardiac arrhythmia and conduction disorder, age > 69 and/or CC	30.24
127 Heart failure and shock	31.72
Pulmonary	
97 Bronchitis and asthma, age 18–69 w/o CC	9.28
96 Bronchitis and asthma, age > 69 and/or CC	16.98
88 Chronic obstructive pulmonary disease	21.16
87 Pulmonary edema and respiratory failure	22.70
89 Pneumonia and pleurisy, age > 69 and/or CC	28.35
82[a] Respiratory neoplasms	35.06
Oncology	
403 Lymphoma or leukemia, age > 69 and/or CC	12.97
410 Chemotherapy	25.66
257 Total mastectomy, age > 69 and/or CC	27.53
413 Other myeloprolif disorder, age > 69 and/or CC	28.54
203 Malignancy of hepatobiliary system or pancreas	29.30
82[a] Respiratory neoplasms	35.06
10[a] Nervous system neoplasms, age > 69 and/or CC	70.59
Neurology	
5 Extracranial vascular procedures	20.17
15 Transient ischemic attacks	21.73
14 Specific cerebrovascular disorder, except TIA	38.65
10[a] Nervous system neoplasms	70.59
Miscellaneous	
39 Lens procedure	12.19
162 Inguinal femoral procedures, age 18–69	13.90
294 Diabetes, age 36 or greater	18.73
183 Esophagitis, gastroent., age 18–69 w/o CC	19.19
182 Esophagitis, gastroent., age 69 and/or CC	20.20
243 Medical back problems	20.50
174 GI hemorrhage, age 69 and/or CC	32.24
296 Nutritional and metabolic disorder, age > 69 and/or CC	43.26

[a]These DRGs appear twice, grouped both by speciality and disease process.

Figure 2
Nursing Workload by Length of Stay for DRG 294

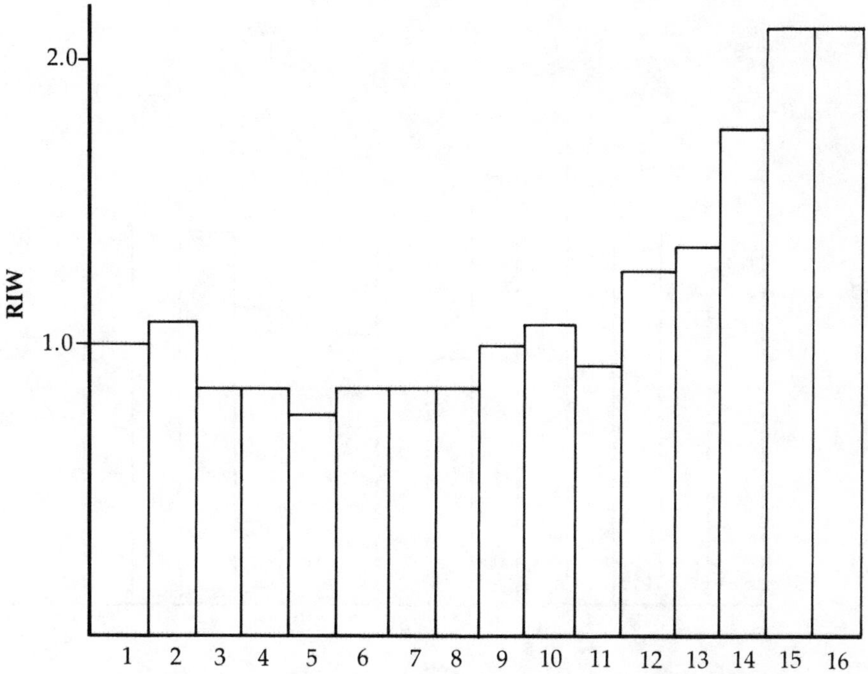

would appear to be a cost-effective service. However, the unusually high costs for nursing care in certain DRG categories need to be explored.

To apply the information derived from this study to administrative and clinical practice, four recommendations are offered.

1. Each individual agency should identify the nursing care costs associated with their high-volume DRGs. As noted previously, there are essentially three methodologies for determining nursing care costs: the per diem method, RIMs, and an acuity-based classification system. Although somewhat more complicated, costs should be calculated based on actual patient acuity. There are two reasons for this. First, as hospitals make adjustments in response to the prospective payment system, patient acuity will fluctuate. For example, during the first six months of operating under DRGs, patient acuity increased significantly in many hospitals, largely because of a decreased length of stay. If an institution begins admitting surgical patients the same day that their surgery is scheduled and shifts many surgical procedures to an outpatient basis, the acuity on the surgical units will increase. Thus, the actual nursing

Figure 3
Nursing Workload by Length of Stay for DRG 257

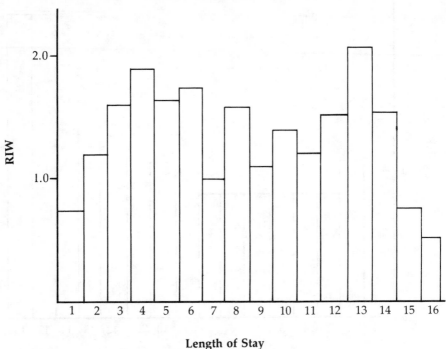

Length of Stay

demands generated by patients may fluctuate both within and between hospitals. Second, if we in nursing are to maintain quality patient care, patient demand must be matched with nursing supply. This can only be done by measuring the patient's nursing care needs, or acuity.

Identification of nursing care costs for high-volume DRGs will help to ensure that inappropriate reductions are not made in the nursing budget. Many hospitals utilize a "fair share" concept in response to declining admissions and patient days. Under this philosophy, each department is required to reduce costs their "fair share" in order to lower overall operating costs. If a nursing department reduces personnel at the same time that patients' requirements for nursing care increase, the quality of patient care may be compromised. Nursing's "fair share" may actually be to increase personnel, but without data on patient acuity and nursing costs, there is no way to validate this.

Information on nursing costs is helpful in additional ways. Analyzing the cost of high-volume DRGs will help in defining an institution's patient mix, developing the appropriate inservice and orientation programs, identifying policy and procedures that need to be updated, identifying the standards of nursing care that have the highest priority for development, and even evaluating usage of supplies and equipment. Most important, this information is crucial for evaluating the effectiveness of nursing practice.

2. Nursing departments should develop intervention strategies for their high-cost DRGs. Once the DRGs with the highest nursing costs are identified, a cost-benefit analysis of each of these DRGs should be done. The goal of this analysis is to ensure quality patient care in the most cost-effective manner. Each DRG needs to be analyzed to determine patient requirements and the common patterns of nursing practice. Methods for delivering nursing care in a more efficient manner can then be designed.

Intervention may not be appropriate in some DRG categories, while in others it may be extremely beneficial. For example, if a cardiac DRG carries a high nursing cost that is found to be associated with monitoring, the benefit might justify the cost. Intervention strategies, if any, might focus on more efficient ways of monitoring or on accurate identification of patients who require monitoring. On the other hand, a high-cost oncology DRG might be associated with the provision of individual emotional support or health teaching. A potential strategy for intervention might be the formation of support groups or classes for patient education. Follow-up could be done on an individual basis to ensure that this method of intervention was effective.

Appropriate intervention strategies can best be determined by clinical task forces involving the professional nurses who provide the actual patient care. Input from clinical specialists can be very helpful, since they are aware of pertinent clinical research and the appropriate nursing standards. It is essential to document the outcome of any intervention strategy, in terms of both cost and quality.

3. Nursing care costs should form the basis for nursing care charges. For a number of years the nursing profession has discussed the need to separate the cost of professional nursing services from hospital charges for room and board. The time is ripe for this. Consumers of health care are becoming much more aware of the costs of health care. The health care bill needs to be itemized so that consumers can understand what they are paying for. Professional nursing services, provided in response to patients' needs, is a major item.

A beneficial by-product of this process is that the nursing department becomes a revenue-generating department, rather than a hospital expense. Since patients are hospitalized in order to receive nursing care, this seems most appropriate.

4. Factors that affect the cost of providing nursing care must be identified. To provide quality patient care in the most cost-effective manner, additional information is needed about factors that affect the cost of care. In general, such factors can be divided into three classifications: patient related, nurse related, and environmental.

Patient-related variables include age, diagnosis, and admitting physician. In addition, the patient's value system and socialization can affect cost. For example, a patient who values independence might put greater effort into recovery than the individual who regards a hospitalization as an opportunity to rest. A patient's level of knowledge will influence his or her receptiveness to and the effectiveness of health teaching. The resources available to a patient, such as family members, financial resources, and resources available in the community can also potentially affect length of hospitalization and recovery.

The nurse-related variables include education, experience, and level of skill. In addition, personal motivation and productivity can affect efficiency and consequently the cost of providing care.

Finally, numerous environmental variables can modify the cost of nursing care. The organizational structure, in terms of the number of personnel in various categories, has direct consequences for costs. Information is needed about which variables should be considered in determining the most effective organizational structure for a nursing department. The question of centralization versus decentralization affects both the quality and timeliness of decision making, with subsequent implications for costs. The philosophy of nursing care delivery (functional, team, total care, or primary nursing) also needs to be considered in terms of cost-benefit analysis. The cost-effectiveness of specialty nursing units needs to be explored. Decisions on staffing patterns, such as the percentage of registered nurses in a unit, the hours of care provided, and staffing ratios have implications for both quality and cost. Resources available to the nurse and even such factors as leadership can potentially affect nursing costs.

Although nursing cannot exert much control over the patient-related variables, the nurse-related and environmental variables can be manipulated. Additional information must be generated through research to determine the most effective means of accomplishing this.

In summary, the goal of the prospective payment system is to provide health care in a cost-effective manner. To accomplish this, the nursing profession must first understand our product and its price. Calculating the cost of nursing care within DRGs is the first step in determining if we are utilizing nursing resources in a way that will maximize quality and minimize cost.

REFERENCES

Curtin, L. L. (1984, October). DRG creep, DRG weights, and patient acuity (Editorial). *Nursing Management, 15*(10), 7–9.

Caterinicchio, R. P. (1983, May). A debate: RIMs and the cost of nursing care. *Nursing Management, 14*(5), 36–41.

Grimaldi, P. L., & Micheletti, J. A. (1982, December). DRG reimbursement: RIMs and the cost of nursing care. *Nursing Management, 13*(12), 12–22.

Joel, L. A. (1984, January–February). DRGs and RIMs: Implications for nursing. *Nursing Outlook, 32*(1), 42–49.

Severity of Illness and Nursing Intensity as Predictors of Treatment Costs

Kathleen Lucke and Joseph Lucke

The federal government has adopted a prospective payment system based on diagnosis related groups (DRGs) in place of the less efficient and more expensive cost-based system of health care reimbursement. If the prospective payment system continues to force health care providers to operate more efficiently and reduce costs, other third-party payers may be interested in adopting a similar system. This could affect virtually all consumers of health care in the nation. It is imperative that a prospective payment system accurately predict necessary treatment costs without causing a reduction in the quality of health care.

Hospitals in New Jersey have been using a prospective reimbursement system since 1981, and the number of patient days and the costs of care have indeed declined. Based on the New Jersey results, it is predicted that there will be a $3.5 billion national savings of hospital costs for Medicare patients over the next three years. But despite the fact that the prospective payment system in New Jersey has been successful in reducing costs, several problems have surfaced. First, about 20 percent of patients were outliers (that is, unusually long or costly cases involving extra payments to the hospital), while the system allows for only 5 to 6 percent. Second, a small percentage of DRGs accounted for a large

The authors wish to thank Judy Aronson and Carol Gagnon, Research and Publication Support Services, for their editing and technical assistance in the preparation of this manuscript.

percentage of patients. Third, patients within a DRG were found not to be homogeneous; a wide disparity existed in consumption of resources. Finally, case mix changed as hospitals attempted to minimize the financial impact of prospective reimbursement (Grimaldi, 1981).

Two major deficiencies exist in the way current prospective reimbursements are derived: severity of illness is inadequately reflected, and intensity of nursing care is ignored. The purpose of this study was to develop and test a method for incorporating measures of severity of illness and nursing intensity into the existing DRG system and to evaluate the extent to which a combination of these measures predicted treatment costs more accurately than the DRG classification system.

SEVERITY OF ILLNESS

Severity of illness is determined not only by the patient's baseline health status, stage of illness, or response to therapy, but also by the quality of care received and access to health care resources. (Grimaldi & Micheletti, 1983; New Jersey State Department of Health, 1982; Schweiker, 1982). DRGs do not take into account all of these factors. The system only narrowly reflects the patient's response to treatment and baseline health status by taking into account certain complications, discharge status, secondary diagnosis, and age.

Other dimensions that constitute the severity-of-illness construct and contribute to resource consumption and treatment costs are not considered in the determination of DRG categories. For example, in addition to secondary diagnosis and age, baseline health status also includes the individual's degree of independence in physical functioning related to the debilitating effects of disease (New Jersey State Department of Health, 1982; Special Committee on Aging, 1983). Depending on the stage of illness, resource consumption may also vary. Newly diagnosed individuals may require more diagnostic studies and education, whereas individuals with chronic or terminal illness may require supportive or maintenance care (Grimaldi & Micheletti, 1983). Response to therapy also varies, depending on the presence of other disease or chronic health conditions, the treatment the individual may be undergoing for the present condition (for example, immunosuppressed patients), available support systems, and the effectiveness of coping strategies.

The thoroughness and timeliness of health care, the number of patients treated with similar diagnoses, and services available within the health care facility all affect the severity of illness (Schweiker, 1982). Yet, for the urban and rural poor, access to the best resources is limited, which may compound the severity of illness for these groups (Muller, 1983; New Jersey State Department of Health, 1982).

SEVERITY-OF-ILLNESS SCALES

Several severity-of-illness scales have been developed for various purposes. Disease-specific scales with prognostic capabilities exist for cardiac, burn, and trauma patients (Feller, Tholen, & Cornell, 1980; Fuchs & Scheidt, 1981; Gustafsen et al., 1983). Horn and others (Horn, Chachich, & Cropton, 1983; Kreitzer, Loebner, & Roveti, 1982) have developed an index of severity for medical patients that compares physicians' practices and evaluates length of stay and costs. They demonstrated that heterogeneity within DRGs is significantly reduced by the addition of a severity index (Horn, 1981). They were able to explain more variance in resource consumption using their severity-of-illness index than when using DRGs alone (Horn & Sharkey, 1983; Horn, Sharkey, & Bertram, 1983).

Knaus, Draper, Wagner, and Zimmerman (1984) developed the Acute Physiology and Chronic Health Evaluation (APACHE) system, a severity-of-illness classification system used initially to study appropriate utilization of beds in intensive care units and to predict patient outcomes. Recently Wagner, Wineland, and Knaus (1983) used the APACHE system to study resource consumption in an intensive care unit for two DRGs. A significant divergence was found between bed charges and costs of nursing care for the two DRGs, indicating that current data used to determine appropriate prices for DRG categories was inadequate because of "substantial variation in inter-hospital severity of illness within DRG categories" (Knaus, 1983). The APACHE system was chosen as the severity-of-illness measure for the current study for several reasons: (1) it is a prospective classification system; (2) it is an objective scale; (3) a high degree of validity and reliability has been established for the scale; and (4) it is easy to use.

NURSING INTENSITY

Intensity of nursing care required by hospitalized patients is not included in the assignment of DRGs. Yet, a primary reason that patients require hospitalization is their need for professional nursing care (Halloran, 1981), and that care constitutes a significant portion of resource consumption (Knaus, 1983). An individual's baseline health status, response to treatment, stage of illness, quality of care, and access to resources will determine the intensity of nursing care that patient requires. In addition, the patient's nursing diagnoses will indicate the amount and type of nursing care required.

Nursing intensity may vary each day for every patient within a DRG. On the day preceding and the day of a diagnostic or operative procedure, nursing intensity increases. The individual's chronic health problems, ability to contribute to self-care, response to therapy, and ability to cope and the presence or absence of support systems to assist the patient after discharge all affect the intensity of nursing care required. The variety of needs for nursing services cause inconsistencies in both the length and cost of hospitalization within DRGs.

RELATIVE INTENSITY MEASURES

The New Jersey State Department of Health initiated the Relative Intensity Measures Studies (RIMs) in 1975 to develop an alternative to the patient day as a means of distributing nursing costs among the DRGs (Caterinicchio & Kinney, 1980). These studies brought about national recognition of nursing care costs as a significant factor in treatment costs. The studies produced interesting results, but further work and refinement are necessary before the relative intensity measures can be incorporated into the DRG reimbursement mechanism. Findings from the New Jersey studies demonstrated that nursing costs account for as much as 90 percent of the total average costs within certain DRGs, and an average of 60 percent of the total average costs within all DRGs (New Jersey State Department of Health, 1983). These studies, however, were not without problems in design, methodology, and empirical results.

Two methodological errors occurred in the RIMs studies. First, case-mix variables were used to group patients into meaningful categories according to consumption of nursing resources. (New Jersey State Department of Health, 1982). Therefore, patient's length of stay was the only variable found to affect nursing time significantly. Instead, variables used to group patients meaningfully according to nursing care required should be factors related to nursing diagnoses, such as immobility, incontinence, impaired skin integrity, or knowledge deficit. The absence of homogeneity within the nursing resource clusters was probably the result of attempting to link nursing intensity with medical conditions, a goal which is counterintuitive.

The second methodological problem in the RIMs studies was the per diem method of allocating nursing costs. Even though the RIMs studies set out to find an alternative to the per diem method, the total costs for each nursing resource group were divided by the average length of stay. This method of allocating costs is again counterintuitive, as evidenced by the estimated patterns of intensity for the nursing resource clusters. According to the results of the RIMs studies, intensity of nursing care rises continuously throughout the entire hospitalization. But in the system these studies used to allocate costs, patients with extremely long

Figure 1
Relationship of Nursing Intensity, Severity of Illness and Length of Stay to Hospital Costs

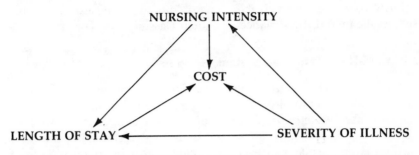

Adapted from S. Kreitzer, E. S. Loebner, and G. C. Roveti, "Severity of Illness: The DRG Missing Link?" *Quality Review Bulletin* (May 1982), 21–34.

hospitalizations would use the same nursing resources on each day of hospitalization as would the patient with an average length of stay.

Although the New Jersey studies were not without problems, they linked measures of nursing intensity with the prediction of costs within DRGs. Combining measures of either severity of illness or nursing intensity with DRGs increased the accuracy of prediction of treatment costs. Nevertheless, a sizable portion of costs remained uncaptured when using these measures separately. Therefore, using severity of illness and nursing intensity together with DRG predictors should improve the prediction of hospital costs.

The relationship between treatment costs, severity of illness, nursing intensity, and length of stay are illustrated in Figure 1. Severity of illness contributes to length of hospitalization, resource consumption, and, consequently, treatment costs that are inadequately reflected by DRGs. Severity of illness also contributes to the intensity of the nursing care required, which in turn contributes to increased length of hospitalization and cost of treatment. Treatment costs vary with the length of hospitalization, which is determined by the intensity of nursing care required and the severity of illness. Thus, any method of predicting treatment costs should reflect both severity of illness and nursing intensity.

CORRELATIONAL STUDY

This correlational study, with a sample size of 135, included all patients admitted to the critical care department of a midwestern public teaching hospital over a one-month period. Multiple-regression analysis determined the extent to which severity of illness, nursing intensity, and DRG length of stay predicted actual treatment costs. The dependent variables were length of stay and treatment costs. The independent variables were severity of illness and two measures of nursing intensity: the within-subject mean and the variance in patient classification scores.

APACHE-II Classification System

The APACHE-II severity of illness classification system, which consists of the patient's acute physiology score, age, and chronic health evaluation, was used to determine severity of illness (Knaus et al., 1984). Physiological parameters in this scoring system are determined by the values farthest from normal on 12 variables obtained during the first 24 hours following admission: temperature, heart rate, mean blood pressure, respiratory rate, arterial oxygenation, arterial pH, serum sodium and potassium, hematocrit, white blood cell count, and the Glasgow Coma Score. Points are also assigned for age. The chronic health evaluation takes into consideration whether the patient has chronic severe insufficiency of a body system, is immunocompromised, or requires emergency rather than elective surgery.

Previous studies have shown a high degree of reliability for the APACHE system because of the objective nature of the scale. Interrater reliability is reported at .96 in several studies (Knaus, Draper, & Wagner, 1983; Knaus et al., 1984; Wagner, Knaus, & Draper, 1983). Validity of the APACHE system has been established using data from 6,100 admissions to intensive care units in 15 U.S. hospitals. Severity of illness and age were significantly related to survival. APACHE allowed accurate estimates of death rates for groups of patients whose mortality at hospital discharge varied from 3 to 80 percent (Wagner, Knaus, & Draper, 1983).

Research applications of APACHE have thus far been limited to bed utilization, prediction of patient outcomes, and risk-benefit calculations concerning invasive diagnostic procedures for critical care patients.

Patient Classification System

A patient classification system (PCS) developed by the critical care department of the midwestern public teaching hospital, was used as the nursing intensity measure for this study. The measure is a weighted system consisting of 14 categories of professional nursing activities. Each nursing activity was weighted based on the amount of time usually required to perform that aspect of patient care, determined after careful study. Points were assigned to each activity by reducing the weight by a factor of 5 to allow faster and more accurate calculation (Schreiber, 1982).

The total of direct and indirect nursing care requirements for each patient constituted the nursing intensity measure. Direct care was calculated by multiplying the total number of PCS points assigned in a 24-hour period by a factor of 5. Indirect care was calculated based on the total PCS points using a regression equation (Lucke, 1984). The nursing intensity measure was collected for each day during the critical care stay. The mean and variance of nursing intensity was determined for each patient. The mean reflected the overall level of nursing intensity for the patient, and the variance reflected the variability in nursing intensity for the patient. A stable patient would have a lower variance than an unstable patient.

Reliability was initially established by education and training of all nurses in the critical care department. The initial interrater reliability for 25 patients was .98. Monthly reliability surveys over 34 months in five critical care units resulted in an average reliability of .97. Validity of the patient classification system was established by comparing the results with the actual direct and indirect care provided patients in five critical care nursing units (Lucke, 1984; Schreiber, 1982).

Variables

The response (dependent) variables were hospital length of stay (HLOS) and hospital cost of stay (HCOS) converted to base 10 logarithms (LHCOS). (The conversion of the cost data to logarithms is a standard statistical procedure for correcting two problems inherent in economic data. First, economic data tend to be skewed to the right; the logarithmic transformation renders their distributions more symmetrical. Second, effects on economic variables tend to be multiplicative; the logarithmic transformation renders them additive.) Two predictor (independent) variables were the DRG-predicted length of stay (PLOS) and the DRG-predicted cost of stay (PCOS), likewise converted to logarithms (LPCOS). Two more predictor variables were age and the APACHE score (APS). The final two predictor variables were the mean score on the patient classification system (MPCS) and its variance (VPCS), generated from the patient classification scores obtained during the patient's stay in critical care.

Data Collection

Data were collected at a 670-bed midwestern public teaching hospital. The average patient population consisted of approximately 25 percent Medicare, 25 percent Medicaid, 25 percent partial-paying, and 25 percent nonpaying patients. This hospital had converted to the prospective payment system on January 1, 1984. The five critical care units were surgical, medical, cardiac care, progressive care, and adult burn intensive care.

The principal investigator obtained data for the APACHE determination for all except burn patients within 24 hours of their admission. Data for burn patients were collected within 72 hours of their admission (Feller, Tholen, & Cornell, 1980). Determinations of nursing intensity for each patient were made by the staff nurses in each of the intensive care units three times a day. Each patient's DRG assignment was obtained from the medical records department following discharge. The length and cost of the hospital stay was obtained from the financial department.

Statistical Methods

The regression models for hospital length of stay and cost of stay were determined by the sequential testing procedure (Bock, 1975). This procedure requires that the predictor variables be arranged in order of importance and tested in ascending order, stopping at the first significant predictor. Only after the predictor variables are selected are their respective regression coefficients estimated. This procedure has three distinct advantages. First, the procedure tests the predictive contribution of new variables above and beyond that of previously established predictors—the new predictors must prove their mettle. Second, unlike many procedures for selecting variables, the statistical tests are valid and mutually independent, allowing control over the type I error rate. And third, the procedure does not capitalize on chance characteristics of the selected sample. The main disadvantage of this procedure is that the variables must be ordered. If no clear ordering is present, multiple orderings can be analyzed, but a large number of reorderings vitiates the advantages of the procedure.

The analyses were conducted with the Statistical Package for the Social Sciences using the multivariate linear model procedure MANOVA and the regression procedure NEW REGRESSION. The type I error rate for each individual statistical test was set at .01 to yield an approximate overall error rate of .05.

RESULTS

Table 1 displays the mean and standard error of the variables age, length of stay, cost of stay, APACHE score, and nursing intensity. The mean age was 55.39 years, and the mean length of stay was 12.89 days. The average cost of stay was $14,956.16. The mean APACHE score was 12.13, carrying a mortality rate of approximately 25 percent. Mean nursing intensity was 91.53, representing nearly eight hours of direct nursing

Table 1
Mean and Standard Error of Variables

Measure	Age	Hospital Length of Stay (days)	Hospital Cost of Stay	APACHE Score	Mean PCS Score
Mean of sample	55.39	12.89	$14,956.16	12.13	91.53
Standard error of sample	1.50	.80	1,508.16	.61	3.95

:are required daily. In comparison, the mean predicted length of stay from DRGs was 8.93 days and the mean predicted cost of stay was $5,906.53.

Supporting the findings of the original DRG research and the RIMs studies, a high correlation ($r = .727$) was found between length of stay and log cost of stay (see Table 2). A similar correlation ($r = .656$) was found between nursing intensity (patient classification score) and treatment costs (LHCOS). There was a somewhat lower correlation ($r = .501$) between predicted (LPCOS) and actual treatment costs (LHCOS). The correlation between length of stay (HLOS) and nursing intensity (MPCS) ($r = .470$) was higher than for actual and DRG-predicted length of stay ($r = .445$).

The first regression analysis was conducted on hospital length of stay, with the predictors arranged as predicted length of stay ($p < .0000+$), age ($p < .29$), APACHE score ($p < .13$), mean PCS score ($p < .0000+$), and variance of PCS score ($p < .052$). Thus, variance in nursing intensity was eliminated immediately as a predictor of length of stay. A second ordering, with age and APACHE score placed last and next to last, respectively, revealed that neither age ($p < .70$) nor APACHE score ($p < .32$) made significant contributions to the model, and they were likewise eliminated as predictors of length of stay. The final estimated model for length of stay was then

$$\text{Estimated hospital length of stay} = -2.30 + .82 \times \text{predicted length of stay} + .094 \times \text{mean PCS score}$$

This regression model has an R^2 of .377 ($p < .0000+$), an estimated population R^2 of .363, and an estimated expected cross-validated R^2 of .358.

The second regression analysis was conducted on log hospital cost of

Table 2
Correlations among Variables

Variable	Hospital Length of Stay	Predicted Length of Stay	Log Cost of Stay	Log Predicted Cost of Stay	APACHE Score	Mean PCS Score	Age
Hospital length of stay	1.000						
Predicted length of stay	.445	1.000					
Log cost of stay	.727	.460	1.000				
Log predicted cost of stay	.460	.870	.501	1.000			
APACHE score	.490	.760	.235	.133	1.000		
Mean PCS score	.470	.180	.656	.258	.492	1.000	
Age	.127	.122	.148	.150	.134	.144	1.000

stay with the predictors arranged as log predicted cost of stay ($p <$ .0000+), age ($p < .20$), APACHE score ($p < .0059$), mean PCS score ($p <$ .0000+), and variance of PCS score ($p < .13$). Thus, VPCS was again immediately eliminated as a predictor. A second ordering with age placed last revealed that it made no contribution to the model ($p < .73$) and was also eliminated. The final estimated model for log hospital cost of stay was then

Estimated LHCOS = 1.18 + .64 × LPCOS − .0069 × APACHE score
+ .0056 × mean PCS score

This model has an R^2 of .559 ($p < .0000+$), an estimated population R^2 of .549, and an estimated expected cross-validated R^2 of .542. To estimate actual costs, rather than their logarithms, the following equation was used:

$$\text{Estimated cost of stay} = 10^{\text{est. LHCOS}}$$

To demonstrate the improvement in prediction using our model, we chose one DRG, number 88 (chronic obstructive pulmonary disease), which had 12 subjects, and we compared actual versus predicted costs (using actual dollar amounts). Figure 2 presents the actual costs, arranged in increasing order, compared with the costs predicted by the model (estimated HCOS). Also included is the cost predicted by DRGs, which is a constant $4,134. The prediction equation could perhaps be improved, as it appears to overestimate low costs in subjects 2 through 5 and seriously underestimate the extremely high cost of subject 12. Nevertheless, as it stands, our prediction equation represents a substantial improvement over using DRGs alone in predicting costs. For these 12 patients, operating under the costs predicted by DRG 88, the hospital would have sustained a loss of $48,422, roughly $4,035 per patient. Operating under costs predicted by the equation developed from our model, the overall loss would have been $2,381, roughly $198 per patient.

Because of the small sample size within a given DRG, it was impossible to study the relationship among costs, nursing intensity, and severity of illness within individual DRGs. Since patients with the highest APACHE scores did not always have the highest cost or the greatest length of stay, it was suspected that a nonlinear relationship existed between severity of illness and treatment costs. To test this, the patients were divided into four groups by severity-of-illness score, and the relationship of scores with hospital costs was examined (see Fig. 3). A curvilinear relationship was in fact found between severity of illness and costs for the sample.

Figure 2
Comparison of Actual and Predicted Costs for DRG 88

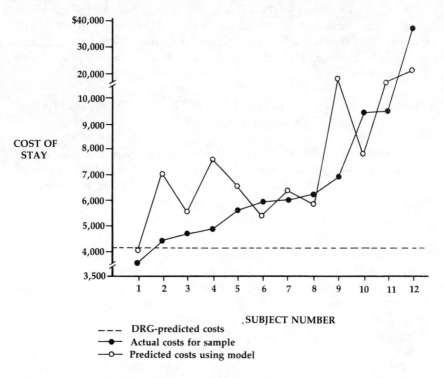

Costs increased for the first three groups of severity scores; however, costs decreased for the group with the highest severity score. Six of the nine patients in the fourth group died the first day of hospitalization, incurring average costs of only $4,000. This accounted for the nonlinear relationship between costs and severity of illness.

DISCUSSION AND CONCLUSIONS

As expected, DRG predictors were significant in predicting hospital length of stay and costs for the sample of critical care patients. Nursing intensity, however, was just as important in predicting hospital costs as were DRG factors. The inclusion of a nursing measure with DRG predictors significantly improved the prediction of length of stay and hospital costs for the sample studied.

A very high correlation existed between the nursing intensity measure used and the severity-of-illness index. In fact, there may have been some overlap in an aspect that was measured by both. This overlap was prob-

Figure 3
Relationship of Cost of Stay and Severity of Illness

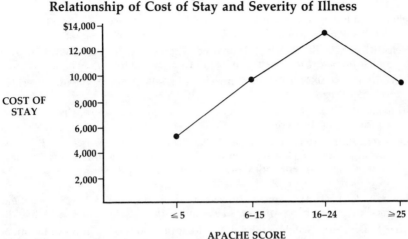

ably due to interdependent or physician-ordered nursing activities which were determined by the patient's physiological status. Other patient needs not accounted for by a severity-of-illness index may include self-care education, emotional and psychological support, and preparation of the patient and significant others for discharge. A nursing intensity measure is the only way to account for these other important aspects of health care required by hospitalized patients. Nursing intensity, therefore, improves the prediction of overall resource utilization by critical care patients over that of DRG predictors and severity of illness.

Although the findings of this exploratory study are not generalizable since all data are from one institution, the results are encouraging. The results are similar to those found in other studies using different indices of severity of illness and nursing intensity. Although a limitation of this study is the testing of the prediction equation on the sample from which it was derived, future prospective studies should test the predictive ability of models that include measures of nursing intensity and severity of illness together with DRG predictors. This and other studies clearly indicate that an improvement in the prediction of hospital costs over that based solely on DRGs can be accomplished by including measures for severity of illness and nursing intensity.

REFERENCES

Bock, R. D. (1975). Multivariate statistical methods in behavioral research. New York: McGraw-Hill.

Caterinicchio, R. P., & Kinney, J. M. (1980). *Developing a case-mix sensitive measure of resource use for the allocation of inpatient nursing costs.* Trenton: State of New Jersey Department of Health.

Feller, I., Tholen, D., & Cornell, R. G. (1980). Improvements in burn care. *Journal of the American Medical Association, 244*(18), 2074–2078.

Fuchs, R., & Scheidt, S. (1981). Improved criteria for admission to cardiac care units. *Journal of the American Medical Association, 246*(18), 2036–2041.

Grimaldi, P. L. (1981). DRG reimbursement in New Jersey: Some initial results. *Hospital Progress.*

Grimaldi, P. L., & Micheletti, J. A. (1983). *Medicare's prospective payment plan.* Chicago: Pluribus Press.

Gustafsen, P., Fryback, D. G., Rose, J. H., Prokop, C. T., Detmar, D. E., Rossmessl, J. C., et al. (1983). An evaluation of multiple trauma severity indices created by different index development strategies. *Medical Care, 21* (7), 674–691.

Halloran, E. J. (1981). Analysis of variation in nursing workload by patient medical and nursing condition. *Dissertation Abstracts International, 41,* 3385B.

Horn, S. D. (1981). Validity, reliability, and implications of an index of inpatient severity of illness. *Medical Care, 19* (3), 345–362.

Horn, S. D., Chachich, B., & Cropton, C. (1983). Measuring severity of illness. *Medical Care, 21* (7), 705–714.

Horn, S. D., & Sharkey, P. D. (1983). Measuring severity of illness to predict patient resource use within DRGs. *Inquiry, 20,* 314–321.

Horn, S. D., Sharkey, P. D., & Bertram, D. A. (1983). Measuring severity of illness: Homogenous case-mix groups. *Medical Care, 21* (1), 14–25.

Joel, L. A. (1985). DRGs and RIMS: Implications for nursing. In M. Beyers (Ed.), *Perspectives on prospective payment.* Rockville, MD: Aspen.

Knaus, W. A. (1983). The use of intensive care: New research initiatives and their implications for national health policy. *Milbank Memorial Fund Quarterly, 61* (4), 561–583.

Knaus, W. A., Draper, E. A., & Wagner, D. P. (1983). Toward quality review in intensive care: The APACHE system. *Quality Review Bulletin, 9* (7), 196–204.

Knaus, W. A., Draper, E. A., Wagner, D. P., & Zimmerman, J. E. (1984). APACHE-II: Final form and national validation results of a severity of disease classification system. *Critical Care Medicine: Proceedings of Annual Meeting, 12* (3), 213.

Kreitzer, S., Loebner, E. S., & Roveti, G. C. (1982, May). Severity of illness: The DRG missing link? *Quality Review Bulletin,* 21–34.

Lucke, K. T. (1984, July). *Patient classification system: Indirect care.* Technical report, Wishard Memorial Hospital, Indiana University Medical Center, Indianapolis.

Muller, C. (1983). Paying hospitals: How does a severity measure help? *American Journal of Public Health, 73* (1), 14–15.

New Jersey State Department of Health (1982). *Relative intensity measures (RIMs).* Trenton: State of New Jersey Department of Health.

New Jersey State Department of Health (1983). *The RIM: A new concept for nursing management.* Trenton: State of New Jersey Department of Health.

Schreiber, M. J. (1982, June). *Patient classification system.* Technical report, Wishard Memorial Hospital, Indiana University Medical Center, Indianapolis.

Schweiker, R. S., (1982, December). *Report to Congress: Hospital payment for Medicare.* Washington, D.C.: U.S. Department of Health and Human Services.

Special Committee on Aging (1983, March). *Prospects for Medicare's Hospital Insurance Trust Fund.* U.S. Senate, 98th Congress, 1st session.

Wagner, D. P., Knaus, W. A., & Draper, E. A. (1983). Statistical validity of a severity of illness measure. *American Journal of Public Health, 73* (8), 878–884.

Wagner, D. P., Wineland, T. D., & Knaus, W. A. (1983). The hidden costs of treating severely ill patients: Charges and resource consumption in an intensive care unit. *Health Care Financing Review, 1* (5), 81–86.

Determining Nursing Costs:
The Nursing Intensity Index

Janet S. Bailie

Health care costs have increased alarmingly over the last 20 years. Health care costs paid by the federal government have risen from $13.9 billion in 1965 to $99.6 billion in 1980—an increase of 716 percent. The federal government pays for more than 50 percent of the nation's bill for health care, mostly through its Medicare and Medicaid programs (Davis, 1985). Government, business, and other third-party payers are seeking new payment systems to control and even reduce current costs for health care.

The prospective reimbursement system has shifted financial reimbursement for health care from a cost-per-diem system to a fixed prospective payment system. The diagnosis related group (DRG) is assigned on the basis of the patient's principal diagnosis, secondary diagnosis, surgical procedure, age, complications, and comorbidity. The hospital's reimbursement for the care of each patient in a given DRG is the same, regardless of the patient's length of stay or the costs incurred. Therefore, hospitals will suffer losses unless costs can be maintained at or below the fixed reimbursement rate.

The author acknowledges the support of Dr. Jane H. Kordana, Director of Graduate Studies, University of South Alabama, College of Nursing and the generosity of Dr. Judy Reitz, The Johns Hopkins University, in allowing the use of the Nursing Intensity Index and providing the necessary education sessions. This research project was partially funded by Sigma Theta Tau, Zeta Gamma Chapter.

At present, the prospective payment system does not directly affect reimbursement for nursing services. Nursing care costs are included in the DRG payment, which includes all hospitalization charges. However, the effective management of patient care resources under the prospective payment system requires nursing managers to identify nursing care hours and associated costs within the DRG reimbursement system. Although nurses have demonstrated their ability to provide quality care to patients, nursing administrators increasingly are called on to quantify this care to justify departmental needs, productivity levels, and personnel expenses. Hospitals are currently reducing labor and supplies in line with decreasing numbers of patient days. However, it is difficult to cut nursing labor costs when the intensity of nursing care required per patient has increased. Typically, hospital nursing services constitute the largest single component of the hospital employees, representing nearly 50 percent of the total hospital labor budget. Moreover, nursing care continues to be the major reason for admitting patients to the hospital. Almost all other services can be provided safely on an outpatient basis. Because of the central importance of nursing in the acute-care setting, control of health care costs means control of nursing costs (Brewer, 1984; Reitz, 1985a).

In light of the new health care environment, hospitals are having to make difficult decisions about resource allocation based on the integration of financial and clinical data. To obtain an accurate picture of the utilization of nursing care resources, it is necessary to correlate DRGs, a medical classification system, with a nursing patient classification system that indicates the nursing care costs required to meet patients' health care needs. Thus, the study to be reported in this paper investigates the relationship between selected DRGs and patient classification data for determining nursing costs.

PATIENT CLASSIFICATION SYSTEMS

The nursing process must be the starting point for developing a data base for managing nursing resources for several reasons. First, the nursing role is continuous; that is, the nurse provides care 24 hours a day to the patient in the acute-care setting. Second, the patient's condition may change frequently and drastically during a hospital stay. Therefore, the intensity of nursing services, and thus nursing costs, will vary according to the patient's needs. Finally, although the nurse considers each patient unique, the study of many patients over time reveals patterns of their needs for nursing care, which can then be categorized or grouped.

One method for quantifying nursing care is a patient classification system. These systems have been developed in nursing to measure differences between patients that account for nursing workload fluctuations. Because industrial engineering time-and-motion studies have served as the primary foundation for patient classification systems in nursing, they generally have centered around the physical tasks performed on and for the patient (Giovannetti & Mayer, 1984). This approach to patient classification is currently being challenged on the grounds that patient care situations require not simple, discrete tasks, but a continuous intellectual process. The patient classification tool used in the author's study, the Nursing Intensity Index (Reitz, 1985a), uses the nursing process as the framework to quantify nursing care requirements of individual patients over the course of their hospitalization. It differs from the engineering models because it measures such important aspects of contemporary nursing practice as patient education and psychosocial interventions, based on patients' needs.

QUANTIFYING NURSING CARE

Historically, nursing administrators have had difficulty determining the true costs of nursing services in quantifiable terms. According to Higgerson and Van Slyck (1982), the major factor contributing to this difficulty is the cost-accounting methods and reimbursement formulas currently utilized by the hospitals' fiscal service departments. The hospital day has been the unit of measure, rather than the intensity of care that individual patients receive. Patients with serious health problems who receive intensive nursing care pay the same amount for a day of nursing care as patients who require less intensive care on the same nursing unit. The daily rate for room and board needs to be separated into its component parts: nursing service, room (bed and shelter), and food and dietary services.

Shaffer (1984) states that nursing power will come from making nursing the vital link between cost and quality. Nursing administrators must have an in-depth knowledge of budgeting, marketing, and financial operations to compete in the patient care marketplace. Nursing's power will be established when the itemized cost of nursing services is stated on the patient's bill. Piper (1983) has discussed the need for nursing administrators to quantify the nursing resources used within DRGs as the criterion for pricing patient care. However, few studies have been done on the relationship of DRGs and nursing services.

One such study was conducted at Stanford University Hospital to obtain information regarding nursing service costs related to DRGs (Mitchell, Miller, Welches, & Walker, 1984). A time-based patient classification system was used to determine the hours of nursing care required. Using a formula, total hours of nursing care were then translated into costs. The findings demonstrated that the DRGs studied varied considerably in use of nursing resources and did not take into account severity of illness. Therefore, the range of costs varied significantly. Several other similar descriptive studies have reported the same findings.

Sovie, Tarcinale, VanPutte, and Stunden (1985) designed and conducted a descriptive correlational study of nursing patient classification data, DRGs, and total costs of patient care. Their data represented 92.8 percent of the hospital's total patient days for one year. A patient classification tool was used to measure the relative nursing effort required in the care of a patient once every 24 hours, using four categories of nursing acuity. The average nursing intensity per patient per hospitalization was then calculated. Based on a 92 percent RN staff, direct nursing care costs were calculated to constitute only to 18 to 24 percent of the average room cost. These researchers again found that the nursing needs of patients were variable within given DRGs.

NURSING INTENSITY INDEX

Most previous studies relating DRGs and nursing costs, such as the ones just described, were conducted using task-oriented patient classification instruments. Reitz (1985b) had similar findings using a classification scheme based instead on the nursing process.

Reitz (1985a) developed and tested a generic nursing intensity measure that identified subgroups of patients who were homogeneous with respect to intensity of nursing care requirements. The Nursing Intensity Index measures the differences in patients' health problems according to their use of nursing resources. The instrument is intended to reliably indicate actual nursing care requirements of individual patients over the course of hospitalization.

The tool uses a prototype design and a four-point ordinal scale to quantify nursing care requirements of individual patients over the course of their hospitalization (see Fig. 1). The index is based on two primary dimensions of biophysical and behavioral health. These are subdivided into 11 functional health parameters, which contribute to the variable magnitude of a patient's requirement for nursing care (see Fig. 2). These functional health parameters operationalize nursing input into patient care.

This tool incorporates several important features for quantifying nursing care: The patient is the unit of analysis rather than discrete nursing interventions. The nursing process is operationalized to serve as the fundamental framework for the design of the tool. The tool measures more than discrete nursing tasks; it also measures such important aspects of nursing practice as planning for patient care, evaluation of patient care outcomes, psychosocial interaction between patient and nurse, and patient education.

The tool is applied retrospectively upon a patient's discharge, based on the medical record, rather than during every shift or 24-hour period of a patient's hospital stay. This enhances reliability, since fewer nurse raters are actually involved in the classification process (Reitz, 1985a). The 11 functional parameters are applied to the completed medical record, and an acuity level of from 1 to 4 is assigned for each category. The overall acuity score is then derived from an average of these levels.

The tool was tested by Reitz (1985c) for reliability and validity at the Johns Hopkins Hospital in all major clinical departments, representing 800 discharges, approximately 9,381 patient days. The average inter-rater agreement across all clinical departments was 84 percent, with a range of 77 percent in the Department of Medicine to 93 percent in the Department of Ophthalmology.

Reitz (1985b) found that nursing intensity, as measured by her tool, showed strong positive correlations with total hospital charges to the patient ($r = .30$), radiology charges ($r = .27$), laboratory charges ($r = 23$), and pharmacy charges ($r = .22$), at a .001 significance level. Regression analysis was used to predict the power of each of the 11 functional parameters of the Nursing Intensity Index. The emotional response parameter demonstrated the greatest power ($R^2 = .419$). The best three parameters in combination were emotional response, elimination, and circulatory function ($R^2 = .646$).

Reitz (1985b) also examined the distribution of nursing intensity within DRGs. Of the 239 cases found in the study population, 64 percent (153 cases) were classified at only one level of nursing intensity; 31 percent (74 cases) had two levels of nursing intensity; 5 percent (10 cases) had three levels; and 1 percent (3 cases) had four levels. DRGs related to mental diseases appeared to be least homogenous for nursing intensity. DRGs related to disorders of the eye were most homogenous.

DESCRIPTIVE STUDY

The current descriptive study used the Nursing Intensity Index to examine the relationship between DRGs and patient classification data for determining average nursing care hours and associated costs. This study was conducted at a 450-bed regional medical center in northwest Florida that serves a three-state area. The nursing staff mix at the hospital is 70 percent registered nurses, 25 percent licensed practical nurses, and 5 percent nursing assistants and technicians. A total patient care nursing care delivery system is practiced throughout the inpatient settings. In this system, licensed practical nurses and registered nurses

Figure 1
Nursing Intensity Index Rating Summary

Patient code no. _____ Pt. location _____ _____ F.U. _____ Nsg. unit _____

Admission date _____ Rater's name _____ Date scored _____

Discharge date _____

	Functional health parameters	Levels			
		1 Minor	2 Moderate	3 Major	4 Extreme
Biophysical health	Nutrition	mild/no deficits	impairment present/ some assistance	significant deficit/ complex plan of care	catastrophic deficits/ life-sustaining therapies
	Elimination	mild/no deficits	deficit present/some assistance, special equipment	uncompensated deficits/ complex plan of care	catastrophic deficits/life-sustaining therapies
	Sensory Function	mild/no deficits	impairment present/ some assistance	significant uncompensated deficits/complex plan of care	senses nonfunctional/ constant monitoring
	Protection	physiologic barriers intact	alteration in barriers/ noncomplex intervention	physiologic barriers significantly compromised/complex therapies	physiologic barriers nonfunctional/extraordinary intervention
	Neurological function	mild/no deficits	impairment/present noncomplex intervention	significant deficits/ complex plan of care	catastrophic deficits/ constant monitoring
	Circulatory function	mild/no deficits	impairment present/ noncomplex therapeutic intervention	significant deficits/ complex plan of care	catastrophic deficits/ constant monitoring
	Respiratory function	mild/no deficits	impairment present/ noncomplex intervention	significant deficits/ complex plan of care	catastrophic deficits/ constant monitoring

		1	2	3	4
Behavioral health	Emotional response	independent adaptation	some maladaptive behaviors/noncomplex intervention	significant maladaptive behaviors/complex plan of care	dangerous to self, others/constant observation
	Social system	intact/supportive	some disorganization present/noncomplex intervention	significantly disorganized resources/complex plan of care	nonfunctional/continuous external support required
	Cognitive response	mild/no deficits	impairment present/noncomplex intervention	significant deficits/complex plan of care	severe impairment/continuous intervention
	Health management pattern	highly adaptive health practices	inconsistent practices/noncomplex intervention	significant maladaptive health practices/complex plan of care	destructive health practices/continuous intervention

Intensity rating (circle one) _____ 1   2   3   4

Principle diagnosis _____

Time start _____ Time stop _____

DO NOT USE WITHOUT COMPLETE DESCRIPTIONS OF HEALTH PARAMETERS

Figure 2
Parameters for Nursing Intensity Index

BIOPHYSICAL FUNCTIONAL HEALTH PARAMETERS

Biophysical health	State of physiologic independence where body systems are performing to an optimal level of functioning.
Nutrition	Intake of nutrients and metabolic processes.
Elimination	Excretion of waste products from the body.
Sensory function	Use of senses to include proprioception, taste, smell, hearing, vision, and an individual's perception of pain.
Structural integrity	Protective, physiologic defense mechanisms.
Neurologic/cerebral function	Integration and direction of body regulatory processes related to reception of and response to stimuli. This includes level of consciousness as well as mental status.
Circulatory function	Supply of blood to body tissue via the cardiovascular system.
Respiratory function	Transfer of gases to meet ventilatory needs.

BEHAVIORAL FUNCTIONAL HEALTH PARAMETERS

Behavioral health	Verbal and nonverbal responses to an altered state of health.
Emotional response	Behavioral outcomes and expression of feelings based on an individual's perception of self (mind, body) as it interfaces with a change in health status. It includes the capacity for adaptive behaviors needed to maintain or regain homeostasis in response to life stressors.
Social system	Interpersonal relationships with family and community that determine the use of resources and services in the maintenance of health.
Cognitive response	Intellectual processes which enable an individual to receive, process and transmit (feedback) information and is influenced by his developmental, educational, and physiological capabilities.
Health management pattern	Motivation to manage personal health-related activities. It includes a person's perception of his own health status, and his motivation to strive for an optimal level of wellness, as demonstrated by follow through with therapeutic treatment plan.

provide all necessary nursing care to the patients. Each nurse is responsible for the assigned patients on a given shift, with a registered nurse functioning as the charge nurse on each unit during each shift.

Sample

A convenience sample of all prospective payment system Medicare patients discharged from January 1 to December 31, 1984, was utilized to determine the ten most common DRGs in the medical center. One medical DRG and two surgical DRGs with the highest volume of patients were selected from that list for the study. Psychiatric cases were excluded because this category of Medicare patients is currently exempt from the DRG method of reimbursement at the hospital. Pediatric patients were also excluded because the sample was too limited.

DRG 39, lens procedures, had the highest volume of admissions, 157 patients, with an average length of stay of 1.33 days. The government averages for this DRG were 2.80 days, with a reimbursement of $1,403. DRG 182, digestive disorders, ranked second, with an average length of stay of 6.20 days. The government averages were 5.40 days, with a reimbursement of $2,088. DRG 209, major joint procedures, was the second highest surgical category with 80 admissions. The average hospital length of stay in this category was 14.83 days versus the government average length of stay of 17.10 days and reimbursement of $7,235.

Randomization was used to obtain a proportionate sample of 20 cases per DRG category, yielding a final sample of 60 cases. The medical records of these 60 cases were reviewed retrospectively for the study.

Data Collection

Data was collected by a registered nurse with demonstrated competence in clinical nursing, experience in performing standard chart review, and expressed interest in the research subject. This nurse completed a 16-hour education program, conducted by Dr. Judy Reitz, the author of the Nursing Intensity Index.

Interrater reliability of the Nursing Intensity Index was examined by computing agreement statistics. A sample of five cases was used to compare the nursing intensity scores assigned by the principal investigator with the scores assigned by the expert panel at Johns Hopkins University. In all five cases, the Nursing Intensity Index scores were the same.

The Nursing Intensity Index was applied to all medical records in the sample to determine the patient classification per patient per hospitalization. Other data was also obtained during data collection: patient's length of stay in days, total hospital charges per patient, and total DRG

Table 1
Nursing Intensity Scores of Top Medical and Surgical DRGs

DRG	Number of Cases	Nursing Intensity			
		Mean	Median	Mode	SD
39	20	1.15	1	1	0.366
182	20	2.05	2	2	0.759
209	20	2.40	2	2	0.598

payment by the federal government. Consultation was used to develop the statistical package and analyze the data. The SAS computerized statistical software package was used for data analysis.

RESULTS

Patient classification data, DRG, and total costs of patient care were obtained for the sample of 60 patients, representing 477 patient days. Table 1 presents the measures of central tendency computed for the patient classification data for each DRG.

DRG 39, lens procedure, had the lowest mean nursing intensity—1.15 on the Nursing Intensity Index, with a standard deviation of 0.366. DRG 209, major joint procedures, had the highest mean nursing intensity, 2.4, and the second highest standard deviation, 0.598. One case out of the 20 studied in DRG 209 had a nursing intensity of 4. DRG 182, gastrointestinal disorders, had a mean nursing intensity of 2.05 and the highest standard deviation of the three DRGs studied, which was 0.759.

Data was also analyzed to determine the percentage distribution of nursing intensity within selected DRGs (see Table 2). The average nursing intensity for all patients studied was 1.866 ($SD = 0.791$), with a range of 1.0 to 4.0. Of the 60 patients in the study population, 36.67 percent were recorded at level 1 in nursing intensity, 41.6 percent at level 2, 20 percent at level 3, and 1.67 percent at level 4.

Table 2
Percentage Distribution of Nursing Intensity Scores by DRG

DRG	Number of Cases	Nursing Intensity Scores (percentage)			
		Level 1	Level 2	Level 3	Level 4
39	20	85	15	0	0
182	20	25	45	30	0
209	20	0	65	30	5

The nursing needs of patients were variable within and between DRGs studied. DRG 39, lens procedures, was the most homogeneous in terms of nursing acuity. Patients in this DRG had two levels of nursing intensity, with the majority of cases (85 percent) having level 1 nursing acuity. DRG 182, digestive disorders, had an even distribution of cases in three categories of nursing intensity, ranging from level 1 to level 3. The majority of cases in DRG 209, major joint procedures, fell into level 2 in nursing acuity.

The final examination of the data compared nursing intensity scores to hospital length of stay and use of hospital resources. Use of resources was measured by total charges to the patient and specifically charges for room and board, laboratory, radiology, and pharmacy (see Table 3). Nursing intensity showed a strong positive relationship with hospital length of stay and total charges. DRG 39, with the lowest average nursing intensity of 1.15, had average charges of $1,849, and length of stay of 1.6 days. DRG 182, with the next highest nursing intensity of 2.05, had average charges of $3,314, and length of stay of 7.8 days. DRG 209, major joint procedures, had the highest average nursing acuity, 2.4, average charges of $10,464, and average length of stay of 14.4 days. The total charges for DRG 209 were over two times greater than the reimbursement for this DRG, even though the average length of stay was three days less than the government's designated length of stay.

DISCUSSION

The major objective of this study was to determine the relationship between selected DRGs and patient classification data for determining nursing costs. Like Reitz's (1985a) study, this analysis found that nursing intensity varied widely within and between selected DRGs. Both studies found that DRG 39 was the most homogeneous for nursing intensity and total hospital charges. In two of the DRGs explored, DRG 182 and DRG 209, the level of nursing intensity level varied widely. These findings support the assumption that patients with different diagnoses require different types and quantities of nursing care. Moreover, since the per diem method of reimbursement for nursing care does not adequately reimburse the hospital for its cost in providing quality patient care, if nursing labor costs vary significantly per patient and per diagnosis, measurement of actual costs per patient is the only effective means of addressing the problem.

The average nursing intensity of this study population was 1.86, while Reitz's (1985a) study found an average of 2.00. Since both studies examined similar DRGs, these findings support the reliability of the Nursing Intensity Index as a measure of nursing intensity that can be used

Table 3
Mean and Range of Nursing Intensity Scores and Hospital Charges

Variable	DRG 39			DRG 182			DRG 209		
	Mean	Minimum	Maximum	Mean	Minimum	Maximum	Mean	Minimum	Maximum
Nursing Intensity Index	1.15	1.0	2.0	2.05	1.0	3.0	2.4	2.0	4.0
Length of stay	1.6	1.0	3.0	7.8	3.0	28.0	14.4	9.0	28.0
Charges									
Total[a]	$1,849	$1,401	$2,651	$3,314	$1,275	$10,269	$10,464	$6,452	$18,560
Room and board	270	158	507	1,260	474	2,896	2,242	1,598	3,211
Laboratory	77	31	460	494	169	1,763	509	250	978
X-ray	139	114	159	257	35	1,473	196	45	710
Pharmacy	90	56	172	579	11	2,558	1,267	850	2,123
Operating room	504	276	903	169	124	295	2,058	822	5,996

[a]Total includes additional charges other than those specified.

to calculate nursing care hours and associated costs, key factors in obtaining adequate reimbursement rates for particular diagnoses under the prospective payment system. Using this model, costs of nursing services can be established according to nursing intensity level. A system of variable billing for nursing services would promote high-quality, cost-efficient patient care by providing adequate reimbursement to support sound nursing staffing patterns; changing current cost-accounting practices to allow justification of the true costs of hospital care; and providing the appropriate level of skilled nursing services to specific patient population groups.

Lack of information on the representativeness of the sample in this study limits its generalizability. Data was collected only at one proprietary community hospital on a limited number of DRGs. Therefore, the findings of this study cannot be generalized to other settings and population groups. It is not known whether the study would produce similar results in other settings, such as an inner-city teaching hospital.

Although comparisons of this study with other reported studies are also limited because of differences in definitions, methodologies, and patient classification tools, other investigators reported similar results. For example, Mowry and Korpman (1985) reported an average nursing intensity of 1.91 (in a 4-point system) for DRG 182, and an average nursing intensity of 1.43 for DRG 39. The similarity of these results to the findings of the current study supports the notion that a generic patient classification tool can be developed that is transferrable among hospitals on a national basis.

An examination of the financial data within the selected DRGs demonstrated variability in patient charges and hospital lengths of stay. Differences in physicians' practices can affect nursing practices, resulting in differences in nursing intensity and costs of nursing care. Nurses need to determine what practices promote positive patient outcomes, and assist with standardizing patient care for specific diagnoses. Hospitals can no longer afford to employ health care professionals who perform unnecessary procedures and overutilize hospital services. The nurse's role in providing continuous care allows the nurse to monitor all patient care activities. Nursing can play a significant role in managing patients' care to achieve cost-efficient, high-quality health care (Piper, 1983).

CONCLUSIONS AND RECOMMENDATIONS

The current study has demonstrated that present cost-accounting methods for nursing services are not adequate for hospitals to obtain reimbursement for the costs of providing quality nursing care to patients.

The DRG reimbursement system does not adequately address patients' nursing care needs. The costing out of nursing services by nursing acuity levels is a means for nursing to receive adequate reimbursement for services rendered. The Nursing Intensity Index is a useful patient classification tool that can be utilized to account for the cost of nursing services per DRG.

The prospective payment reimbursement system has affected professional nursing in the roles of practice, teaching, and research. Clinical practice has been affected by an increase in patient acuity with a concurrent decrease in nursing resources. Obtaining reimbursement per patient by diagnosis and acuity level would promote quality clinical nursing practices. In the educational arena, there is an increased need for academically well-prepared nurses to handle this new health care environment. However, less money is available in hospitals for continuing education for nurses. In nursing research, much more work is needed in the areas of staff mix, delivery models, and patient care outcomes. The nursing profession is in the position to demonstrate its impact on patient care outcomes.

This study and others have demonstrated that a patient classification tool can be used to measure the costs of nursing care by patient acuity level. On a national basis, however, nursing leaders and researchers need to agree on a standard, objective method for classifying patients' nursing care requirements within the nursing profession.

The following recommendations are made as a result of this study:

1. The Nursing Intensity Index should continue to be tested in many more hospitals across the country, so that the tool can be accepted on a national basis as the standard method for quantifying patients' nursing care requirements.

2. Many specific DRGs need to be analyzed, utilizing the same patient classification tool, to better assess the homogeneity of DRGs for nursing intensity.

3. Further studies need to be done to identify the DRGs with the highest nursing intensity. Specific DRGs need to be examined to determine if particular International Classification of Diseases (ICD-9-CM) diagnoses are similar in respect to their nursing resource use.

REFERENCES

Brewer, C. (1984, January/February). Variable billing: Is it viable? *Nursing Outlook, 32*, 38–41.

Davis, R. G. (1985, Winter). Congress and the emergency of public health policy. *Health Care Management Review, 10*, 61–72.

Giovannetti, P., & Mayer, G. G. (1984, August). Building confidence in patient classification systems. *Nursing Management, 15*, 31–34.

Higgerson, N. J., & Van Slyck, A. (1982, June). Variable billing for services: New fiscal direction for nursing. *Journal of Nursing Administration, 12*, 20–27.

Mitchell, M., Miller, M., Welches, L. W., & Walker, D. D. (1984, April). Determining cost of direct nursing care by DRGs. *Nursing Management, 15*(4) 29–32.

Mowry, M. M., & Korpman R. A. (1985, July/August). Do DRG reimbursement rates reflect nursing costs? *Journal of Nursing Administration, 15*, 29–35.

Piper, L. R. (1983, November). Accounting for nursing functions in DRGs. *Nursing Management, 14*, 46–48.

Reitz, J. A. (1985a). *Development of nursing intensity index.* Technical report, The Johns Hopkins Medical Institutions, Baltimore.

Reitz, J. A. (1985b). *The Nursing Intensity Index: A valid and reliable instrument for patient classification.* Technical report, Johns Hopkins Medical Institutions, Baltimore.

Reitz, J. A. (1985c). *Reliability and validity testing of a nursing intensity index.* Technical report, Johns Hopkins Medical Institutions, Baltimore.

Shaffer, F. (1984, June). Nursing power in the DRG world. *Nursing Management, 15*, 28–30.

Sovie, M. D., Tarcinale, M. A., VanPutte, A., & Stunden, A. (1985, March). Amalgam of nursing acuity, DRGs and costs. *Nursing Management, 16*(3) 22–42. Reprinted in this volume, pp. 121–148.

Building a Base for Management of Costs: A Research Program

Lynne H. Cheatwood and Patricia A. Martin

Nursing as a profession has been cost conscious from the time of Nightingale (Woodham-Smith, 1951). With increasing formal education, particularly master's and doctoral course work in nursing management, the 1980s find hospital-based nurse leaders aware of the need for sound fiscal responsibility. Nurses who have planned change in their curricula from undergraduate programs forward cannot fail to appreciate the power of knowledge. They know that they need data to best address the increasing complexity of the forces having an impact on their areas of responsibility today. An ongoing research program at Miami Valley Hospital is attempting to provide such a base for managing nursing costs in this era of prospective payment. This program uses data from a variety of sources already available but not correlated in the present data management system.

NEED FOR NURSING DATA

Hospitals in this country now operate under the federal government's prospective payment system. This is a form of prospective reimbursement in which hospitals are paid a fixed rate that is calculated in advance and does not change for a predetermined period of time, usually a year. Under this system, a predetermined reimbursement fee is prescribed according to the resources allocated to a diagnosis related group (DRG) rather than based on the actual resources consumed for a particular patient. It is a system designed to work by a process of cost averaging;

213

that is, the user of more resources is balanced by the user of less. These resources include the nurses who provide the nursing care. It is known that nursing care may vary from patient to patient, even though their diagnoses fall within the same DRG (Cheatwood & Martin, 1985). What is not known is the pattern of nursing resource use within a DRG.

If the nurses required to provide the nursing care for a particular patient are fewer than anticipated, the hospital will have money left for other resources or for profit. If more nurses than anticipated are required to provide the nursing care, the hospital will have to use fewer resources in other areas to compensate, or the hospital will experience a decreased profit margin. Both situations interfere with efficient planning for the distribution of the resources allocated to a health care setting.

Categorizing patients by DRGs was an attempt to identify and define a product for the health care industry (Shaffer, 1983). Defining a product helps to delineate the resources needed to maintain the industry and the tasks to be accomplished to demonstrate its efficiency. The question remains as to whether or not the DRG category is an appropriate indicator of the similarity of nursing resource needs and, therefore, an appropriate criterion for planning the efficient allocation of nursing resources.

The percentage of a hospital's budget that is used for nursing care has been variously reported to be 14 to 60 percent (Davis, 1983; Staley & Luciana, 1984; Walker, 1983). According to Edwardson (1985), it is the largest single cost in any hospital's budget. Jones (1984) has stated that "nursing requirements may be a strong predictor of total resource consumption for a hospital episode" (p. 316). If these authors are accurate, then the knowledge of the precise proportion of resources used in providing needed nursing care is critical information.

This information has a special significance not only to nurses and hospital administrators but to all health care consumers as well. In 1983, the federal government established the Prospective Payment Assessment Commission (ProPAC) to recommend annually to the Department of Health and Human Services appropriate changes needed in DRG payments and the DRG classification system. ProPAC "seeks assistance from the nursing community in defining prospective payment issues relative to nursing, in determining the availability and content of data sources and in identifying nursing research currently being conducted related to prospective payment and the DRG classification system" (Young, 1984, p. 130). As Williams (1984) notes, nursing data will not guarantee success in tying nursing care needs to the DRG system, but the lack of data will seriously compromise nursing's influence on reimbursement policy.

In addition to the need for quantitative information on nursing care, there is a need for qualitative or descriptive information as well. Nursing diagnoses are descriptors of needed nursing care, just as medical diagnoses are descriptors of needed medical care. DRGs are based on medical diagnoses and therefore take into consideration the medical care of those patients. They are not based on nursing diagnoses, however, and may not take into consideration patients' nursing care needs. As Lang and Clinton (1984) point out, "It is noteworthy that no investigations assessing the quality of nursing care used nursing diagnosis to classify patients" (p. 142). They express hope that as the theoretical emphasis on nursing diagnosis increases, the empirical studies based on nursing diagnosis will also increase.

A baseline of both quantitative and qualitative measures of nursing care is needed to allow nursing to evaluate its relationship to DRGs. Questions have been raised about the consistency of nursing care required by patients categorized within a DRG. Information regarding this baseline and its consistency is needed to make efficient changes in the delivery of nursing care or the criteria used in the determination of DRGs.

MIAMI VALLEY HOSPITAL RESEARCH PROGRAM

Miami Valley Hospital is a 772-bed tax-exempt urban regional referral center located in the East North Central region for DRG reimbursement. Nursing diagnosis has been used there since the beginning of primary nursing in 1976. The hospital's active involvement in the Fifth and Sixth National Conferences on Nursing Diagnosis was a major step toward increased sophistication in the use of nursing diagnosis. Paralleling the evolution of skills in nursing diagnosis was the development of a staffing system based on actual need for nursing care. The staffing system is a computerized patient classification system which was implemented hospitalwide in 1979. Initially, it was an Ohio Hospital Management Services system, but the system has achieved additional levels of sophistication through increased sensitivity to individual patient care needs. A resident expert continually monitors and fine tunes the system to maintain its reliability and organizational effectiveness.

The Division of Nursing at Miami Valley Hospital has been cost conscious for many years. The budget is decentralized to the nursing unit level. The division has its own financial analyst, and a number of nurses within the division have attended formal and informal classes on budgeting, costing, and general health care financial management. These are some of the internal forces that served as the impetus for a research program for costing nursing care. The overall objectives for this research program are as follows:

1. To determine a methodology for identifying the cost of providing nursing care to specific groups of patients (that is, by DRG or product line).
2. To identify the influence of specific demographics (such as nursing diagnosis and age) on the nursing care hours required.
3. To describe commonalities of nursing diagnosis by specific groups.

FRAMEWORK FOR THE STUDY

Several concepts, definitions, and assumptions underlie the research program at Miami Valley Hospital. These will be reviewed briefly along with the limitations that affect the current study.

Measuring Efficiency

Efficiency is classically defined as the ratio of input to output (Alford, 1924; Riggs & Felix, 1983). Gibson (1980) defines efficiency as the amount of resource input used relative to the degree to which an organization is able to achieve its goals. Expressed another way, "efficiency refers to the ratio between resources allocated to a task and the task to be accomplished" (Kaluzny, Warner, Warren, & Zelman, 1982, p. 31). When the efficiency ratio is confined to units of production, the term used is *productivity* and the ratio is resources consumed to goods and services produced (Riggs & Felix, 1983). Edwardson (1985, p. 9) states that "productivity is a measure of efficiency," and the ratio is between labor, material, and equipment used on the one hand, and the goods and services produced on the other. Whether the term *efficiency* or *productivity* is used, the relationship of the input of any resource to the output of tasks, services, or goods is the same. Thus, the general equation or ratio used to represent efficiency is:

$$\frac{\text{Efficiency}}{\text{(Productivity)}} = \frac{\text{Output or tasks to be accomplished}}{\text{Input or resources allocated}}$$

A study of efficiency in a human service system is difficult because the traditional expectation in these systems is to be "all things to all people" (Budde, 1979). Nursing fits well into this tradition. Even though it is difficult to measure subjective factors such as human services, however, it is still critical.

In the current study, efficiency establishes the input or resource allocated as payment, which is represented by the DRG. This payment covers the hospital stay for all patients who have been determined to fall within the same DRG. The output or task to be accomplished is the nursing care provided to these patients. Nursing care can be subdivided into quantitative and qualitative measures. One quantitative measure is the total hours of nursing care provided to each patient during that patient's hospitalization and one qualitative measure is the nursing diagnoses selected and documented for each of those patients during their hospitalization. Consequently, the specific equation used to represent efficiency in this study is the following:

$$\text{Efficiency} = \frac{\text{Nursing Care} \begin{cases} \text{Quantitative (Total hours of care)} \\ \text{Qualitative (Nursing diagnoses)} \end{cases}}{\text{DRG (determinant for prospective payment)}}$$
(Productivity)

(This equation was used to produce the tables of findings in the current study showing hours of care by DRG and nursing diagnoses found in patients grouped by DRGs.)

This model depicts efficiency as a relationship between nursing care and the DRG at a given point in time. To improve the efficiency of this relationship, nursing must provide a greater amount of nursing care for the same DRG payment or provide the same amount of nursing care for a lesser DRG payment. To accomplish this task, nursing must first know how much nursing care is provided in relation to the current DRG payment.

Diagnosis Related Group (DRGs)

For this study, DRGs are defined as "a classification system of patients according to their hospital resource use" (Joel, 1983, p. 560). Much has been written about the input or resources allocated part of this model (Feldman & Goldhaber, 1984; Grimaldi, 1983; Joel, 1983; Shaffer, 1983, 1984). Because prospective payment is a national model, everything that has been written is relevant to all hospitals.

Dowling (1979) summarizes the concept of prospective rate setting in four steps:

1. An authority outside health care establishes the charges or payment rates.
2. Rates are determined in advance.
3. Patients pay the predetermined rate rather than the actual cost.

4. Hospitals absorb either the loss or the surplus.

There are currently some exceptions to the flat-fee DRG payment. Hospital capital costs and the cost of medical education are examples of items that are paid separately from and in addition to the patient's hospitalization payment (Davis, 1984). Rates are calculated separately for urban and rural hospitals. There is also a process of phased implementation over a four-year period, with the 100 percent national rate beginning in October 1986. Pediatric, psychiatric, rehabilitation, and long-term care units and hospitals are currently exempted from the DRG system.

As the resources allocated for health care become more scarce, the competition for use of those resources increases and the questions of what services will be maintained and at what level become more important. The services of nursing are carefully scrutinized because they consume such a large part of the budget and account for such a large portion of the existing positions. As Etheridge (1985) has emphasized, however, "nursing practice departments are the most important marketing source of any health care institution" (p. 39).

Nursing Care: Quantitative Measure

Nursing care hours are defined as the total number of hours of actual nursing care required by a patient during that patient's entire hospitalization. These are calculated using a computerized patient classification system. Such systems have been in the design stage for years. They are attempts to quantify specific nursing interventions and to establish categories of patients based on the nursing effort required (Alward, 1983). In the 1985 *Accreditation Manual for Hospitals*, published by the Joint Commission for the Accreditation of Hospitals, they restate their position that the "nursing department/service shall define, implement and maintain a system for determining patient requirements for nursing care on the basis of demonstrated patient needs, appropriate nursing interventions and priority for care" (p. 98). The basic premise of a patient classification system is that patient care activities can be defined behaviorally and converted to time standards (Nyberg & Wolff, 1984).

The patient classification system used at Miami Valley Hospital for this series of studies allows patient care elements to be selected from a computer screen located at the nursing station. The selection of appropriate elements of care for each patient is made every eight hours by the patient's primary nurse. Each element has a weighted time value and a designated minimum level of skill required—registered nurse (RN), licensed practical nurse (LPN), or trained attendant (TA). In addition to the time calculated for selected elements of care, there is a variable of base hours of care that is calculated per patient according to the type of unit the patient is on (critical care, advanced care, renal transplant, and so forth) and the number of hours of care calculated from the specific elements for that patient. That is, the greater the number of hours of care required by a specific patient according to selected elements, the greater the number of base hours of care. Base hours are always additional RN hours. Audits of the system are done on a regular basis to ensure a high level of reliability. The patient classification system has been in place for eight years and is reviewed, fine tuned, and updated semiannually for each unit. Staffing of the patient care units is done according to the patient classification system.

Although patient classification systems have been used for a number of years and have credibility, there are variables that differ from hospital to hospital that inhibit the transfer of a system from one institution to another, including philosophy, standards, care delivery system, skill mix, medical staff demands, physical plant and design, equipment, and supporting services (Alward, 1983). Thus, while the resources allocated for nursing care according to DRGs fit a national standard, the tasks to be accomplished are not standardized even between any two institutions. Nevertheless, as Edwardson (1985) notes, patient classification data are widely advocated as the variable for determining the cost of nursing. Herzog (1985) points out that whatever way we eventually choose to determine the cost of nursing, patient classification systems are essential.

Nursing Care: Qualitative Measure

As part of the nursing process of assessment, plan, implementation, and evaluation, nursing diagnoses are developed by analysis of the assessment data and synthesis of multiple elements to determine a patient problem that nursing can independently address. Nursing diagnosis is a qualitative measure of the tasks to be accomplished based on the nursing interventions that are suggested by the diagnosis. These have some element of standardization as a result of the work of the North American Nursing Diagnosis Association to develop an internationally standardized nomenclature of nursing diagnoses, each operationalized with an established set of signs and symptoms and probable etiologies (Kim, McFarland, & McLane, 1984). Other authors have also published books on nursing diagnosis to assist the practitioner with the articulation of patient problems and appropriate nursing interventions (Carpenito, 1983; Gordon, 1984–85).

Patient care standards at Miami Valley Hospital are written based on nursing diagnosis and state the expected care to be administered for each of those diagnoses. These standards have been written for a predominantly RN primary care nursing delivery system with the belief that this is the most efficient system. With the changes in health care and the constrained economic environment, the value of the RN is increased as the RN role becomes more flexible and able to accommodate functions once covered by specialty roles (Sovie, 1985). Curtin (1984) states that professionals' services add up to more than the sum of their tasks and the hours they spend. The manner and method in which they convey and apply knowledge is involved. The nursing diagnosis, expected patient outcomes, and plan of intervention for that diagnosis are documented on the nursing care plan. This plan is a permanent part of the patient's medical record.

A minimal number of studies have reviewed nursing diagnosis in relation to DRGs. A study by Halloran in 1980 "indicated that DRGs accounted for only 26 percent of the variance in nursing workload, while nursing diagnoses, primitive as they are in their present stage of development, accounted for 52 percent" (Jacox, 1984, p. 45). Halloran and Kiley (1984) further state that "the nursing diagnosis is among the most theoretically sound methods of describing patient problems in nursing terms" (p. 40). A study recently published by the American Nurses' Association (1985) explored the relationship between nursing diagnoses and nursing resources within specific DRGs.

Assumptions

Two basic assumptions affected the current study. The first was that the patient classification system used gave an accurate measure of the required hours of nursing care. As noted, the elements of the patient classification system are studied and updated semiannually to maintain them as accurately as possible. The second assumption was that nursing diagnoses are a qualitative measure of nursing care. Patient care standards are written based on nursing diagnoses and state the expected care to be administered for each specific nursing diagnosis. At present, these are the best measures we have to determine both the quantitative and qualitative nature of nursing care.

Limitations

One limitation imposed on the study concerns the mismatch of the patient population studied to develop DRGs and the patient population now using them. DRGs were determined using a cross section of all patients with a particular medical diagnosis. However, the patients whose stays are currently being determined and reimbursed according to DRGs are the elderly and chronically ill (Medicare) and the indigent (Medicaid). Nyberg and Wolff (1984) found that Medicare patients required 10 percent more nursing resources per day, and Presgrove (1985) found that the nursing hours required for indigent Medicaid patients increased from 5.76 hours per patient day in 1981 to 6.61 hours per patient day in 1982. Thus Miami Valley Hospital's program of study may demonstrate more nursing care hours per patient than would be found in the total population of patients with the same medical diagnosis.

Generalizability of the findings may be limited by such factors as use of only one hospital, data collection confined to short time frames (five months being the longest), and use of contrived rather than natural systems both to capture nursing care hours (patient classification system) and to describe the nursing care needed (nursing diagnosis). The studies need replication both in the same hospital at another time and in other settings with their own patient classification tools to determine generalizability.

RESEARCH PROGRAM DEVELOPMENT

As noted, the current study is based on several previous studies carried out at Miami Valley Hospital, which will be summarized here.

Maternity Study

The first study in this research program was conducted in the spring of 1983 and had as its purpose the identification of perinatal nursing costs (McNamee & Martin, 1984). A convenience sample of maternity patients and newborn infants, taken during a 30-day period, was determined by the nurse administrator to be representative for that clinical area. The acuity system was used to identify hours of direct care. These hours, multiplied by nurses' salary midpoints, yielded the direct care costs. Unit management costs were calculated per patient day to include salaries of unit clerk-receptionists and clinical nursing coordinators. Nursing administrative costs per patient day included the maternity nursing director's salary and a proportion of other administrative and support salaries. Because nursing costs were included in room charges, the costs were examined in relationship to both overall and room charges. These findings are presented in Table 1.

Nursing Diagnosis–Medical Diagnosis

A study by Martin and York (1986) reviewed 20,309 records for the relationship between nursing diagnosis and primary medical diagnosis.

Table 1
Findings of Maternity Studies

Patient Category	Percentage of Room Charge	Percentage of Total Charge
Maternity patients	47	16[a]
Female infants	54	46
Male infants	52	40
Total infants	53	43

[a]Acuity did not capture labor-delivery nursing costs.

The study was retrospective, using medical records abstracts in which nursing diagnosis and medical diagnosis were numerically represented. Pain was the most prevalent nursing problem, with 3,035 patients having this nursing diagnosis, but only 7 percent of the patients could be accounted for by the two most commonly shared medical diagnoses of spinal disc displacement (4 percent) and back pain (3 percent). The rest of the findings further supported the contention that nursing diagnoses are not well matched to any medical diagnoses.

Methodology Refocused

The authors refined the methodology for capturing direct care costs in order to be able to analyze findings within a DRG framework (Cheatwood & Martin, 1985). An ex-post-facto descriptive correlational design was used to look at all Medicare patients admitted to four similar general medical-surgical units over a two-week period. Acuity was used as the quantitative measure and nursing diagnoses as the qualitative measure of nursing care needed.

The study demonstrated satisfactory methodology, but the findings related to DRGs were very limited. In the 55 patients there were 32 different DRGs and the largest group (heart failure and shock) had only 10 patients. Two trends were identified that need further study: (1) the young old (aged 65 to 79) used less resources than the old old (aged 80 to 95), and (2) only a few nursing diagnoses were held in common within the DRG subsample.

Orthopaedic Study

Martin and Kelly (1986) examined the cost of nursing care on the orthopaedic unit. They found that immobility played a major role in increasing nursing care time. They also found that overall, orthopaedic patients' nursing care costs (direct and indirect) accounted for less than

20 percent of a patient's total charges (the range was 8.3 to 17.9 percent of total charges).

THREE MOST PREVALENT DRGs

Population and Sample

The authors' present study consisted of a convenience sample of patients whose bills were paid by Medicare or Medicaid and who were admitted with the three most prevalent diagnoses for Miami Valley Hospital. These diagnoses were DRG 127, heart failure and shock; DRG 14, specific cerebrovascular disorders except TIA (transient ischemic attack); and DRG 373, pregnancy without complications. Cases were followed to postdischarge DRG assignment, and only those cases assigned one of these three DRG numbers remained in the study. There were 33 patients in DRG 127, 31 patients in DRG 14, and 40 patients in DRG 373.

Data Collection

Medicare or Medicaid patients with initial diagnoses that would potentially be classified into one of these three DRG categories were identified on admission. Individual data sets were compiled that included the patient's DRG, age, length of stay (LOS), required RN hours, required LPN hours, required TA hours, required base hours, and required total hours of nursing care time, as calculated using the patient classification system.

In addition to this information, a record was made of the nursing diagnoses that were selected and documented by the primary nurse for each patient on that patient's nursing care plan. Nursing diagnoses are usually selected from the list in the *Classification of Nursing Diagnoses* proceedings that comes out every two years (see Kim, McFarland, & McLane, 1984) or from the *Manual of Nursing Diagnosis* by Gordon (1984–85). However, if the primary nurse feels that none of the diagnoses listed are appropriate, she is free to choose one of her own design.

Findings

The first objective of the overall program for management of nursing care costs was to determine a methodology for identifying those costs in specific groups of patients. The methodology tested in previous studies was used in the present study to determine the range, mean, and median age, length of stay, and total nursing care hours per patient within a DRG category. These findings are shown in Table 2. Although costs

Table 2
Patient Variables for Three DRGs

DRG	Age (years)	Length of Stay (days)	Total Nursing Care Hours
DRG 127—Heart failure and shock (N = 34)			
Range	57–95	3–17	24–187
Mean	77	7	65
Median	77	6	52
DRG 014—Specific cerebrovascular disorders except TIA (N = 31)			
Range	58–92	1–30	12–387
Mean	78	11	107
Median	79	10	89
DRG 373—Pregnancy without complications (N = 40)			
Range	15–36	1–4	3–27
Mean	23	2	14
Median	21	2	14

were calculated at Miami Valley Hospital, they are not reported because of the variance in salaries among institutions, and hours of care were considered the finding of more general interest.

The standard deviation of nursing care hours for DRG 127 was 25. Seventeen patients fell within one standard deviation of the mean, with nine below and eight above. However, a few patients with extensive nursing care requirements raised the mean nursing care hours well above the median. The standard deviation of nursing care hours for DRG 14 was 84. Two of the 31 patients were well above two standard deviations from the mean, while two patients were only slightly beyond one standard deviation below the mean. This accounted for the large discrepancy between mean and median nursing care hours for DRG 14. The standard deviation of nursing care hours for DRG 373 was five. Twenty-nine patients fell within one standard deviation, with six below and five above. The low variance in nursing care hours for this DRG may reflect nursing's perspective that normal pregnancy is not an illness requiring extensive nursing care, but a normal, healthy event that requires information and support.

The other objectives of the study were to describe commonalities in nursing diagnosis by patients within specific DRGs (see Tables 3, 5, and 7), and to identify the influence of the number of nursing diagnoses on the nursing care hours needed (see Tables 4, 6, and 8).

For DRG 127, heart failure and shock, the numbers of patients in each category of nursing diagnosis were small, making generalizations difficult (see Table 3). It is interesting to note that two nursing diagnoses,

Table 3
Effect of Nursing Diagnosis on Nursing Care Hours for DRG 127

Nursing Diagnosis	Number of Patients	Mean Nursing Care Hours
Potential for injury	7	63
Impaired skin integrity	7	97
Intolerance to activity	4	90
Self-care deficit	2	67
Health maintenance alteration: potential	2	46
Alteration in comfort: pain	2	51
Ineffective breathing patterns	2	71
Alteration in cardiac output	2	71
Anxiety	1	56
Home maintenance alteration: potential	1	51
Alteration in breathing patterns	1	52
Impaired physical mobility	1	176
Alteration in bowel elimination	1	176
Decreased activity	1	29
Alteration in communication	1	92
No nursing diagnosis	12	58
Total	33	65

impaired skin integrity and intolerance to activity, had much higher mean hours of nursing care than the overall mean for patients in DRG 127. The interventions for these two nursing diagnoses often require long blocks of time and may even require the services of more than one nurse. Although the number of nursing care hours increased with additional diagnoses (see Table 4), the mean number of hours of care for patients with no nursing diagnosis was 58, which is higher than for patients with one nursing diagnosis.

The total numbers of patients in DRG 14 were again too small to make any generalizations (see Tables 5 and 6). The patients with the two most commonly used nursing diagnoses (potential for injury and impaired

Table 4
Effect of Number of Nursing Diagnoses on Nursing Care Hours for DRG 127

Number of Nursing Diagnoses	Number of Patients	Range	Mean	Median
1	10	29–63	50	51
2	8	28–187	77	53
3	2	62–176	119	94
4	1	—	92	—

Table 5
Effect of Nursing Diagnosis on Nursing Care Hours for DRG 14

Nursing Diagnosis	Number of Patients	Mean Nursing Care Hours
Potential for injury	13	132
Impaired skin integrity	12	137
Alteration in communication	5	72
Alteration in bowel elimination	4	128
Impaired physical mobility	3	94
Ineffective airway clearance	3	211
Self-care deficit	3	91
Alteration in nutrition	3	92
Ineffective family coping	2	181
Alteration in tissue perfusion	2	121
Potential for hemorrhage	2	105
Alteration in cardiopulmonary tissue function	1	55
Potential for aspiration	1	387
Alteration in pattern of urinary elimination	1	150
Sleep pattern disturbance	1	41
No nursing diagnosis	3	44
Total	31	107

skin integrity) required more nursing care hours than the mean, indicating interventions of safety measures and skin care. The required number of nursing care hours increased with additional nursing diagnoses until the level of four or more. However, the influence of the few patients who used large amounts of nursing care time was again illustrated by the considerable discrepancy between the means and medians.

Patients in DRG 373, pregnancy without complications, were the most similar in terms of nursing care hours and nursing diagnosis (see Tables

Table 6
Effect of Number of Nursing Diagnoses on Nursing Care Hours for DRG 14

Number of Nursing Diagnoses	Number of Patients	Range	Mean	Median
1	8	22–118	70	76
2	15	29–348	110	89
3	3	165–387	246	197
4 or more	2	55–197	126	92

Table 7
Effect of Nursing Diagnosis on Nursing Care Hours for DRG 373

Nursing Diagnosis	Number of Patients	Mean Nursing Care Hours
Potential alteration in health maintenance	17	16
Knowledge deficit	9	15
Potential alteration in parenting	6	11
Compromised family coping	2	17
Potential for growth in family coping	1	20
Disturbance in self-concept in role performance	1	10
Teen parenting	1	10
Anxiety	1	12
No nursing diagnosis	10	13
Total	40	14

7 and 8). Numbers of patients with diagnoses of potential alteration in health maintenance and knowledge deficit were slightly above the total mean, but the number with potential alteration in parenting was well below the total mean. The postpartum units at Miami Valley Hospital have stickers with a nursing diagnosis and a choice of potential etiologies and interventions appropriate to those etiologies. Primary nurses choose the nursing diagnosis sticker and then check or write in their selection of the etiology and interventions. This may have accounted in part for some of the similarity in this DRG.

No definite patterns in relation to nursing diagnosis and nursing care hours were identified by this study. Nursing diagnoses listed were defined earlier as those selected and documented by the primary nurse. Perhaps there are reasons, other than the patient's need, for documenting or not documenting a nursing diagnosis for a patient. The expectation of the supervisor for a written care plan, the overall time available to the nurse on any given day to write on the care plan, and

Table 8
Effect of Number of Nursing Diagnoses on Nursing Care Hours for DRG 373

Number of Nursing Diagnoses	Number of Patients	Range	Mean	Median
1	21	3–27	15	14
2	5	8–20	14	14
3	4	10–20	15	15

the comfort level of the nurse in documenting nursing diagnoses are all potential influences.

An additional objective of the study was to identify the influence of age on nursing care hours. The young old (aged 65–79) and the old old (80–95) are shown with range, mean, and median nursing care hours and length of stay (see Table 9).

The range of nursing care hours for the young old was much wider than that for the old old. The two patients who were well over two standard deviations above the mean both fell in the young-old category. When those two patients were not considered, the mean nursing care hours for the young old dropped to 74 and the median to 52. None of the patients in the old-old category were so skewed in their nursing care requirements, which made the old old appear more consistent in their high use of resources. The similarity between the young old and old old in mean length of stay indicates that the number of hours of nursing care required by the old old were not inflated due to a longer hospital stay. This finding leads to the conclusion that, in general, the young old used less nursing care hours per day of stay than the old old.

FUTURE DIRECTIONS

The program of building a research base for management of costs will continue at Miami Valley Hospital over the next few years with an improved computerized data collection system. The new system will be programmed to do some of the time-consuming steps now done by hand. For example, the labor and delivery unit is trying a system in which the indicators on the acuity screen are Gordon's health care patterns, as indicated by the nursing diagnosis etiology clauses. In addition, the pa-

Table 9
Effect of Age on Nursing Care Hours and Length of Stay

Variable	Young-Old (57–79) (N = 39)	Old-Old (80–95) (N = 26)
Nursing Care Hours		
Range	12–387	32–197
Mean	89	80
Median	60	62
Length of Stay		
Range	1–30	3–17
Mean	9	8
Median	6	7

tient classification system is always being improved. It may be changed to calculate required nursing care time as an automatic by-product of computer-entered physician's orders, as well as computer-selected nursing diagnosis, etiologies, and interventions.

The next step anticipated in the research program involves the addition of bedside terminals for nurses' charting. This would allow nurses to document that the required nursing care was actually administered. It may even be possible to document the actual time spent in providing the needed care.

IMPLICATIONS

The prospective payment system has forced nursing to develop methodologies for collecting baseline data on nursing care costs per DRG. Only when we know what we currently use in nursing resources per DRG can we identify ways to reduce that cost. As stated earlier, patient classification systems and their time values are essentially unique to each institution. This requires that a large amount of data be collected nationwide in large and small, urban and rural, teaching and nonteaching hospitals in order to have a data base of sufficient size to assure confidence in the conclusions reached. Continued research on the influence of individual nursing diagnosis on the cost of nursing care is also needed. Age is currently a factor in the DRG decision tree, but research may continue to show that the young old and the old old require different amounts of nursing care for the same DRG.

Many ongoing studies are trying to capture the real cost of nursing. The one in existence the longest is New Jersey's Relative Intensity Measures (Grimaldi & Micheletti, 1982). Johns Hopkins Medical Center is developing a system called the Nursing Intensity Index (Reitz, 1985). One of these systems may work well for placing patients in a cost category that is sensitive to real variance in patient situations. Developing a workable methodology is certainly the first step.

The question remains, however, if the American public is unwilling or unable to pay for current nursing care, how do we as nurses renegotiate the care that the patient wants and is able to pay for? The nursing profession is leading the way by providing a research base for responsible decision making.

REFERENCES

Alford, L. P. (1924). *Management's handbook*. New York: Ronald Press.

Alward, R. R. (1983). Patient classification systems: The ideal vs. reality. *Journal of Nursing Administration, 13*(2), 14–19.

American Nurses' Association. (1985). DRGs and nursing care. Kansas City, MO: American Nurses' Association.

Budde, J. F. (1979). *Measuring performance in human service systems—Planning organization and control.* New York: American Management Associates Communication.

Carpenito, L. J. (1983). *Nursing diagnosis: Application to clinical practice.* Philadelphia: Lippincott.

Cheatwood, L., & Martin, P. (1985). Descriptors for nursing care under DRGs. In B. Minckley & L. Young (Eds.), *Thriving or surviving? Managing pro-active environments for nursing* (pp. 95–101). Indianapolis, IN: Midwest Alliance in Nursing.

Curtin, L. (1984). Reconciling pay with productivity (Editorial). *Nursing Management, 15*(2), 7–8.

Davis, C. K. (1983). The federal role in changing health care financing. *Nursing Economics, 1,* 98–104, 146.

Davis, C. K. (1984). The status of reimbursement policy and future projections. In C. A. Williams (Ed.), *Nursing research and policy formation. The case of prospective payment* (pp. 17–23). Kansas City: MO: American Academy of Nursing.

Dowling, W. L. (1979). Prospective rate setting: Concept and practice. *Topics in Health Care Financing, 6*(1), 15–23.

Edwardson, S. R. (1985). Measuring nursing productivity. *Nursing Economics, 3,* 9–14.

Etheridge, P. (1985). The case for billing by patient acuity. *Nursing Management, 16*(8), 38–41.

Feldman, J., & Goldhaber, F. (1984). Living with DRGs. *Journal of Nursing Administration, 14*(5), 19–22.

Gibson, C. (1980). *Managing organizational behavior.* Homewood, IL: Richard S. Irvin.

Gordon, M. (1984–85). *Manual of nursing diagnosis.* New York: McGraw-Hill.

Grimaldi, P. L. (1983). New Medicare DRG payment calculations issued. *Nursing Management, 14*(11), 19–23.

Grimaldi, P. L., & Micheletti, J. (1982). DRG reimbursement: RIMs and the cost of nursing care. *Nursing Management, 13*(12), 12–22.

Halloran, E. J., & Kiley, M. (1984). Case mix management. *Nursing Management, 15*(2). 39–45

Herzog, T. P. (1985). Productivity: Fighting the battle of the budget. *Nursing Management, 16*(1), 30–34.

Jacox, A. (1984). Prospective payment: Focus on clinical nursing research. In C. A. Williams (Ed.), *Nursing research and policy formation. The case of prospective payment* (pp. 40–55). Kansas City, MO: American Academy of Nursing.

Joel, L. (1983). DRGs: The state of the art of reimbursement for nursing services. *Nursing & Health Care, 4*(10), 560–563. Reprinted in F. A. Shaffer (Ed.), *DRGs: Changes and Challenges* (pp. 57–64). New York: National League for Nursing, 1984.

Joint Commission on Accreditation of Hospitals (1985). *Accreditation manual for hospitals.* Chicago: Joint Commission on Accreditation of Hospitals.

Jones, K. R. (1984). Severity of illness measures: Issues and options. *Nursing Economics, 2*(5), 312–317.

Kaluzny, A. D., Warner, D., Warren, S. G., & Zelman, W. N. (1982). *Management of health services.* Englewood Cliffs, NJ: Prentice-Hall.

Kim, M. J., McFarland, G., & McLane, A. M. (Eds.) (1984). *Classification of nursing diagnoses: Proceedings of the fifth national conference.* St. Louis: Mosby.

Lang, M. N., & Clinton, J. F. (1984). Assessment of quality of nursing care. In H. H. Werley & J. J. Fitzpatrick (Eds.), *Annual review of nursing research,* Vol. 2 (pp. 135–163). New York: Springer.

Martin, P. A., & Kelly, P. A. "Identifying Orthopaedic Nursing Costs." In this volume, pp. 243–258.

Martin, P. A., & York, K. (1986). Relationship among nursing diagnoses and between medical and nursing diagnoses. In M. Hurley (Ed.), *Classification of nursing diagnosis: Proceedings of the sixth national conference,* (pp. 425–437). St. Louis: Mosby.

McNamee, S. M., & Martin, P. A. (1984). Identification of prenatal nursing costs: Essential element of decision making. Abstracted in *Journal of Obstetric and Gynecologic Nursing, 13*(1), 58.

Nyberg, J., & Wolff, N. (1984). DRG panic. *Journal of Nursing Administration, 14*(4), 17–21.

Presgrove, M. (1985). Indigent patients: More nursing on less revenue. *Nursing Management, 16*(1), 47–51.

Riggs, J. L., & Felix, G. H. (1983). *Productivity by objectives.* Englewood Cliffs, NJ: Prentice-Hall.

Reitz, J. A. (1985). Toward a comprehensive nursing intensity index. Part I: Development. *Nursing Management, 16*(8), 21–30.

Shaffer, F. A. (1983). DRGs: History and overview. *Nursing & Health Care, 4*(7), 388–396. Reprinted in F. A. Shaffer (Ed.), *DRGs: Changes and challenges* (pp. 15–34). New York: National League for Nursing, 1984.

Shaffer, F. (1984). Nursing power in the DRG world. *Nursing Management, 15*(6), 28–30.

Staley, M., & Luciana, K. (1984). Eight steps to costing nursing services. *Nursing Management, 15*(10), 35–38.

Sovie, M. (1985). Managing nursing resources in a constrained economic environment. *Nursing Economics, 3*(2), 85–94.

Walker, C. (1983). The cost of nursing care in hospitals. *Journal of Nursing Administration, 13*(3), 13–18.

Williams, C. A. (Ed.) (1984). *Nursing research and policy formation: The case of prospective payment* (pp. 1–3). Kansas City, MO: American Academy of Nursing.

Woodham-Smith, C. B. (1951). *Florence Nightingale.* New York: McGraw-Hill.

Young, D. A. (1984). Prospective payment assessment commission: Mandate, structure and relationship. *Nursing Economics, 2*(5), 309–311.

Comorbidity and Length of Stay: A Case Study

Lois Grau and Chris Kovner

Since the advent of Medicaid and Medicare in 1965, health care costs in the United States have escalated. Although a range of cost-containment measures have been publicly debated in recent years, one of the most radical proposals—the Medicare prospective payment system—was quietly implemented in 1983 with little protest or comment from nursing or other health professionals.

The prospective payment system radically changed the financing of hospital care. Previous systems reimbursed hospitals retrospectively, on the basis of the costs incurred during a patient's course of hospitalization. Prospective payment, in contrast, pays hospitals a fixed fee based on the patient's discharge diagnosis, creating an incentive for earlier discharge and other ways of reducing the consumption of costly hospital resources.

The implementation of this system raises two questions. The first is concerned with the classification system itself; that is, the extent to which classification categories (diagnosis related groups, or DRGs) reflect resource consumption, and the degree to which the system is clinically relevant (Jencks, Dobson, Willis, & Feinstein, 1984). The issue for nursing is whether reimbursement rates based on DRGs accurately reflect the kind and amount of nursing care required by patients classified within the same DRG.

The second question addresses the major reason for implementation of prospective payment—hospital cost containment. The issue is whether the system is sufficiently sensitive to the complex reasons for medically unnecessary days spent in the hospital and overutilization of other hos-

233

pital resources. Clearly, the misuse and overuse of hospital services fail to make medical or economic sense; however, the factors that underlie the excessive use of costly hospital resources are complex and include, in addition to administrative inefficiencies and the voluntary overuse of expensive technology, a hospital's need to provide basic custodial and nursing care because of inadequate or inaccessible community and institutional long-term care. Limiting hospital stays to those that are medically necessary, may compromise the appropriateness of disposition decisions made by nurses and others involved in discharge planning.

This paper discusses both questions in relation to a pilot study of the length of hospital stay of Medicare patients with hip fractures. The study's purpose was to examine the relationship of comorbidity (a secondary discharge diagnosis of somatic or mental illness) to hospital length of stay among patients classified in the same DRG. The reimbursement rate for this DRG, like many others, does not take comorbidity into account for patients over the age of 69 in its reimbursement rate. This study tests the assumption of the prospective payment system that, after a certain age, comorbidity is not a significant predictor of hospital resource consumption. This assumption suggests that patients with comorbid conditions are no different than others with respect to need for nursing care and other hospital services.

BACKGROUND OF THE PROBLEM

On October 1, 1983, hospitals in all but four states (New York, New Jersey, Maryland, and Massachusetts) began receiving reimbursement for Medicare-covered hospital costs through the Medicare prospective payment system. Rates are paid on a per discharge basis, the amount of payment being determined by which of 468 DRGs the discharge is assigned to. Discharges are assigned a diagnostic group based on data abstracted from the inpatient record, including age, sex, principal diagnosis, up to four complications or comorbidities, and surgical procedures performed.

Although the specifics of the reimbursement system are complex, payment is basically the product of a dollar rate and the weight assigned to the particular DRG. The dollar rate represents a combination of the hospital's historic costs and the federal/regional rate. Special adjustments in the dollar rate are made for cancer hospitals, regional referring hospitals, teaching hospitals, and sole community hospitals. The DRG weight is an index representing the relative resource use for inpatient services. For example, the weight for open heart surgery is substantially higher than the weight for hernia surgery.

The purpose of the prospective payment system is to create economic incentives to reduce hospital resource consumption and length of stay. Cases that are outliers with respect to cost or length of stay (1.94 standard deviations from the mean or 20 days greater than the mean) are reimbursed at 60 percent of the hospital's per diem rate after outlier status is attained. On the other hand, cases that have less than average costs or lengths of stay create surpluses for the hospital.

As a practical matter, discharge cases are first classified into one of 23 major diagnostic categories based on body systems. Cases are then classified into one of the 468 DRGs. Some DRGs use only the primary discharge and age as inclusion criteria; others, however, include age, comorbidity, and type of treatment. For example, hip fracture is represented by three DRGs, each of which pays the hospital a different rate. If a hip fracture patient does not have a surgical procedure, the case is put into DRG 236, regardless of the patient's age. If the patient has surgery, is 69 or under, and has no complications or comorbidity, the case is placed into DRG 211. If the patient has surgery but is age 65 or over and has a coexisting condition or complications, or if the patient is simply over 69, the case is placed into DRG 210 (American Medical Association, 1984). Thus, a 70-year-old with no complications is in the same DRG as an 83-year-old with comorbidity and complications. These criteria reflect a number of assumptions; first, that surgical treatment requires additional hospital resources, regardless of the patient's age; and second, that comorbidity, in contrast, requires additional hospital resources only for patients who fall between the ages of 65 and 69. Presumably, after the age of 69 the presence or absence of one or more comorbid conditions has no effect on the consumption of hospital resources.

Proponents of the prospective payment system argue that as a result of the law of large numbers, overall consumption of resources within a DRG will average out—costly cases will be canceled out by those that result in surpluses for the hospital. Others suggest that the system lacks clinical relevance because its case-mix classification scheme is insufficiently sensitive to severity of illness and comorbidity (Horn, Horn, & Sharkey, 1984; Rieder & Kay, 1985; Smits, Fetter, & McMahon, 1984; Young, 1984). Some have expressed concern that particular groups of patients, such as the mentally ill with medical problems, may be jeopardized under the prospective payment system (Office of Technology Assessment, 1985) because it fails to adequately predict resource consumption and resulting hospital costs. It has also been suggested that some hospitals, particularly in urban areas, get a disproportionate share of sicker patients within a particular DRG.

An additional concern has been the omission of nursing time needed for patient care as a factor in estimating the relative weights of DRGs

(Halloran & Halloran, 1985; McKibbin, Brimmer, Clinton, Galliher, & Hartley, 1985; Smits, Fetter, & McMahon, 1984). The failure to monitor and project intensity of nursing care results in exclusion of from 20 percent to 30 percent of the costs of care from hospitals' cost-control models (Thompson, 1984).

A final concern is that sicker patients will be prematurely discharged from hospitals in an effort to decrease resource consumption and hospital expenditures. Thus, home health care agencies may be overtaxed by the increasing acuity of clients' conditions. It is also likely that families will be confronted with the need to pay for or to themselves provide needed personal care and related services that are not covered by Medicare.

STUDY OF LENGTH OF STAY

Because of the concerns over the accuracy and the effects of prospective payment, it is important to examine the similarities and differences among patients that influence their consumption of hospital resources. A relatively accurate and widely accepted indicator of hospital resource consumption is a patient's length of stay in the hospital, the variable of interest in the present study. To measure the influence of patient characteristics such as comorbidity on length of hospital stay, however, it is necessary to eliminate the potentially intervening effects of the economic incentives inherent in the prospective payment system. This was accomplished by selecting a research site in New York State prior to the state's mandated implementation of the prospective payment system in January 1986.

Retrospective analysis of hospital discharge records was undertaken to explore the relationship of somatic and mental comorbidity to hospital length of stay among Medicare patients with hip fractures. Hip fracture was chosen because it is a common problem among the elderly and one in which the primary medical intervention—surgery—is relatively clear-cut. The outcome of treatment is subject to the influence of the individual patient's health status prior to the fracture, however, suggesting that comorbidity might also influence length of hospital stay.

The study sample consisted of all cases of hip fracture admitted to a major medical center during 1983 and 1984 that met the following criteria: (1) the patient received surgical treatment of the fracture; and (2) the patient was age 65 to 69 with comorbidity or complications, or was older than 69, regardless of the presence or number of comorbid conditions. These criteria are identical to those for DRG 210, allowing comparison of actual consumption of hospital resources with those allotted for this particular DRG under the prospective payment system.

The final sample consisted of 225 patients—176 women (78 percent) and 49 men (22 percent)—who met these criteria. The average age of both male and female sample members was 80, and the average length of hospital stay for the entire sample was 42 days (the median was 29 days). Of these patients, 116 (52 percent of the sample) had no comorbidity, as evidenced by a lack of any secondary discharge diagnosis; 89 sample members (40 percent) had one or more secondary discharge diagnoses of a somatic disorder; and 20 sample members (9 percent) had a secondary discharge diagnosis of some type of mental disorder. These three groups did not differ significantly in age or sex.

Data were analyzed using descriptive statistics and multiple regression techniques. The regression equation included age, comorbidity and discharge disposition as independent variables. Comorbidity and discharge disposition were constructed as dummy variables (physical comorbidity, mental comorbidity, or no comorbidity; and death or discharge to home, to home care, or to a nursing home).

FINDINGS

Both discharge to nursing home and presence of somatic comorbidity were significantly related to log length of stay ($p < .001$). The relationship of mental comorbidity to log length of stay approached significance ($p = .067$) (see Table 1). (Log length of stay is used to reduce skewness of the distribution).

Length of stay for patients in this study varied widely, with a range of 2 to 465 days. Patients with somatic comorbidity remained in the hospital the longest—an average of 54 days. This was followed by patients with mental comorbidity, whose average length of stay was 49 days. Patients with neither somatic nor mental comorbidity had the short-

Table 1
Relationship of Comorbidity to LogLength of Stay

Independent Variables	LogLength of Stay[a]		
	b	Beta	Significance
Logage	0.91144	0.109866	.0964
Discharge to home care	0.38116	0.26632	.0938
Discharge to nursing home	0.87580	0.49072	.0002
Discharge to home	0.38633	0.25727	.0914
Mental comorbidity	0.29431	0.11832	.0677
Physical comorbidity	0.32338	0.22338	.0007

[a]Constant = -1.15142; adjusted R^2 = .14620; overall F = 7.39283.

Table 2
Coexisting Disorders and Discharge Disposition

Coexisting Disorders	Discharge Disposition[a]									
	Home		Home Care		Nursing Home		Death		Total	
	N	%	N	%	N	%	N	%	N	%
Mental disorder	7	3.1	10	4.4	1	.4	2	.9	20	8.9
Somatic disorder	28	12.4	32	14.2	23	10.2	6	2.7	89	39.5
No disorder	40	17.8	54	24.0	20	8.9	2	.9	116	51.6
Total	75	33.3	96	42.6	44	19.5	10	4.5	225	100.0

[a]Chi-square = 10.41878; df = 6; p = .1081.

est average hospital stay—32 days. These data are in sharp contrast with the national mean length of stay for DRG 210 of 20.6 days (Grimaldi & Micheletti, 1985). Although this finding is of concern because of its radical deviation from national norms, it is consistent with the tendency of patients hospitalized in medical centers to experience longer stays than their counterparts in community hospitals.

Cases discharged to nursing homes had by far the longest length of stay—an average of 72 days. The average lengths of stay for patients discharged home either with home care or without home care were the same—34 days. The ten individuals who died during the course of hospitalization had an average stay of 48 days.

The four discharge disposition groups did not differ significantly in sex or age, nor was there any significant association between discharge disposition and presence of somatic or mental comorbidity (see Table 2). Hence, it would appear that comorbidity and discharge disposition were independently related to hospital length of stay.

DISCUSSION

The findings of this exploratory study suggest that comorbidity, particularly secondary somatic illnesses, are significantly related to hospital length of stay. Investigation of only one DRG in a single hospital can, of course, only suggest the problem. The findings do, however, conform with those of other, larger studies. For example, a study of 32,000 Medicare patient discharges found severity of illness and comorbidity to be more important than age in explaining treatment costs (Conklin, Lieberman, Barnes, & Louis, 1984). Use of Horn's severity-of-illness index significantly reduces variance in hospital resource consumption (Horn, Horn, & Sharkey, 1984).

Accuracy of DRGs

These and related investigations represent a new generation of case-mix classification studies that address the first question raised at the outset of this paper: whether the DRG case-mix system is clinically relevant and accurately reflects resource consumption. However, only a relatively small number of studies consider nursing care as a variable in case-mix determination. In one such study, the New Jersey State Department of Health (1983) attempted to link the intensity of nursing services to DRGs through the development of the relative intensity measures (RIM) classification scheme. The importance of this problem is suggested by the work of Berki, Ashcraft, and Newbranger (1984) in which a proxy of nursing intensity was found to be significant in explaining intra-DRG variation, and by the recent findings of Halloran and Halloran (1985) that nursing diagnoses better explained variability in nursing care than did selected DRG inclusion criteria. In addition, Arndt and Skydell (1985) found wide variation in the nursing care requirements of patients within several DRGs. However, as noted by Thompson (1984), such studies tend to focus only on the volume of nursing care, ignoring the level of skill involved.

Furthermore, the DRG classification system fails to include the dementias, the most common mental disorder of the elderly, as acceptable comorbid conditions. This omission raises questions in light of findings that associate dementia with outlier length of hospital stay (Meiners & Coffey, 1985) and the need for additional nursing care (Halloran & Halloran, 1985). The present study did not find coexisting mental disorder to have a significant association with hospital length of stay; however, this may be the result of the relatively small number of cases that fell into this group. Moreover, a review of 50 hospital charts randomly drawn from the sample of cases with no secondary discharge diagnoses revealed that 50 percent contained data which indicated the presence of mental disorder. Within this subsample there was a significant difference in hospital length of stay between patients with coexisting mental disorder and patients who gave no indications of somatic or mental comorbidity. This finding suggests that mental comorbidity may be underreported in discharge medical records.

The limitations of the present study precluded measurement of nursing time and intensity; but other studies as well as clinical experience point to the impact coexisting conditions have on the need for nursing care. For example, Halloran and Halloran (1985) found that a patient's mental status was a significant predictor of nursing workload. The memory loss and confusion associated with dementia reduce the patients' self-care abilities, thus increasing dependence on the nursing staff. Somatic comorbid conditions, such as diabetes and cerebral vascular disease, require additional nursing time in and of themselves, and they may also retard recovery or necessitate more intensive restorative care.

Unnecessary Hospital Days

The strong positive relationship found between discharge to a nursing home and hospital length of stay carries implications for the second question posed earlier; that is, whether the prospective payment system reflects the factors that account for medically unnecessary or questionable hospital days. In the present study, discharge to a nursing home was not significantly related to comorbidity, age, or sex. The lack of relationship to these risk factors for nursing home placement may be a function of the underreporting of coexisting mental disorder, as previously discussed, or of the problem of "hospital backup," in which patients are retained because of difficulty in implementing appropriate discharge plans. Barriers to discharge may include the reluctance of nursing homes to accept Medicaid patients, those who require intensive nursing care, or those who exhibit behavioral problems as a consequence of dementia or psychiatric disorders. Although patients who are retained in the hospital for these reasons may not require the intensive medical resources of the hospital, they do require ongoing nursing care. Moreover, this care necessarily includes the thought and time involved in planning for discharge disposition and preparing the patient for it. Nurses may become caught between the economic imperative of the hospital to discharge the patient quickly, regardless of the appropriateness of the disposition, and their professional imperative to ensure that the discharge plan is in the best interests of the patient and his or her family.

The availability of and access to home health care services also influences hospital utilization. Adequate and affordable services make early discharges possible and, in many cases, desirable, while inaccessible or limited community services lead to unnecessary human suffering and increase the likelihood of rehospitalization or nursing home placement.

Medicare, the major health benefit program for the elderly, expends less than 2 percent of its total annual revenues on home health care services (House Select Committee on Aging, 1985) and continues to limit these services to individuals who are "homebound" and require "intermittent skilled nursing care." Similarly, Medicaid spent roughly $500 million on home care in 1984, about 1 percent of its total budget. Medicaid mandates only intermittent skilled nursing and home health aide coverage for the categorically needy. Presumably, as hospital stays shorten, the demand for home care will continue to exceed the resources of the Medicaid and Medicare programs.

Home health care agencies are currently reporting an increase in the acuity of their client populations as a result of earlier hospital discharges. As a result, these agencies must provide more intensive and skilled nursing care, taxing their resources under current reimbursement levels. This is occuring at a time when community nursing has made strides in implementing programs to address the long-term care needs of elderly patients. Earlier discharges from the hospital will not reduce the need for long-term community nursing care, but will add to it the need to care for acutely ill elderly patients who, in the future, may also require long-term nursing and other home care services.

IMPACT OF PROSPECTIVE PAYMENT

The economic and human costs of the prospective payment system for the elderly who rely on federal programs for basic subsistence and health care has yet to be determined. This study found wide variations in the length of hospital stay of patients treated for hip fracture at one medical center; this variation is explained in part by comorbidity and discharge disposition. If these patients were to be hospitalized under prospective payment, this variation would presumably be reduced in the direction of shorter hospital stays, with unknown consequences for discharge disposition and subsequent health outcomes.

The impact of prospective payment on nursing will be felt both in the hospital and in the community. Whether hospitals will attempt to contain costs by reducing expenditures on nursing care is not yet known. However, the potential for such cuts is large and can only be reduced by demonstrating the need for and impact of nursing care for different categories of patients. Community nursing is likely to experience increased demand for services, particularly for care of acutely ill patients. This demand, coupled with the ongoing need for long-term community care, may strain the economic resources of agencies, which may find it necessary to expand recruitment and training efforts to meet new demands for service.

The problem of hospital cost containment requires consideration of the community context in which hospitals exist and, in particular, the need for and sources of nursing care. When cost-containment efforts are directed at the elderly, as is the case with prospective payment, medical care is only a part of the issue. The many physical and psychosocial needs of elderly patients require comprehensive attention from nurses and other health care providers who are attuned to the need for coordinated care within the hospital and after discharge.

REFERENCES

American Medical Association (1984). *DRG's and the prospective payment system: A guide for physicians.* Chicago: American Medical Association.

Arndt, M., & Skydell, B. (1985). Inpatient nursing services: Productivity and cost. In F. A. Shaffer (Ed.), *Costing out nursing care: Pricing our product* (pp. 135–153). New York: National League for Nursing.

Berki, S. E., Ashcraft, L. F., & Newbranger, W. C. (1984). Length of stay variations within ICDA-8 diagnosis related groups. *Medical Care, 22,* 126–142.

Conklin, J., Lieberman, J., Barnes, C., & Louis, D. (1984). Disease staging: Implications for hospital reimbursement and management. *Health Care Financing Review,* annual supplement, 13–22.

Grimaldi, P., & Micheletti, J. (1985). *Prospective payment: The definitive guide to reimbursement.* Chicago: Pluribus Press.

Halloran, E., & Halloran, D. (1985). Exploring the DRG/nursing equation. *American Journal of Nursing, 85,* 1093–1095.

Horn, S. D., Horn, R. A., & Sharkey, P. D. (1984). The severity of illness index as a severity adjustment to diagnosis-related groups. *Health Care Financing Review,* annual supplement, 33–45.

House Select Committee on Aging, U.S. Congress (1985). *Building a long term care policy: Home care data and implications.* Washington, D.C.: U.S. Government Printing Office.

Jencks, S. S., Dobson, A., Willis, P., & Feinstein, P. H. (1984). Evaluating and improving the measurement of hospital case mix. *Health Care Financing Review,* annual supplement, 1–12.

McKibbin, R., Brimmer, P., Clinton, J., Galliher, J., & Hartley, S. (1985). *DRG's and nursing care.* Kansas City, MO: American Nurses' Association.

Meiners, M., & Coffey, R. (1985). Hospital DRG's and the need for long term care services: An empirical analysis. *Health Services Research, 20,* 360–384.

New Jersey State Department of Health (1983, August). *A prospective reimbursement system based on patient case mix for New Jersey Hospitals, 1976–1983: The "RIM"—A new concept for nursing management.* Trenton: State of New Jersey Department of Health.

Office of Technology Assessment (1985). *Medicare's prospective payment system: Strategies for evaluating cost, quality, and medical technology.* Washington, D.C.: U. S. Congress.

Rieder, K. A., & Kay, T. L. (1985). Severity of illness within DRGs using a nursing patient classification system. In F. A. Shaffer (Ed.), *Costing out nursing care: Pricing our product* (pp. 85–99). New York: National League for Nursing.

Smits, H. L., Fetter, R. B., & McMahon, L. F., Jr. (1984). Variations in resource use within diagnostic related groups: The severity issue. *Health Care Financing Review,* annual supplement, 71–78.

Thompson, J. (1984). The measurement of nursing intensity. *Health Care Financing Review,* annual supplement, 47–56.

Young, W. (1984). Incorporating severity of illness and comorbidity in case management. *Health Care Financing Review,* annual supplement, 23–31.

Identifying Orthopaedic Nursing Costs

Patricia A. Martin and Patricia A. Kelly

Given the current mood of both consumers and regulators, health care costs are nearing the acceptable ceiling. In 1983, the nation's expenditure for health care reached $354.5 billion, roughly 10.7 percent of the gross national product. This represented a 10 percent increase over the previous year, while the inflation rate over that same time period was less than 4 percent (American Nurses' Association, 1985). Experts forecast that health care expenditures could reach $1 trillion per year by 1992 unless drastic measures are initiated to control these costs (Curtin & Zurlage, 1984).

In none of the various industries in the United States that are undergoing dramatic change have factors such as deregulation, competition, new technology, and new payment systems come together as rapidly as in the hospital industry. In a short period of time, several major changes have had their impact on health care: the prospective payment system, under which hospitals are reimbursed a predetermined amount per patient diagnosis instead of retrospective payment for reasonable charges; new types of competitors, such as free-standing outpatient surgery centers, health maintenance organizations, and preferred provider organizations; and deregulation of the construction of new hospitals and outpatient facilities. These changes come amid declines in hospital use and increases in the costs of labor and supplies.

In this new fiscal environment, it is the low-cost provider who will survive the competition. For many health care institutions, cost containment has taken the form of decreasing the number of employees, particularly those devoted to the provision of care. For example Humana, Inc., the investor-owned corporation of about 200 hospitals, has decided to concentrate on reducing costs by decreasing staff. Humana hospitals averaged only 2.7 or 2.8 employees per bed in 1983, compared to 3.3 in hospitals nationwide (Coddington, Palmquist, & Trollinger, 1985). The question arising from the ranks of nursing is, How can health care workers be eliminated without compromising the quality of care?

The time is right for the nursing profession to identify its value to health care delivery. In the past nurses have stated that nursing care affects patient outcomes, but they have not specified that impact in measurable, financial terms. Nursing must justify its contribution to the margin between price (DRG allocation) and cost (required nursing hours) (Reschak & Holm, 1985). Nursing must know what care is currently provided and at what cost as a baseline in order to explore how the same or better care can be delivered more efficiently. Protocols, plus analysis of patient outcomes, may eliminate some of the sacred cows of care delivery while preventing change for the sake of change alone. Although nursing has a reputation for being reactive, the profession must now act quickly and responsibly, before the system acts for it.

The development of measurements that are rational for nursing (such as hours of nursing care rather than simply length of stay), the identification of more specific cost allocations, and the refinement of clinical delineations to include the patient's nursing care needs can finally give nursing the opportunity to go beyond mere words to demonstrate the significant financial results of nursing care.

Because of this change in focus, the nursing administrator of today must choose to be "consciously competent"—that is, responsive to three audiences: the consumer, the nurse, and the government (Veninga, 1982). These three audiences have spoken: the consumer has said, "lower the rate of cost increase in health care;" nurses have urged, "maintain the quality of patient care;" and the government through legislation has demanded, "become more cost-conscious and efficient." These values are qualitative in nature. In order to respond to them, the nursing administrator needs quantitative as well as qualitative data to form a baseline from which to make management decisions. Quantitative data are needed to lessen uncertainty, to plan for changes, and to provide a baseline for evaluation of those changes.

Historically, budgeting and subsequently staffing have been carried out using the archaic method of predicting patient days and the nursing care required. Under this system, assessment and individualized care by a nursing staff are frequently viewed as too costly. This method does not take into consideration the influence on the cost of nursing care of fluctuating acuity or the individual nature of desired patient outcomes. Until recently, few cost-accounting and reimbursement procedures have involved serious efforts to identify nursing care requirements using a patient classification system. Under the prospective payment reimbursement system, the patient's medical diagnosis, medical complications, and age determine the parameters for length of stay and resources available for hospital care. Absent from these determinations are considerations of the intensity and kinds of nursing care each condition may require throughout the hospitalization (Curtin, 1985).

Hospitals are labor-intensive service organizations, and nursing is the most labor-intensive component of the hospital. The percentage of a hospital budget that is allocated for nursing care is reported, depending on the author, to be anywhere from 14 to 21 percent (Walker, 1983) to 30 to 60 percent (Davis, 1983). This makes the nurse executive responsible for the largest cost center within the hospital. The prospective payment system has forced nurse executives to develop methodologies for collecting data on nursing care costs per diagnosis related group (DRG). Only when we know what we currently use in nursing resources per DRG can we identify ways to reduce that cost.

The nurse executive needs accurate cost analysis data to make the economically wise decisions that ensure a balance between cost containment and the delivery of safe, quality nursing care. Both qualitative and quantitative data, describing a valid baseline, plus periodic reassessment are necessary for progressive management. The data provided can answer two relevant questions: What is the cost of the program that the professionals prescribe for quality care? How much of the price tag belongs to nursing? With data of this nature, health care providers and planners can begin to determine the answers to the ethical and economic questions asked so often today: Who is entitled to health care? How much care can be provided within the budget that the consumer is able and willing to allocate for health care? How can the views of the consumer and professional be reconciled?

The new federal regulations will not affect direct reimbursement for nursing services at present, but there is considerable evidence that hospital nursing departments will be required to justify the cost for nursing services according to the patient's acuity, which, in turn, must correlate with the patient's DRG. The costing out of nursing services is generally viewed as advantageous for the profession and as a means for nursing eventually to receive its fair share of the health care dollar.

CONCEPTUAL FRAMEWORK

The conceptual framework for the study presented in this paper is Arndt and Huckabay's (1980) view of the health care organization as a structural sociotechnical system. The composite administrative process is one of five subsystems, with its main concern being overall administration. In the past nursing has mainly been concerned with the technical level of administration—the delivery of direct patient care. Recently, the realm of most nursing administrators has expanded to the organizational level, where coordination of technical care takes place. The nursing administrator of today is more involved in the institutional level of administration, which puts the nursing administrator in a position for continuous interaction with the external environment. The responsibility of actively confronting an ever-changing external environment mandates that the nursing administrator seek relevant measurements of both the process and outcomes of the system in order to build a firm base for decision making. The study to be described is a response to the nursing administrator's need for additional organizational "vital signs" in order to be responsive to the previously described environment of rapidly expanding technology, tightening economic times, and very vocal audiences.

Beyond specific research findings, the actual involvement of the nursing department in research sets the stage for change. The facilitator of change must be viewed as knowledgeable by those to be influenced. Research activities help to highlight the nursing administrator's knowledge and build credibility during the process of expanding that knowledge. The nursing administrator can use a research approach to establish the flow of objective data needed for decision making. In small organizations, the research role may be only one facet of the administrator's job. In a larger organization with a staff of nurse researchers, the administrator must still participate actively in the process. It is the administrator who can identify the validity of the questions and the meaningfulness of the methodology. The conceptual clarity that accompanies the development of a well-thought out study builds the administrative researcher's knowledge base about the content area long before the findings are completed. Ultimately, the findings provide the proof necessary to make people more receptive to the changes decided on by the nursing administrator.

The traditional view of hospital nursing services limits the effective execution of the responsibility to be proactive in our increasingly demanding environment. The descriptive study being reported here was conducted to enhance the understanding of the nursing costs currently hidden by traditional accounting practices. Nursing has long been viewed as a drain on the hospital economy, while auxiliary services are seen as contributing to revenue. With payment by case or product line, this study enables the nurse administrator of the orthopaedic area to identify a baseline of nursing costs against which proposed efficiency standards can be targeted and strategies evaluated. This study identifies possible benchmarks and verifies methodology for future studies as everyone examines the high cost of hospital care.

DATA SOURCES

The site for the study was Miami Valley Hospital, a 772-bed, tax-exempt, urban regional referral center located in Dayton, Ohio (East North Central region for DRG reimbursement). At this hospital, the nurse administrators receive a monthly statement from the Financial Department containing responsibility costs by nursing unit, nursing department, and Division of Nursing. These data provide a global approach to costs but do not reflect the cost per type of patient (that is, case mix). A system to be implemented by 1986 should merge some of these separate systems.

The monthly statement gives cost figures for resources used divided into categories such as salaries, supplies, services, and the like. Each of these reported categories are moderately specific. Salaries are listed by employee and by job classification. They are separated into the amount allocated for work time and paid time off (vacation, sick leave, and so forth). The report also provides as comparison figures the previous year's expenses and the budgeted expenses. The only output data available on the report are patient days for the reporting period. These figures are generated by the Finance Department but at present cannot be matched with data from accounts payable about revenue generated, data from medical records about medical conditions treated, or data from nursing about intensity of care utilized. Nursing care costs are included in the room charge on patients' bills. Thus, nursing care costs are recovered based on the length of stay and are not differentiated according to the different levels of care delivered within a nursing unit.

The hospital has a factor-based patient classification system, which determines the hours of nursing care required from each job classification to meet patients' needs. In this system, patients are rated by specific elements of care, such as general pulmonary care or complex intravenous therapy. This differs from prototype systems, which rate the patient on an ordinal scale by level of care required, such as self-care or moderate care. Data is entered into the computer system on each shift by the unit-based primary nurse, who identifies each patient's nursing care requirements. At present, these data are used for staffing purposes only. The unit's total nursing care hours include the hours for each job classification—registered nurse (RN), licensed practical nurse (LPN), and trained attendant (TA). The number of personnel needed is computed on each shift.

Although the present system has been available since 1978, it will be some time yet before a new system is available that will marry acuity, care planning, and the budget. In the meantime, several nursing studies have been completed and others are in process to both increase the nursing administrator's awareness of selected comparisons of acuity and patient groupings and to expand the administrator's awareness of the possibilities for data and data analysis to support decision making. (Cheatwood & Martin, 1986).

DATA COLLECTION

The target of analysis in this study was the two orthopaedic units. Patient acuity data were obtained from a computer printout. The current computer system does not calculate total nursing care time per patient for more than an eight-hour time span. The printout for each shift lists the amount of RN, LPN, and TA time required for each patient in hours or partial hours. The total amount of nursing time a patient required was obtained by totaling all the printouts from each shift for the patient's entire length of stay.

The population involved in this study consisted of all patients admitted on two orthopaedic units between May 12 and May 25, 1985, who spent their entire hospitalization on these units and who were discharged by May 31. The sample size was 44. In addition to acuity, the demographic data of age, sex, admitting diagnoses, and total charges were also collected. Demographic data on each new patient and patient acuity were collected concurrently on a daily basis. The total charges for each patient were obtained from the Department of Patient Accounts after discharge. Data collection took approximately 30 hours over a three-week span.

DATA ANALYSIS

Both direct and indirect nursing care costs were calculated for the study. Direct nursing costs (variable costs) are monetary values attached to the activities involved in the provision of nursing care to an individual patient. These costs vary and are directly proportional to a patient's level of need, which defines the caregiver (RN, LPN, or TA) and amount of time needed for care. Nursing activities include all aspects of the nursing process performed by unit personnel, regardless of job classification. A financial analyst computed the salary expense figures to preserve confidentiality. One option for calculating hourly salary costs was to use the midpoint of the salary range for each job classification. Although the simplicity of this approach has made it popular, several factors limit its accuracy: the average length of employment; distribution of nursing personnel on the unit, such as the proportion of primary nurse Is and IIs; the presence or absence of LPNs; the distinction between LPNs who are and are not allowed to pass medications; and the presence of TAs. Because of these limitations, the approach taken was to calculate the average hourly salary specific to the orthopaedic areas for each of the three types of caregivers. Because the staff on the orthopaedic unit was very experienced, the average salary was higher than the midpoint for the RN salary range. The average hourly salary figure was multiplied by the total nursing care hours for each patient to derive the direct nursing care costs on an individual patient basis (for example, an RN average salary of $10 an hour multiplied by 30 hours of care for one patient equals $300 of RN care for that patient).

Indirect nursing costs (fixed costs) are all costs of resources necessary for the provision of nursing care. These costs include activities such as administration, supervision, overhead, and patient and staff education, plus other fixed costs (costs that do not vary with patient census or acuity) that are ascribed to nursing. These were calculated at three levels: unit costs, department costs, and Division of Nursing costs. These indirect costs were translated into cost per patient day. Although it is known that some patients require more indirect care time, the factors and methodology for this have yet to be addressed.

Unit costs included the salaries of the clinical nursing coordinator (head nurse) and the unit clerk (unit receptionist) and unit supplies and services. The unit cost of orthopaedic technicians utilized on the units was calculated by taking 80 percent of their salaries (because 80 percent of their time is spent on the orthopaedic units and 20 percent of their time is spent in the Emergency Trauma Center). These expenses for the month of data collection were divided by the number of patient days on the unit for that same month to arrive at a cost per patient day.

Nursing department costs included the salaries of the director of nursing, her secretary, and the cost of related supplies. The previous four months' data were used to obtain an average figure, because monthly fluctuations in these costs are not related to the patient population. These total costs were first divided by the number of areas for which the director of nursing is responsible to arrive at a cost for the orthopaedic areas. The orthopaedic costs were then divided by the number of patient days on the unit to arrive at a department expense per orthopaedic patient day.

Division of Nursing costs included overhead and the salaries of the assistant vice-president, staffing office, nursing research, enterostomal therapy, the Department of Nursing Education and Resources (which includes clinical nurses, clinical specialists, and education coordinators), discharge planning, utilization review, and the IV Therapy Department. This total was divided by the total number of patient days for the hospital to produce costs per patient day. Calculations were based on the time period from January to April 1985 to stabilize these figures. The final calculation of indirect care costs was as follows:

Unit costs	$26.71/patient day
Department costs	.88/patient day
Division costs	16.66/patient day
	$44.25/patient day

The cost of direct nursing care and the indirect costs for each patient were combined and averaged to provide a total nursing care cost.

Data for each orthopaedic patient (including direct and indirect nursing care costs, total charges, length of stay, age, and sex) were grouped based on the patient's medical diagnoses into six general categories or subproduct lines by anatomical proximity to the area being treated. These categories and the number of patients in each were cervical disc disease (4), upper extremity (12), shoulder (3), lumbar-thoracic region (14), hip (3), and lower extremity (8).

FINDINGS

Demographics of Sample

The participants in the study were 21 males and 23 females ranging from 15 to 76 years of age. Nine were less than 30 years of age, 24 were between 30 and 60, and 11 were over 60. The median age was 42.5 and the mean was 45. The distribution was bimodal (three patients each were 30 and 61 years of age).

Nursing Care Required by Type of Worker

The number of hours of nursing care required for each type of worker and for each category of orthopaedic patients are presented in Tables 1–3. The totals for all caregivers are shown in Table 4. How well the sizes of these categories represent the proportion of patients in these groups over longer periods of time is not addressed in this study. When these longitudinal data are known, they will help to determine which categories would be selected for efforts to improve nursing efficiency. The first column in each table shows the total number of hours of care required. During the time of this survey, the lumbar-thoracic category ranked first in total nursing care hours required (see Table 4). As this was the largest category of patients in the sample, this finding was to be expected. Because these data are influenced by number of patients, the next level of analysis was hours of care per patient.

The findings shown in the third column of the tables represent the

Table 1
RN Nursing Care Required

Patient Category	Total RN Hours		N		RN Hours per Patient		Average Stay (days)		RN Hours per Patient Day
Cervical	44.65	÷	4	=	11.16	÷	4	=	2.79
Upper extremity	73.62	÷	12	=	6.14	÷	2	=	3.07
Shoulder	47.29	÷	3	=	15.76	÷	4	=	3.94
Lumbar-thoracic	231.46	÷	14	=	16.53	÷	5	=	3.31
Hip	135.35	÷	3	=	45.12	÷	11	=	4.10
Lower extremity	119.30	÷	8	=	14.91	÷	4	=	3.73

Table 2
LPN Nursing Care Required

Patient Category	Total LPN Hours		N		LPN Hours per Patient		Average Stay (days)		LPN Hours per Patient Day
Cervical	3.18	÷	4	=	0.80	÷	4	=	0.20
Upper extremity	13.87	÷	12	=	1.16	÷	2	=	0.58
Shoulder	16.50	÷	3	=	5.50	÷	4	=	1.38
Lumbar-thoracic	36.02	÷	14	=	2.57	÷	5	=	0.51
Hip	20.38	÷	3	=	6.79	÷	11	=	0.62
Lower extremity	23.31	÷	8	=	2.91	÷	4	=	0.73

Table 3
TA Nursing Care Required

Patient Category	Total TA Hours		N		TA Hours per Patient		Average Stay (days)		TA Hours per Patient Day
Cervical	5.91	÷	4	=	1.48	÷	4	=	0.37
Upper extremity	11.04	÷	12	=	0.22	÷	2	=	0.46
Shoulder	9.16	÷	3	=	3.05	÷	4	=	0.76
Lumbar-thoracic	44.00	÷	14	=	3.14	÷	5	=	0.63
Hip	20.07	÷	3	=	6.69	÷	11	=	0.61
Lower extremity	16.50	÷	8	=	2.06	÷	4	=	0.52

Table 4
Total Nursing Care Required

Patient Category	Total Hours		N		Total Hours per Patient		Average Stay (days)		Total Hours per Patient Day
Cervical	53.74	÷	4	=	13.44	÷	4	=	3.36
Upper extremity	110.45	÷	12	=	9.20	÷	2	=	4.60
Shoulder	72.95	÷	3	=	24.32	÷	4	=	6.08
Lumbar-thoracic	311.21	÷	14	=	22.23	÷	5	=	4.45
Hip	175.58	÷	3	=	58.52	÷	11	=	5.32
Lower extremity	162.06	÷	8	=	20.26	÷	4	=	5.06

mean number of required hours of care per patient over the total stay. The hip category ranked highest, but these patients also stayed the longest (an average of 11 days compared to the next longest average stay of 5 days). Because this data is influenced by length of stay, the third level of analysis was hours of care per patient day of stay, presented in the fifth column of Tables 1–4. Shoulder patients required the most care from both LPNs and TAs. However, RNs devoted more care per day of stay to hip patients than to shoulder patients. The hip category ranked second when the hours of care from all three types of caregivers were totaled (see Table 4).

Nursing Care Costs per Category

It was not surprising that the hip patients consumed the most hours of direct nursing care per patient, had the highest indirect cost, and thereby were the most costly on a per patient basis. This can be directly attributed to these patients' long average stay of 11 days, but even their average cost per day of stay ($99.16) was second only to that of shoulder patients ($108.43) (see Table 5). Upper extremity patients (with an average stay of only 2 days) consumed the least care per patient over the entire length of stay. The cervical patients required the least care per day. A final interesting finding was the relationship between direct and indirect cost of care. For the categories of hip, shoulder, and lower extremity patients, the direct cost was greater than the indirect cost of caring for these patients. This related to the fact that these are the top three categories in intensity of care in terms of hours of care required per patient (see Table 4). Table 5 presents further details on cost per patient by category.

A comparison of nursing care costs and total charges shows that the cost of nursing care for patients in the lumbar-thoracic category was the highest when viewed as a percentage of the total charges per patient (see Table 6). This finding is not surprising since these patients frequently do not undergo surgery, so their non-nursing costs remain comparatively low. The shoulder patients ranked second in percentage of total costs. These are categories in which nursing has the most impact on the cost to the hospital and therefore could most influence the hospital's profit margin.

IMPLICATIONS AND DISCUSSION

The purpose of this study was not to answer the debate on how to charge for nursing care, but rather to identify and clarify the costs of that care. Because most patient classification systems cannot be readily

Table 5
Nursing Care per Patient Category

Patient Category	Nursing Care Costs per Patient			
	Direct[a]	Indirect[b]	Total	Per Diem
Cervical	$140.85	$180.63	$ 321.47	$ 80.37
Upper extremity	84.13	97.08	181.21	90.60
Shoulder	241.99	191.73	433.72	108.43
Lumbar-thoracic	226.86	228.58	455.45	91.09
Hip	604.01	486.70	1,090.71	99.16
Lower extremity	204.15	160.39	364.54	91.13

[a]Direct costs are the total RN hours times salary, the total LPN hours times salary, plus the total TA hours times salary.
[b]Indirect costs were calculated on exact number of shifts of care needed by the sample, transposed into days of care, times the cost per day.

adapted to many different hospitals, the hours of nursing care assigned to each patient category cannot be transferred from one institution to another (Giovannetti, 1979). Each hospital must develop its own workload index and validate its own estimate of average nursing resource requirements for each category and the subsequent costs. The methodology of this study is therefore expected to be more useful for others than the findings.

In this study, the hip and shoulder patients consumed the greatest number of RN hours per day of stay. Therefore, these patients may be targeted by management for further study on how to hold quality and at the same time to decrease the time and subsequent cost. The ability to moderate and control the delivery of care services, adjusting intensity and cost when necessary, will have a definitive impact on costs. The

Table 6
Comparison of Nursing Care Costs to Total Charges

Patient Category	Nursing Care Cost as Percentage of Total Charge
Cervical	8.8
Upper extremity	8.3
Shoulder	15.6
Lumbar-thoracic	17.9
Hip	11.6
Lower extremity	10.1

greatest numbers of patients were found in the lumbar-thoracic, upper extremity, and lower extremity categories. It should be noted that the lumbar-thoracic patients, because of their sheer numbers, required the most nursing care and therefore should have a high priority for further study by nurse administrators.

The costs compiled in this study were only those incurred on the orthopaedic units. No costs for any nursing care in the operating room or recovery room were included, because neither nursing care hours nor cost per case were available as yet for those areas. Further data need to be collected and analyzed to clarify the surgical costs. It is interesting that in this sample, nursing costs accounted for proportionally very little of the consumer charges, especially considering that patients in these categories spend most of their stay in the care of nursing.

Hospitals are viewing themselves in terms of their product lines; and administrators, physicians, and practitioners alike are discovering how efficient they can be in the provision of health care. How well providers and consumers of health care services deal with the revolutionary changes taking place in the industry will have profound implications for every sector of our society in the years ahead. Is it possible to maintain or improve the quality of health care in the face of economic pressures brought on by a fast-changing, highly competitive marketplace? The answer to this question is of paramount importance to health care providers and consumers alike. Research activities provide one avenue for data input into the system. With sound, relevant data, today's well-educated and experienced nurse administrators will be able to handle creatively the opportunities made available by the turbulent, changing environment. Nursing is ready to accept the challenge offered by today's environment for health care delivery.

REFERENCES

American Nurses' Association. (1985). *Environmental assessment: Factors affecting long-range planning for nursing and health care.* New York: American Nurses' Association.

Arndt, C., & Huckabay, L. (1980). Administrative theory within a system's frame of reference. *Nursing Administration: Theory for practice with a systems approach.* (2d ed., pp. 19–47). St. Louis: Mosby.

Cheatwood, L. H., & Martin, P. A. (1986). Building a base for management of costs. In this volume, pp. 213–231.

Coddington, D., Palmquist, L., & Trollinger, W. (1985). Strategies for survival in the hospital industry. *Harvard Business Review, 63*(3), 129–238.

Curtin, L. (1985). Integrating acuity: The frugal road to safe care (Editorial). *Nursing Management, 16*(9), 7–8.

Curtin, L., & Zurlage, C. (1984). *DRGs: The reorganization of health.* Chicago: S-N Publication.

Davis, C. (1983). The federal role in changing health care financing. *Nursing Economics, 1,* 98–104, 146.

Giovannetti, P. (1979). Understanding patient classification systems. *Journal of Nursing Administration, 9*(2), 4–9.

Reschak, G., & Holm, K. (1985). Accounting for nursing costs by DRG. *Journal of Nursing Administration, 15* (9), 15–20, 26.

Veninga, R. (1982). *The human side of health administration.* Englewood Cliffs, NJ: Prentice-Hall.

Walker D. (1983). The cost of nursing care in hospitals. *Journal of Nursing Administration, 13*(1), 13–18.

The Cost-Quality Tradeoff in Productivity Management

Sandra R. Edwardson

When Congress adopted prospective payment as the basis for reimbursement for Medicare, it made several important assumptions. Members of Congress seemed to believe the quality of care received by Medicare recipients was at least acceptable but that the costs were unacceptably high. They knew that previous efforts to reduce costs had not been successful. They also suspected that hospitals use a variety of service models for providing care, some of which are more elaborate or costly than necessary. Therefore, rather than trying to find new regulations to control the use of resources, they chose a new approach—a payment system that gives each hospital an economic incentive to develop its own methods for holding down costs.

The rest is history. Every hospital in the country is going about the task of improving its productivity. This flurry of activity has revealed some confusion about what productivity means and how it can be measured. Although the nursing literature is filled with case studies and a few reports of productivity research, our knowledge about practices that lead to improved productivity is sketchy.

This paper will describe and evaluate selected measures of productivity currently used in hospital nursing. Then several proposals will be made to improve the methods used to measure and achieve productivity.

PRODUCTIVITY MEASURES

As Jelinek and Dennis (1976) demonstrated, a great deal of attention has been focused on variables that can be used to assess the productivity of nursing services, but very little has been done to define the relationship of these variables to one another and to the larger hospital and health care system. They used an open systems model showing the relationship between inputs, processes, and outputs and suggesting the influence of the environment in which the three elements exist (see Fig. 1).

Jelinek and Dennis (1976) proposed the following definition of nursing productivity:

> The concept of productivity encompasses both the effectiveness of nursing care, which relates to its quality and appropriateness, and the efficiency of care, which is production of nursing output with minimal resource waste [p. 3].

This formulation is consistent with standard economic definitions of productivity, yet also takes into account some of the special characteristics of nursing services. Chief among these is the increasing tendency to incorporate both efficiency and effectiveness into the operational definition of the output of health care organizations (American Management Sciences, 1980).

Effectiveness of the hospital's output refers to the safety, appropriateness, and excellence of care and encompasses the issues of changes in health status, patient outcomes, and patient satisfaction (American Management Sciences, 1980). *Efficiency*, on the other hand, occurs whenever the combination of inputs used in the process produces the maximum feasible output and results in a positive relationship between the marginal costs incurred and benefits realized (Pauly, 1970).

Figure 1
Nursing Productivity Framework

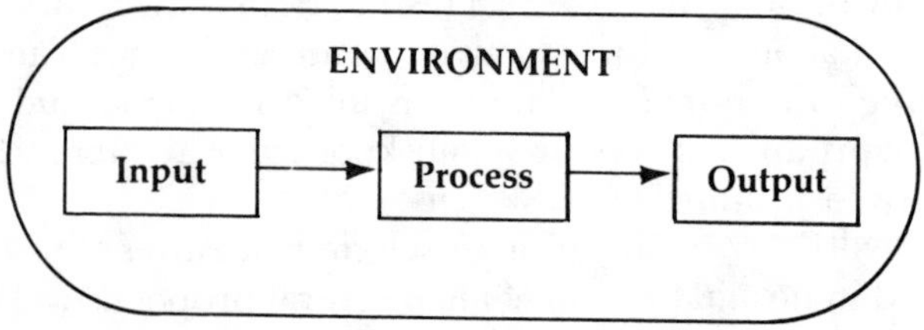

Adapted from R. C. Jelinek and L. C. Dennis, *A Review and Evaluation of Nursing Productivity* (Bethesda, MD: Health Resources Administration, 1976), 14.

Resources Per Patient Day

Many performance measures used in nursing and purporting to be productivity measures concentrate on efficiency but fail to provide a comprehensive assessment of inputs and outputs; they also tend to ignore effectiveness. Nursing hours per patient day, for example, is a commonly used indicator of labor productivity that is simple and easily understood. But it attributes all performance and all changes in performance from one time period to another to a single input—nursing hours. It provides no information on the possible contributions of changes in technology, supplies, and equipment. It also neglects any modifications that may have been made in the skill level of those providing the nursing hours, the type and intensity of patient days being considered, or the quality of the patient days being produced.

A similar measure—nursing salary costs per patient day—has the advantage of implicitly incorporating differences in skill level by using salary differentials as a proxy measure of skill mix, but it also fails to consider characteristics of the patient day.

Both nursing hours per patient day and salary costs per patient day are useful as measures of labor productivity (that is, personnel costs per unit of output), but only if the nature of the patient day is held constant. Categorizing patient days into DRGs, or preferably into DRGs adjusted for severity of illness, would improve the validity of comparisons of nursing hours and nursing salary costs per patient day.

Degree of Occupation

Another very informal productivity indicator in common use is the "busyness scale." What nursing manager has not observed unit staff in a continual flurry of activity or has not been beset by complaints from the staff that they are overworked? There are ways to assess systematically the adequacy of staffing by using measures such as that developed by Williams and Murphy (1979). But the question remains whether a fully occupied staff is also a productive staff. It may simply be that their work is poorly ordered and organized or that they lack the support services and equipment necessary to reduce their effort. Although the staff may be exceedingly busy and understaffed using current models of practice, there may still be room for improving the quantity and quality of care given without increasing costs. This is another example of a question that can be answered only by using an empirical approach.

Utilization Rates

Another well-known performance measure is the one produced by most nurse staffing systems based on patient classification—that is, the ratio comparing targeted with actual full-time equivalent usage of nursing personnel. While this is perhaps the single best day-to-day control monitor available to nursing managers, it is more appropriately called a utilization indicator rather than a productivity indicator unless certain assumptions are made about targeted hours of care.

The actual-required staff ratio is useful as a productivity measure only if the nursing service assumes or has demonstrated that the targeted number of nursing hours can provide the quantity and quality of care that the hospital wishes to provide. To affirm the validity of the number of hours targeted, the nursing department either needs to use the research findings of others or do its own evaluation studies to demonstrate that care of a given level of quantity and quality can be produced by a given number of nursing care hours. In effect, the targeted number of hours of care is used as a substitute for direct measures of the quantity and quality of nursing care output.

Consider a hypothetical example. Assume that the targeted hours of care for a maternity service are five hours of professional and two hours of nonprofessional nursing care during the postpartum period. By a careful evaluation of outcomes, the maternity service has determined that patients are discharged in a timely manner and that the mothers have the needed knowledge and skill in caring for themselves and their infants, are satisfied with the care they received, and have a satisfactory complication rate. Given this level of monitoring of outcomes against the institution's own standards of care, targeted hours of care could quite legitimately be substituted as an indicator of the appropriate quantity and quality of care.

In other words, using staff utilization ratios to judge productivity is based on one very important, but frequently unacknowledged assumption: the standard hours of care used by the patient classification system to calculate required nursing hours are assumed to provide the desired level of service. To the extent that the organization has measured and is satisfied that the target level of staffing produces an acceptable quantity and quality of care, it may be an appropriate substitute for a direct measurement of productivity. But the common expectation that the actual use of staff should be less than 100 percent of the targeted level suggests that the standards used to establish the target are believed to be too high or that the organization is willing to compromise its standards, with unknown consequences.

Unfortunately, most hospitals lack the time, money, and expertise to do the kind of study necessary to establish the links between input and output and are unlikely to find sufficient research evidence in the literature to verify or improve current practices. Alternative methods for justifying the dollars and time invested in nursing care will have to be substituted until sufficient evaluative and research evidence is accumulated.

PRODUCTIVITY GAINS

Having discussed the most commonly used productivity measures, I will now review some of the areas in which productivity gains are possible. There are three general ways in which potential gains can be made: through changes in inputs (such as nursing staff, supplies, equipment, the physical facility, and support services), through changes in practice, and through increased control of demand for services. This discussion will focus on changes in staffing practices and changes in practice.

Changes in Input

Matching Supply with Demand.   Even a cursory review of the literature or survey of workshop topics reveals that nursing managers expect to achieve major gains in productivity by controlling the use of staff. Because nursing is so labor intensive, it is understandable that staffing receives the greatest amount of attention. But because of wide fluctuations in demand for service, it is also the most difficult area in which to achieve economy. Most sectors of the economy can adjust to changing demand for goods and services by hiring new staff or laying off unneeded personnel, stockpiling products, or postponing activities. In contrast, the hospital industry has historically experienced shortages of trained personnel and faces unusual uncertainties in forecasting demand for service. Solutions such as hiring and layoffs have proven to be unwise and too insensitive except in the long run.

Similarly, because the production and consumption of nursing services are simultaneous events, nurses cannot stockpile their "products" during periods of reduced demand for use or sale in periods of increased demand. Nor can most nursing activities be postponed until demand slackens. Furthermore, because health care has a unique status among economic goods, it is difficult to turn away people seeking service. Refusing to render service is not only considered morally questionable, but in today's highly competitive environment, it would probably also be considered the height of foolishness.

Nursing managers have used several strategies for coping with highly variable demand and relative inflexibility in regulating the supply of nursing services. Among the most widely adopted of these strategies is variable staffing based on patient classification systems. The methods used to develop and maintain these systems are sophisticated, and the systems themselves seem to be gaining credibility with policymakers. The challenge ahead for managers is to continually monitor the systems for validity and reliability to ensure that the systems maintain their accuracy and credibility.

Another less obvious potential problem with patient classification data is the temptation to use them for purposes for which they were not designed. Patient classification systems were intended to give a quick and accurate prediction of patient care requirements a few hours hence. As a result, indicators are selected for their ease of measurement and their power as predictors of the time required to care for patients. Indicators were not intended to provide descriptions of all nursing activities or of the skill and conceptual abilities needed to plan and evaluate care activities.

In doing productivity studies, therefore, it is inappropriate to expect patient classification indicators to be used as a comprehensive description of the process of care given or to be proxies for the skill level required, unless the system was specifically designed to perform this dual function. Some of patient classification systems of the factor type attempt to serve as a basis for documenting care given as well as predicting care required. These factor systems provide a more complete description of the process of care than do the prototype systems, but cannot be considered exhaustive.

Staff Substitutions.   Another traditional strategy for improving productivity is to use the principle of staff substitution. From a theoretical point of view, one can argue for and against staff substitution as a method for improving productivity. The empirical evidence is also inconclusive.

Most studies of staffs that are entirely or predominantly made up of registered nurses suffer from methodological problems that reduce their overall credibility and generalizability. Some are uncontrolled case studies (for example, Burt, 1980; Hinshaw, Scofield, & Atwood, 1981; Miller, 1980). Many studies that experimented with increasing the proportion of professional to nonprofessional staff were done in conjunction with the introduction of primary nursing, making it impossible to sort out which of the reported changes are attributable to skill mix and which to the change in the mode of care (Dahlen, 1978; Marram, Barret, & Bevis, 1974; Nenner, Curtis & Eckhoff, 1977; Osinski & Powals, 1980).

Reported advantages of a high proportion of professional staff are greater patient satisfaction (Abdellah & Levine, 1958) and better coordination and quality of care (Georgopoulous & Mann, 1964; Miller &

Bryant, 1965). At least two studies have confirmed the relative costliness of nursing assistants. Nursing assistants have been found to be occupied only 65 to 73 percent of the time, as opposed to registered nurses, who are occupied 92 to 100 percent of the time (Christman, 1978; Clark, 1977). These findings suggest that the unpredictable demand for service in the hospital may temper the theoretical gains to be made from staff substitution.

Given some of the methodological problems in studies of staff substitution, the tentative conclusion is that high ratios of professional to nonprofessional staff appear to be no more costly and are frequently less costly in terms of salaries and turnover rates (Burt, 1980; Corpuz & Anderson, 1977; Dahlen, 1978; Forseth, 1980; Hinshaw, Scofield, & Atwood, 1981; Marram, Barret, & Bevis, 1974; Marram, Flynn, Abaravich, & Carey, 1976; Miller, 1980; Nenner, Curtis & Eckhoff, 1977; Osinski & Powals, 1980).

Changes in the Process of Care

The largest gains in productivity will undoubtedly come from reducing lengths of stay when possible. In order to accomplish this, nurses will either have to do more efficiently what they are doing now, or they will have to do things differently. Happily, many of the activities that are likely to be most successful in reducing lengths of stay are also activities nurses have valued and have wanted to improve for some time. Care planning that had in the past seemed superfluous to many practitioners has become an essential ingredient in selecting and ordering care and treatment activities.

The elusive goal of multidisciplinary health care teams is also within grasp. As many hospitals have learned in choosing product line management strategies for coping with DRGs, this care planning is likely to be most effective when done by all the disciplines involved in the care of patients in a particular DRG. In at least one St. Paul hospital, nurses are not only active members of DRG product teams, but are also the leaders of the group. This role is appropriately filled by a nurse, since nurses are already pivotal in the organization and coordination of all care and treatment activities and have the most comprehensive view of what actually happens to patients in the course of their hospitalizations. Most professionally educated nurses will also have a good understanding of the family and of community services needed by and available to patients.

The possible strategies for reducing costs that are likely to evolve from such interdisciplinary analysis are numerous and familiar. There are already many reports of institutions substituting outpatient preparation and follow-up care for traditional inpatient services, implementing day programs, using case managers to improve coordination and integration of service, and so forth. What is most exciting about the challenge to reduce lengths of stay is the potential for unleashing the creativity of nurses. Unfortunately, however, helping a nursing staff appreciate the creative potential in reducing lengths of stay and cutting costs presents an enormous challenge to management. I will propose an investigative strategy for meeting this challenge, but first I will explore the nature of the challenge.

Competing Value Systems. When faced with cost-reduction measures, nurses' principal concern is the possibility that they will not be able to provide safe, let alone high-quality care. This is a particularly uncomfortable issue because demands to do more with less are in direct conflict with nursing's professional value system.

Mauksch (1966) contrasted the two dominant value systems operating among nurses. On the one hand, nurses have been socialized into the values of a profession in which decision making is based on a knowledgeable assessment of the needs of individual patients, one at a time. Having determined those needs, the nurse then feels an obligation to see that they are met without regard for the patient's ability to pay. On the other hand, nurses as citizens and as employees of bureaucratic institutions are also influenced by an economic value structure. Economic resources are scarce by definition. According to the economic value structure, decisions about the allocation of resources must always be made in light of alternative uses of those resources. All other things being equal, alternatives with the greatest marginal benefit per marginal cost are to be preferred.

Staff nurses and managers alike are caught between these two value orientations. On the one hand, they are drawn by socialization and inherent humanitarian predilections toward the professional value system. On the other, they are drawn toward the economic model because of their awareness of the crisis created by the rising costs of health care and their obligation as citizens to see that other important social needs, such as those for education, defense, social services, and public utilities, are met. Nurses are forced to make tradeoffs between cost and quality.

The prevailing model of cost-quality tradeoffs in health care presumes that there is a direct relationship between these two factors. For every increment in resources invested in health care, an increment in the level of quality of service is expected to follow. Conversely, for every decrease in cost, a commensurate decline in quality is expected.

Given the dilemma outlined, it is time to consider a new conceptual model for cost-quality tradeoffs. Figure 2 presents a model proposed by

Figure 2
Conceptual Cost-Quality Tradeoff Curve

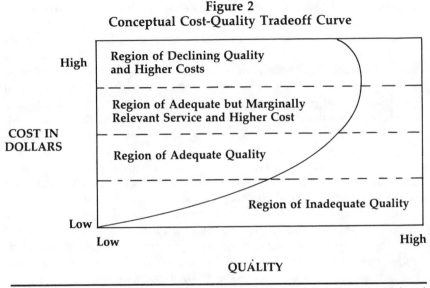

Adapted with permission from R. H. Brook, A. R. Davies, and C. J. Kamberg, "Selected Reflections on the Quality of Medical Care Evaluation in the 1980s," *Nursing Research* (1980), *29*, 127–133. Copyright © 1980, American Journal of Nursing Company.

Brook, Davies, and Kamberg (1980). The model identifies four levels of quality of care—inadequate, adequate, adequate but marginally relevant, and declining. The hypothetical production function represented by the curve suggests that an increase in the quantity of care can be expected to produce comparable increments in quality up to some point. Then the production function enters the region of diminishing returns. In this region, the level of quality remains the same despite increased investments in care. Finally, the curve bends backwards, suggesting that beyond some point, added services actually decrease the benefit realized by the patient. Examples of such counterproductive expenditures include fruitless efforts to prolong life and iatrogenic illnesses.

To summarize the implications of this model, quality costs money since it presupposes an adequate quantity of services and often means more care. But it is also clear that care costs more when it is delivered inefficiently. Finally, excessive but harmful care is most costly but of lower quality. It may result in loss in individual and social benefit because scarce resources are not put to the best use (Brook, Davies, & Kamberg, 1980).

It is crucial, therefore, that each nursing department define what it means by quality care—that is, what its acceptable level of care will be. Such definitions have always been implicit in the design and organization of programs of care. Nursing organizations have never been financially able to do everything that was theoretically possible. Standards of acceptable quality have always been somewhat less than the maximum possible. There have never been enough of the right kind of nurses in the right place at the right time. The difference now is that nursing service organizations are being forced to be much more explicit about identifying a target level of care. Because the resources available are much more limited, the gap between what is possible and what is affordable is greater.

Identifying Levels of Care.   How then does the practicing administrator faced with squeezing out additional efficiency and faced with a reluctant nursing staff identify a target level of care? At the risk of gross oversimplification, there appear to be two basic approaches: the textbook approach and the constrained budget approach.

Using the textbook approach implies an attempt to attain the ideal and is powered by the professional value system. The goal is to achieve the best possible outcomes for the particular client. There are several ways to establish standards of quality using the textbook approach. One is to go to the textbooks and the professional journals for evidence of the kinds of outcomes that can be expected. Frequently, however, practitioners will find that nothing has been written on the subject about which a standard is needed. An alternative is to rely on expert opinion. The experts can be asked to make a judgment about what the expected outcomes should be, or they may be asked about the best process for achieving the desired outcome. When the method is applied properly, experienced nurses can be finely tuned measurement instruments.

Another alternative to empirical evidence is to identify a patient judged to have received good care. Having identified such a patient, the process used to achieve the care or the outcome of the care can then be described and established as a norm.

Under the second major strategy for identifying a target level of quality, the constrained budget model, the goal is to achieve an affordable level of care for all. Two methods for identifying a target level of quality are apparent: analysis of cost-effectiveness and analysis of episodes of illness. Cost-effectiveness analysis is simply a method for comparing the cost of two or more methods for achieving a given outcome. Since it is already widely used, it will not be discussed in greater detail here.

A second approach for identifying a target level of care under a budget constraint is to analyze an episode of illness. The approach is based on the supposition that it is necessary to accept that hospitals can no longer bring all or most of their patients to the optimal level of recovery before discharge.

Under a budget-constraint model, a fundamental change in the role of hospital nurse may be necessary. The focus may have to change from responsibility for bringing patients to a given level of health to identifying ways of bridging the gap to posthospitalization services. The proportion of time spent in providing direct care is likely to decrease, while the proportion of time spent in planning, coordination, and preparing the patient for self-care is likely to increase.

Such a change implies using a new set of quality indicators. In the best of all possible worlds, patient outcomes should be measured when recovery or the optimal level of health has been reached. This implies that patients can be located at that point in time in order to evaluate how well they have fared: Have they been readmitted to the hospital? Have they used any out-of-hospital service? What is their level of functioning? What has been their level of pain, suffering, and distress along the way?

Is this impossible? Systematic long-term evaluation is probably not possible for patients not in health maintenance organizations (HMOs), except in special studies. Researchers could be recruited to plan and execute such studies, but because such research is expensive, it would probably require outside funding. Longitudinal studies of HMO patients, whose care is all within the control of an organized set of providers, are much easier, provided that the HMOs are cooperative.

If longitudinal studies are not possible, some intermediary steps can be taken. At the least, hospital nurses can seek feedback from colleagues in community health nursing, home health agencies, and clinics about how well patients were prepared for discharge and the principal improvements required. Another method may be to do telephone follow-ups of selected patients to assess their functioning and what could have been done to ease their recovery.

Assuming that such information has been gathered and recorded somewhat systematically, the nursing department should be able to make a reasonably informed estimate of when discharge is both safe and can be linked to needed follow-up services. The study may reveal that follow-up services are not available or are available but not adequate. On the other hand, services might be available and of good quality, but the follow-up study might suggest that patients would simply recover more quickly, more fully, or at a lower overall cost if they remained in the hospital another day or two. In either case, the nursing department would have the kind of information needed to influence hospital and public policies about how health care resources should be distributed.

This investigative strategy has real potential for significantly improving productivity for two reasons. First, it seems to be consistent with what we know about the motivation of professional workers. Although the conclusions are tentative, several investigators have found nurses to have higher job satisfaction when their job scope is enlarged (Bechtold, Szilagyi, & Sims, 1980) and when they are afforded greater autonomy (Alexander, Weisman, & Chase, 1982; Dear, Weisman, Alexander, & Chase, 1982).

A second reason for believing that an investigative strategy may help solve some of the potentially explosive problems of doing more with less is that it does away with the traditional practice of dividing accountability for nursing practice. In most instances, responsibility for financial accounting has been assigned almost exclusively to managers, while staff nurses have been given primary responsibility for clinical practice.

This practice is debilitating for a number of reasons. First, it sets up and continually reinforces a "we-they" split between management and "labor." Second, this division of accountability has diminished nurses' ability to discharge our professional responsibility to assure the health care policymakers and the public that we are making the best use of the resources devoted to nursing services. Finally, divided accountability probably has impeded the building of the body of scientific and professional knowledge necessary for advancing the discipline and improving practice.

The split between staff nurses and managers is a natural phenomenon in bureaucratically structured institutions and will probably always be present to a certain degree. But to the extent that the search for the optimal point on the cost–quality tradeoff curve can be a mutual enterprise, this split may be reduced and the deep value conflict experienced by all professionals practicing in bureaucratic structures may be eased.

REFERENCES

Abdellah, F. G., & Levine, E. (1958). *Effects of nursing staffing on satisfaction with nursing care.* Chicago: American Hospital Association.

Alexander, C. S., Weisman, C. S., & Chase, G. A. (1982). Determinants of staff nurses' perceptions of autonomy within different clinical contexts. *Nursing Research, 31,* 48–52.

American Management Sciences. (1980). *Productivity and health.* Bethesda, MD: Office of the Assistant Secretary of Health.

Bechtold, A. E., Szilagyi, A. D., & Sims, H. P. (1980). Antecedents of employee satisfaction in a hospital environment. *Health Care Management Review, 5,* 77–88.

Brook, R. H., Davies, A. R., & Kamberg, C. J. (1980). Selected reflections on the quality of medical care evaluation in the 1980s. *Nursing Research, 29,* 127–133.

Burt, M. L. (1980). The cost of all-RN staffing. In G. Alfano (Ed.), *All-RN Nursing Staff* (pp. 87–90). Wakefield, MS: Nursing Resources.

Christman, L. (1978). A micro-analysis of the nursing division of one medical center. *Nursing Digest, 6* (2), 83–87.

Clark, E. L. (1977). A model of nursing staffing for effective patient care. *Journal of Nursing Administration, 7* (2), 22–27.

Corpuz, T., & Anderson, R. (1977). The Evanston story: Primary nursing comes alive. *Nursing Administration Quarterly, 1* (2), 9–50.

Dahlen, A. (1978). With primary nursing, we have it all together. *American Journal of Nursing, 78,* 426–428.

Dear, M. R., Weisman, C. S., Alexander, C. S., & Chase, G. A. (1982). The effect of the intensive care nursing role on job satisfaction. *Heart and Lung, 11,* 560–565.

Forseth, J. (1980). Does RN staffing escalate medical care costs? In G. Alfano (Ed.), *All-RN nursing staff* (pp. 103–110). Wakefield, MS: Nursing Resources.

Georgopoulous, B. S., & Mann, F. C. (1962). *The community hospital.* New York: Macmillan.

Hinshaw, A. S., Scofield, R., & Atwood, J. R. (1981). Staff, patient, and cost outcomes of all-registered nurse staffing. *Journal of Nursing Administration, 11* (11 & 12), 30–36.

Jelinek, R. C., & Dennis, L. C. (1976). *A review and evaluation of nursing productivity.* (DHEW No. HRA 77–15). Bethesda, MD: Health Resources Administration.

Marram, G., Barret, M. W., & Bevis, E. M. (1974). *Primary nursing: A model for individualized care.* St. Louis: C. V. Mosby.

Marram, G., Flynn, K., Abaravich, W., Carey, S. (1976). *Cost-effectiveness of primary and team nursing.* Wakefield, MS: Contemporary Publishing.

Mauksch, H. O. (1966). The organizational context of nursing practice. In F. Davis (Ed.), *The nursing profession: Five sociological essays* (pp. 109–137). New York: Wiley.

Miller, P. W. (1980). Staffing with RNs. In G. Alfano (Ed.), *All-RN nursing staff* (pp. 91–95). Wakefield, MS: Nursing Resources.

Miller, S. J., & Bryant, W. D. (1965). *A division of nursing labor: Experiment in staffing a municipal hospital.* Kansas City: Community Studies.

Nenner, V. C., Curtis, E. M., & Eckhoff, C. M. (1977). Primary nursing. *Supervisor Nurse, 8* (5), 14–16.

Osinski, E. G., & Powals, J. G. (1980). The cost of all RN staffed primary nursing. *Supervisor Nurse, 11* (1), 16–21.

Pauly, M. V. (1970). Efficiency, incentives and reimbursement for health care. *Inquiry, 7,* 114–131.

Williams, M. A., & Murphy, L. N. (1979). Subjective and objective measures of staffing adequacy. *Journal of Nursing Administration, 9* (11), 21–29.

Part 3
New Uses for Patient Classification

A Patient Classification System for Rehabilitation Nursing

Teri Paradise, Marcel Dijkers, and Marylou Maxwell

Existing well-known patient classification systems are not suitable for use in rehabilitation nursing because rehabilitation patients, rather than being passive recipients of care, are active participants. They get dressed and attend therapy sessions. They go to the dining room to eat and to the recreation area to try out newly learned skills. In addition, many have bowel training programs, require frequent catheterization, or have to be assisted in transfers, such as from bed to wheelchair. Finally, therapeutic communication and teaching are central aspects of rehabilitation nursing.

Starting in 1979, the nursing staff of the Rehabilitation Institute in Detroit, Michigan, has developed, tested, and implemented a patient classification system that is suited to the unique nursing needs of rehabilitation patients and the specific tasks of rehabilitation nurses. At that time, no rehabilitation nursing patient classification tools had been published, and our search did not find evidence that any were in existence, although several have been published since then (for example, Burgher & Hanson, 1980; Jordan & McCoy, 1984; Schuster, 1984). The Rehabilitation Institute system provides a mechanism for measuring the acuity level of all inpatients on a daily basis. Based on the results, staff needs for each of three shifts on all nursing units are determined. A computer program is used to do the necessary calculations and print the results. At the end of each month, the patient classification data are combined with staffing data to generate detailed reports.

The system was developed and implemented in four partly overlapping phases: planning, data collection and analysis, implementation, and evaluation and revision. This paper briefly describes the main elements of the Rehabilitation Institute's classification system, especially as it differs from acuity systems implemented in hospitals elsewhere. We will, however, focus on the nature of the data collected and the management purposes, other than staffing, for which they are used.

PLANNING PHASE

At the start of the project, a departmental committee analyzed various existing classification tools, both published and unpublished, including all of the better known ones: St. Luke's Hospital of Arizona Medical/Surgical tool (Cisarik, Higgerson, & Van Slyck, 1978), PRN 76 classification (Audette, Carle, Simard, & Tilquin, 1978; Tilquin, Audette, Carle, & Lambert, 1978), and various tools designed following GRASP methodology and described in the first GRASP manual (Meyer, 1978).

Each tool was evaluated with respect to content (tasks included and excluded); definition of tasks included; layout and clarity; reliability and validity (if reported); and various aspects of completing the tool, totaling ratings, and so forth. None of these tools were specifically developed for rehabilitation nursing; most were designed for medical-surgical units. They included tasks that did not apply to rehabilitation patients, such as preoperative preparation, while tasks that are central to rehabilitation nursing were either missing, delineated in insufficient detail, or given too low or too high a weight.

The committee had to agree with authors (such as Giovannetti, 1979) who have stressed that each hospital has to develop its own patient classification system, because differences in physical layout, nursing care delivery approach (team versus primary provider), standards of care, personnel mix, common patient diagnoses, and the like make every situation unique. The committee decided that (1) we could not evade the task of developing our own system, and (2) the GRASP approach was the soundest methodology for doing so. In view of later developments, the latter decision was a fortunate one.

A plan for systematic development of a patient classification system was developed at this time, including forms to be used in various studies.

DATA COLLECTION AND ANALYSIS

As a first step, nursing personnel on all units and shifts and of all skill levels and job descriptions were required to keep lists of what tasks they did and how often they did them. These lists were analyzed, and those direct care nursing tasks were identified that accounted for a significant percentage of staff time because of their frequency and/or duration. These tasks were categorized into seven areas of care, such as elimination, treatment, and so forth.

Next, each separate task was analyzed and a definition written. All 86 descriptions were combined in a handbook, which constituted the basis of the later work and eventually became the handbook used by the nurses doing classification. Description and definition made possible standardization of task performance during later time and frequency studies. These studies focused on RNs, LPNs, and rehabilitation nursing aides, but all other categories of personnel, including head nurses, unit clerks, and treatment room technicians, were included.

Personnel were instructed to keep a tally of how many times they performed each specific task during their shift. The data were compiled to determine the percentage of care that was delivered on each shift. The percentage of care rendered per shift was found to vary by unit as a result of differences in the nursing care delivery approach (primary versus team) and the type of patients (for example, spinal cord injury versus rheumatology).

Direct observation time studies were conducted for each task in the handbook. The time studies involved the level of personnel ordinarily assigned to perform the specific task being studied. Prior to performing the task, the staff member reviewed the written steps in the handbook. As she or he performed the function, the staff member was timed by an observer. Although this method of study is costly and time-consuming, it is necessary if the tool is to withstand scrutiny.

Compiling the results from the time studies was a lengthy process. Each task was assigned a standard time based on the average time it took the employees to perform that function during the studies. Once that was done, final assembly of the tool took 28 drafts! Based on frequency and standard time, a total time per day was calculated for each task. Finally, a point value was determined for each task that took into account total time per day, adjustments for direct care tasks not included in the tool, and all indirect care. A fatigue and delay factor was built in by counting each eight hours worked as seven hours available for patient care.

The tool that resulted from this phase looked very much like the one in use today (see Figure 1). It includes 53 tasks in seven areas that encompass the major functions of patient care, including diet, elimination, hygiene, medication, treatment, mobility and transfers, and patient's state and behavior. Each individual task has a point value of from 1 to 12, with each point representing 15 minutes of staff time. Note that the tool does not distinguish between levels of personnel required to perform a task. Some patient classification systems do produce requirements for staff of each level of preparation, either directly or by means

Figure 1
Rehabilitation Institute Patient Classification System

Admission Date: _____
Cognitive Level: _____
Diagnosis (Medical) _____

Check box only if applicable to patient.

DIET	Feeds self	*I&C	1	Comments
	Feeds self with help	*NPO	2	
	Total feed	*Teach	5	
	*Tube feeding q6		6	
	*Tube feeding q4	*Complex total feeding	9	

ELIMINATION	**BOWEL**	Toilets with help	*Incontinent	2
		Bowel training		3
		*Complex bowel care	*Teach	4
	BLADDER	*Self cath	*Urinalysis	1
		*Staff cath q8 or q12	*Foley/Condom	2
		*Staff cath q6		3
		Toilet with help	*Incontinent	4
		*Staff cath q4	*Teach	
		*Complex bladder care		8

HYGIENE	Bathes self with min. assist		2
	Bed bath with mod. assist	Shower chair	3
	Complete bed bath	*Teach	4
	*Complex bath		6

*MEDS	Routine meds	PRN meds	1
	Mult. meds, QID or more	Self meds	2
	Complex meds	Teach	4
	Continuous IV		5

*TREATMENT	Routine V.S. (TPR-BP) &/or Tx.		1
	V.S. q shift or QID &/or Tx.		2
	Dressing change &/or Tx.		3
	Dressing or Tx.	Teach Tx.	4
	Complex dsg.	Tx. or freq. V.S.	

Write in appropriate number 5 to 12. Use *Handbook* for reference.

MOBILITY/ TRANSFERS	Bedrest	Standby assist	1
	Ambulate with help	Min. help with ADL	2
	Moderate help with ADL & transfer	*Teach	4
	*Max. help with ADL		8

STATE/ BEHAVIOR	Other instructional needs	4
	Cognition deficit	6
	Extended nursing care	12
	TOTALS	

*Indicates need for supportive charting.

of a conversion table (for example, Plummer, 1976; Torrez, 1983). It was decided that accounting for level of staff required would complicate the tool without adding any real advantages—what use is it to know that you need to add .13 RN, .14 LPN, and .58 aide to the staff scheduled for a shift, when the only personnel available is one RN?

Also note that while the tool determines the amount of nursing care required for a 24-hour period, it does not indicate how many of those hours have to be available on each of three shifts. On a rehabilitation unit, patient needs for nursing care are slow to change, and the percentage distribution over the hours of the day is quite constant. Therefore, there is no need to classify patients on every shift or more frequently, as is done on most medical-surgical units. Responsibility for classification can be assigned to one nurse who determines the patient's needs for 24 hours as a whole, rather than for each shift. Thus, in our system, the number of hours needed on each shift is not assessed by the nurse doing the classification; it is determined at a later phase, after points have been totaled over all patients on a unit. Standard formulas, based in part on the results of the frequency studies and in part on judgment by the head nurses, are used to split 24-hour staff requirements over three shifts. The formulas differ somewhat between units, depending on the type of patient and nursing care pattern. The closed head injury unit, for example, uses 40 percent for day, 40 percent for evening, and 20 percent for night to allocate staff; on the general physical medicine and rehabilitation units, the percentages are 55 percent, 30 percent, and 15 percent, respectively.

In bridging from data analysis to implementation, the committee needed to pilot test the tool. One unit was chosen for this task, and all nursing personnel on the unit participated in a training session in preparation for a limited trial period. During this trial period some minor revisions were made. Also during this time, it was decided who would classify the patients, tally the units, and report the tally information to the Nursing Office.

After evaluating the data gathered for a large number of patients on the total number of points per patient, the committee decided to divide the entire point range into levels of required care. The point ranges for each level were determined by plotting the classification results for a large number of patients on a graph and dividing them somewhat arbitrarily into five acuity levels. Each level was then assigned the average number of nursing care hours based on the points of the sampled patients in that level (see Table 1). This was done solely to simplify manual calculation of nursing staff requirements. The procedure discards some detail in the information, but when scores are aggregated over an entire nursing unit this does not result in a serious loss of information.

Table 1
Point Range and Estimated Mean Hours of Nursing Care for Five Patient Categories

Category	Points	Average Hours of Care
I	0–6	1.4
II	7–13	2.7
III	14–21	4.3
IV	22–37	7.2
V	38+	11.1

IMPLEMENTATION

After the pilot test, the tool was introduced on the rest of the nursing units. All staff participated in training sessions prior to the implementation of the tool.

Initially, calculation of the staffing needs of each of the hospital's six units was performed by hand. This was a time-consuming and error-prone procedure, even though the five care levels rather than the original point totals were used. Similarly, monthly reports were produced by hand, showing unit trends in number of patient care hours, relationship of hours of care available to hours of care needed, and so forth. Producing even a rudimentary monthly report took close to two working days.

To reduce personnel requirements and increase accuracy of the results, computer programs were written for data entry, data checking,

Table 2
Sample Daily Report:
Number of Patients, Total Care Hours Required, and Staff Required by Shift for Each Unit on 2/23/89

Unit	Number of Patients by Level of Care						Total Care Hours	Staff Required by Shift			
	I	II	III	IV	V	Total		Day	Evening	Night	All
4W	5	5	5	5	0	20	89.0	6.3	3.8	2.5	12.7
4N	6	6	6	6	6	30	173.4	13.6	7.4	3.7	24.7
7W	12	13	14	1	0	40	137.1	10.7	5.8	2.9	19.5
7N	3	3	3	3	3	15	86.7	4.9	4.9	2.4	12.3
3W	10	0	10	0	10	30	180.0	14.1	7.7	3.8	25.7
Total	36	27	38	15	19	135	666.2	49.8	29.7	15.5	95.1

and producing the daily staffing report and the monthly reports. After the nurses classify their patients, a clerk tallies the number of patients per unit in each of the five categories. This information is entered into the computer at about 2 p.m. daily. Immediately, a report is printed (see Table 2) stating the number of full-time equivalent staff (FTEs) required for each shift. This makes it possible to make staff assignments on the next three shifts, starting with the afternoon shift.

Information on the number of staff members actually working on each shift (scheduled staff less those absent, plus floating staff) is entered into the computer after the close of the month. This information, specifying the number of FTEs in all categories of nursing staff on each shift, is combined with the patient classification data to generate a monthly report.

USING THE DATA

A variety of data are generated by the patient classification system that can be used by managers and administrators for a variety of purposes. The monthly report contains four main tables. Each table has information specific to the individual unit plus combined data from all units for an institute total or average. The first table has the following nine areas of information, as shown in Figure 2:

Area 1: The sum over all days of the month of the number of patients classified each day in each acuity level category and total.

Area 2: The number of patients in each category and the total number of patients on the average day during the month calculated by dividing the corresponding figure in area 1 by the number of days in the month.

Area 3: The percentage distribution of patient days produced during the month.

Area 4: The average daily census during the month.

Area 5: The average daily staffing (all personnel on all shifts).

Area 6: The sum over all days of the month of the number of patient care hours required every day by category of patient, calculated by multiplying the corresponding figures in area 1 by the estimated patient care hours required by each category.

Area 7: The number of patient care hours required on the average day during the month in each category and total, calculated by dividing the corresponding figure in area 6 by the number of days in the month.

Figure 2
Sample Monthly Report I
JUNE, 1985
average daily census, average daily staffing,
and
classified patient days, and classified patient care hours:
total, averages and percents

UNIT 3rd	(re-al) adc	ads	total classified census in month						average per day						mean per pat.	percent of total					
			I	II	III	IV	V	total	I	II	III	IV	V	tot		I	II	III	IV	V	tot
patient days	34.7	21.8	168	314	384	177	29	1072	5.6	10.5	12.8	5.9	1.0	35.7		16	29	36	17	3	100
pt care hrs			235.2	847.8	2112.0	1451.4	321.9	4968.3	7.8	28.3	70.4	48.4	10.7	166	4.6	5	17	43	29	6	100

Area 8: The number of nursing care hours needed per 24 hours by the average patient on the average day.

Area 9: The percentage distribution of patient care hours required during the month, calculated by expressing each of the five categories of area 6 as a percentage of the total of area 6.

The second table (see Figure 3) has the following 17 areas of information:

Area 1: The number of patients in each classification level and the total classified census each day.

Area 2: The real census on the unit as of midnight that day.

Area 3: The percentage of patients classified. If this is under 100 percent, some patients on the unit were not classified. If this is over 100 percent, more patients were classified than actually were on the unit. Discrepancies may be due to errors or to a difference in the hour at which the census is determined by the nursing and accounting departments.

Areas 4, 7, 10, and 13: Respectively, the number of patient care hours required during days, afternoons, midnights, and all shifts combined; these figures are calculated by multiplying the number of patients classified in each category by the number of hours of care required, summing over all categories and allocating a percentage of the total hours to each shift.

Areas 5, 8, 11, and 14: The number of hours of care available from nursing personnel (based on actual staffing) during days, afternoons, midnights, and all shifts, respectively, calculated by multiplying the number of FTE personnel by seven hours.

Areas 6, 9, 12, and 15: The percentage of care rendered based on the hours of care available.

Area 16: The number of FTE staff available on all shifts combined.

Area 17: The information given in areas 1 through 16 for the average day in the month.

The third table (see Fig. 4) has twelve areas of information, as follows:

Areas 1, 2, 3, and 4: The number of staff members available for each staff category—RN, LPN, rehabilitation nursing aide (RNA), nursing technician (NT), and unit aide (UA)—and total, on the average day of the month, during days, afternoons, midnights, and all shifts combined, respectively.

Areas 5, 6, 7, and 8: The percentage distribution of staff available on the average day of the month.

Figure 3
Sample Monthly Report II

JUNE, 1985

number of patients (patient days), classified and real
census, and PCH with NCH per shift, each day and ave. month

UNIT 3rd	classified census						real cen-sus-fd	% cls	day shift			evening shift			night shift			all shifts			# of staff
date	I	II	III	IV	V	tot (1)	(2)	(3)	pch (4)	nch (5)	% (6)	pch (7)	nch (8)	% (9)	pch (10)	nch (11)	% (12)	pch (13)	nch (14)	% (15)	(16)
06/01/85	8	6	9	5	1	29	29	100	70.9	63.0	89	38.7	42.0	109	19.3	21.0	109	129.0	126.00	98	18.0
06/02/85	8	6	9	5	1	29	29	110	70.0	56.0	79	44.8	42.0	94	19.3	28.0	125	129.0	126.00	98	18.0
06/03/85	7	7	11	6	1	32	31	106	82.2	77.0	94	44.8	63.0	142	22.4	28.0	126	149.5	147.00	98	21.0
06/04/85	8	8	10	6	1	33	31	106	81.5	77.0	94	44.4	63.0	113	22.2	28.0	113	148.1	168.00	113	24.0
06/05/85	6	7	12	7	1	35	35	106	90.5	91.0	101	49.4	56.0	113	24.7	28.0	113	164.4	175.00	106	25.0
06/06/85	6	9	13	9	1	38	36	104	77.0	77.0	74	56.7	56.0	99	28.4	28.0	99	189.1	161.00	85	23.0
06/07/85	4	10	15	8	0	39	36	108	100.9	84.0	83	55.0	49.0	89	27.5	21.0	77	183.5	161.00	88	23.0
06/08/85	4	10	13	8	1	36	36	100	99.4	56.0	56	54.2	52.5	97	27.1	28.0	103	180.8	129.50	72	18.5
06/09/85	6	14	12	5	0	38	36	109	99.4	56.0	56	54.2	45.5	84	27.1	28.0	103	180.8	129.50	72	18.5
06/10/85	7	15	13	5	0	39	37	105	86.5	77.0	85	49.3	49.0	99	24.6	28.0	114	164.3	154.00	94	22.0
06/11/85	5	15	13	5	0	39	37	105	88.8	84.0	89	47.2	63.0	133	23.6	28.0	119	157.3	168.00	107	24.0
06/12/85	5	16	13	6	0	40	39	103	88.8	84.0	95	48.4	56.0	116	24.2	28.0	116	161.4	168.00	104	24.0
06/13/85	5	13	13	6	0	37	39	100	94.0	84.0	89	51.3	49.0	96	25.6	28.0	109	170.9	161.00	94	23.0
06/14/85	6	11	15	5	0	37	37	100	89.5	77.0	86	48.8	49.0	100	24.4	28.0	115	162.8	154.00	95	22.0
06/15/85	6	11	15	5	0	37	37	100	88.9	56.0	63	48.5	42.0	87	24.2	21.0	87	161.6	119.00	74	17.0
06/16/85	6	12	15	5	0	38	38	100	90.4	56.0	63	49.3	45.5	94	24.2	28.0	116	161.6	129.50	80	18.5
06/17/85	7	12	15	5	0	38	38	100	90.4	84.0	93	49.3	49.0	99	24.6	35.0	142	164.3	168.00	102	24.0
06/18/85	7	12	15	6	0	40	39	103	90.4	84.0	93	49.3	49.0	99	24.6	28.0	114	164.3	161.00	98	23.0
06/19/85	7	11	15	6	0	39	39	100	95.6	91.0	95	52.2	49.0	94	26.1	35.0	134	173.9	175.00	101	25.0
06/20/85	7	11	15	6	0	39	39	100	94.2	98.0	104	51.4	56.0	109	25.7	35.0	136	171.2	189.00	110	27.0
06/21/85	6	9	13	5	0	33	33	118	79.9	84.0	89	51.4	56.0	109	25.7	28.0	109	171.2	168.00	98	24.0
06/22/85	6	9	13	5	0	33	33	100	79.9	56.0	70	43.6	42.0	96	21.8	28.0	128	145.2	126.00	87	18.0
06/23/85	6	13	13	6	2	37	35	106	99.6	77.0	77	54.3	56.0	103	21.8	28.0	128	145.2	126.00	87	18.0
06/24/85	2	10	13	6	3	34	33	103	101.1	91.0	90	55.1	56.0	102	27.6	35.0	129	181.1	168.00	93	24.0
06/25/85	4	12	12	6	3	35	34	103	99.6	84.0	84	54.3	49.0	90	27.2	28.0	103	183.8	182.00	99	26.0
06/26/85	3	10	12	6	3	34	35	97	98.8	77.0	78	53.9	56.0	104	27.0	28.0	104	179.7	161.00	90	23.0
06/27/85	4	11	12	6	3	36	32	113	101.1	84.0	83	55.1	56.0	102	27.6	28.0	101	183.8	168.00	91	24.0
06/28/85	2	10	11	5	3	31	31	100	90.5	52.5	58	49.4	45.5	92	24.7	28.0	113	164.6	126.00	77	18.0
06/29/85	2	11	11	5	3	31	31	100	90.5	52.5	58	49.4	45.5	92	24.7	31.5	128	164.6	129.50	79	18.5
06/30/85	2	10	11	5	3	31	31	100	90.5	52.5	58	49.4	45.5	92	24.7	31.5	128	164.6	129.50	79	18.5
mean or %	5.6	10	13	5.9	.97	35.7	34.7	103	91.1	74.0	81	49.7	50.3	101	24.8	28.6	115	165.6	152.8	92	21.8

17

Figure 4
Sample Monthly Report IV

AUGUST, 1985
number of staff available, average per day
absolute and percentages, by shift and category
and
average nursing care hours available per patient
by shift and category

UNIT 3rd	day shift						evening shift						night shift						all shifts					
	rn	lpn	rna	nt	ua	tot	rn	lpn	rna	nt	ua	tot	rn	lpn	rna	nt	ua	tot	rn	lpn	rna	nt	ua	tot
averages	1.39	2.35	5.87	.387	0.00	10.0	.59	1.89	4.03	.152	0.00	7.66	1.03	.645	2.06	.355	0.00	4.10	4.01	4.89	12.0	.894	0.00	21.8
percents	14	24	59	4	0	100	21	25	53	2	0	100	25	16	50	9	0	100	18	22	55	4	0	100
nch/pat	.29	.49	1.23	.08	0.00	2.09	.33	.40	.84	.03	0.00	1.61	.22	.14	.43	.07	0.00	.86	.84	1.02	2.51	.19	0.00	4.56

Areas 9, 10, 11, and 12: The number of nursing care hours available per average patient, from each category of staff and the total, on the average day of the month, during days, afternoons, midnights, and all shifts combined, respectively.

Area 12: The total—the number of nursing care hours available per patient in 24 hours for the average day of the month.

The fourth table (see Fig. 5) contains 15 areas of information.

Areas 1, 2, 3, and 4: The number of personnel available in each category (RN, LPN, RNA, NT, UA) and the total for days, afternoons, midnights, and all shifts combined, respectively, for each day of the month.

Area 5: The total number of personnel available per shift for every day of the month.

Areas 6, 7, 8, and 9: The average number of personnel available for days, afternoons, midnights, and all shifts, respectively, for the month.

Area 10: The average total number of personnel available for days, afternoons, and midnights, respectively, for the month.

Areas 11, 12, 13, and 14: The average percentage distribution of nursing care hours available per category of personnel.

Area 15: The percentage distribution of staff over each shift on the average day.

These monthly summaries are distributed to nursing department administrators, supervisors, and managers and to hospital administrators. Depending on their interests and scope of responsibility within the organization, they will focus on different aspects. For example, a head nurse will want to focus on the report shown in Figure 4 to determine whether there are any patterns or trends regarding patient acuity and census in relationship to days of the week. If she determines that there are peak admission days or peak discharge days, she might want to change the pattern or adjust the staffing patterns to meet the needs. This table also makes it easy for the manager to compare, between shifts, the care that is needed versus the care that is available in relationship to the days of the week. She can make adjustment in the work assignments between shifts or can adjust staffing to meet the needs.

A head nurse might also want to focus on the report depicted in Figure 5, which presents the number of nursing personnel (FTEs) per category that worked per shift each day of the month. The head nurse, while monitoring the personnel mix per shift, can also compare the numbers of existing personnel to the budgeted positions in each category of per-

Figure 5
Sample Monthly Report IV

JUNE, 1985
number of FTE in each category, by shift and total
for each day and mean and percentage, whole month

unit 3rd		day shift						evening shift						night shift						all shifts						all levels		
date		rn	lpn	rna	nt	ua	tot	rn	lpn	rna	nt	ua	tot	rn	lpn	rna	nt	ua	tot	rn	lpn	rna	nt	ua	tot	day	eve	nite
06/01/85		1.0	2.0	6.0	0	0	0	9.0	1.0	1.0	4.0	0	0	0	6.0	1.0	0	0	2.0	0	0	0	3.0	3.0	3.0	12	0	0	0	18	9.0	6.0	3.0
06/02/85		2.0	2.0	5.0	0	0	0	8.0	1.0	1.0	4.0	0	0	0	6.0	2.0	0	0	2.0	0	0	0	4.0	4.0	3.0	11	0	0	0	18	8.0	6.0	4.0
06/03/85		1.0	3.0	7.0	0	0	0	11.0	1.0	1.0	4.0	0	0	0	6.0	1.0	1.0	2.0	0	0	0	4.0	4.0	4.0	13	0	0	0	21	11.0	6.0	4.0
06/04/85		1.0	3.0	7.0	0	0	0	9.0	3.0	1.0	4.0	0	0	0	9.0	1.0	1.0	2.0	0	0	0	4.0	5.0	4.0	13	0	0	0	24	11.0	9.0	4.0
06/05/85		2.0	3.0	8.0	0	0	0	13.0	2.0	1.0	5.0	0	0	0	8.0	1.0	1.0	2.0	0	0	0	4.0	5.0	5.0	15	0	0	0	25	13.0	8.0	4.0
06/06/85		2.0	3.0	7.0	0	0	0	11.0	2.0	1.0	5.0	0	0	0	8.0	1.0	1.0	2.0	0	0	0	4.0	5.0	5.0	14	0	0	0	23	11.0	8.0	4.0
06/07/85		2.0	3.0	7.0	0	0	0	12.0	2.0	2.0	4.0	0	0	0	7.0	1.0	1.0	2.0	0	0	0	4.0	4.0	6.0	13	0	0	0	23	12.0	7.0	4.0
06/08/85		1.0	2.0	5.0	0	0	0	8.0	1.0	1.5	5.0	0	0	0	7.5	1.0	1.0	1.0	0	0	0	3.0	3.0	4.5	11	0	0	0	19	8.0	7.5	3.0
06/09/85		1.0	2.0	5.0	0	0	0	8.0	1.5	1.0	4.0	0	0	0	6.5	1.0	1.0	1.0	0	0	0	3.0	3.5	4.0	11	0	0	0	19	8.0	6.5	3.0
06/10/85		2.0	2.0	7.0	0	0	0	11.0	2.0	1.0	4.0	0	0	0	7.0	1.0	1.0	2.0	0	0	0	4.0	5.0	4.0	13	0	0	0	22	11.0	7.0	4.0
06/11/85		2.0	2.0	7.0	0	0	0	12.0	2.0	1.0	5.0	0	0	0	8.0	1.0	1.0	2.0	0	0	0	4.0	5.0	4.0	14	0	0	0	24	12.0	8.0	4.0
06/12/85		2.0	2.0	8.0	0	0	0	12.0	2.0	1.0	5.0	0	0	0	8.0	1.0	1.0	2.0	0	0	0	4.0	5.0	4.0	15	0	0	0	24	12.0	8.0	4.0
06/13/85		1.0	2.0	5.0	0	0	0	8.0	1.0	1.0	5.0	0	0	0	7.0	1.0	1.0	1.0	0	0	0	3.0	3.0	4.0	11	0	0	0	22	11.0	7.0	3.0
06/14/85		2.0	2.0	7.0	0	0	0	8.0	1.0	1.0	4.0	0	0	0	7.0	0	1.0	2.0	1.0	0	0	4.0	3.0	4.0	13	1.0	0	0	23	11.0	7.0	4.0
06/15/85		1.0	2.0	5.0	0	0	0	8.0	1.0	2.0	4.0	0	0	0	6.0	0	1.0	2.0	0	0	0	3.0	3.0	4.0	10	0	0	0	17	8.0	6.0	3.0
06/16/85		2.0	2.0	8.0	0	0	0	8.0	1.0	1.5	4.0	0	0	0	6.5	1.0	0	3.0	0	0	0	4.0	3.5	4.0	11	0	0	0	19	8.0	6.5	3.0
06/17/85		2.0	2.0	8.0	0	0	0	12.0	2.0	1.0	4.0	0	0	0	7.0	0	2.0	2.0	1.0	0	0	4.0	4.0	5.0	14	1.0	0	0	24	12.0	7.0	4.0
06/18/85		2.0	2.0	8.0	0	0	0	12.0	2.0	2.0	3.0	0	0	0	7.0	1.0	1.5	2.0	0	0	0	5.0	5.0	5.0	15	0	0	0	25	12.0	7.0	5.0
06/19/85		2.0	2.0	9.0	0	0	0	13.0	2.0	2.0	4.0	0	0	0	8.0	2.0	0	3.0	0	0	0	5.0	5.0	6.0	16	0	0	0	27	13.0	8.0	5.0
06/20/85		2.0	3.0	9.0	0	0	0	14.0	2.0	2.0	4.0	0	0	0	8.0	0	1.0	3.0	1.0	0	0	5.0	4.0	5.0	15	1.0	0	0	24	12.0	8.0	5.0
06/21/85		1.0	3.0	8.0	0	0	0	8.0	2.0	2.0	4.0	0	0	0	6.0	2.0	0	3.0	0	0	0	4.0	5.0	5.0	11	0	0	0	18	8.0	6.0	4.0
06/22/85		1.0	2.0	5.0	0	0	0	8.0	1.5	1.0	3.5	0	0	0	6.0	2.0	0	2.0	0	0	0	4.0	3.5	3.0	11	0	0	0	18	8.0	6.0	4.0
06/23/85		1.0	2.0	5.0	0	0	0	8.0	1.5	1.0	3.0	0	0	0	6.0	1.0	0	2.0	0	0	0	4.0	3.5	3.0	11	1.0	0	0	24	11.0	8.0	5.0
06/24/85		1.0	2.0	5.0	0	0	0	11.0	1.0	3.0	4.0	0	0	0	8.0	1.0	1.0	3.0	0	0	0	5.0	3.0	4.0	13	0	0	0	24	11.0	8.0	5.0
06/25/85		2.0	3.0	8.0	0	0	0	13.0	1.0	3.0	4.0	0	0	0	8.0	1.0	3.0	1.0	0	0	0	5.0	4.0	7.0	15	0	0	0	26	13.0	8.0	5.0
06/26/85		2.0	3.0	8.0	0	0	0	13.0	1.0	2.0	4.0	0	0	0	7.0	1.0	0	1.0	1.0	0	0	4.0	4.0	5.0	14	1.0	0	0	24	13.0	7.0	4.0
06/27/85		2.0	2.0	7.0	0	0	0	11.0	2.0	2.0	4.0	0	0	0	8.0	0	2.0	2.0	0	0	0	4.0	4.0	6.0	13	0	0	0	23	11.0	8.0	4.0
06/28/85		2.0	2.0	8.0	0	0	0	12.0	2.0	3.0	3.0	0	0	0	8.0	2.0	0	2.0	0	0	0	4.0	4.0	5.0	14	0	0	0	24	12.0	8.0	4.0
06/29/85		1.0	2.0	5.0	0	0	0	7.5	1.5	1.0	4.0	0	0	0	6.5	2.0	0	2.0	0	0	0	4.0	4.5	3.0	11	0	1.5	0	18	7.5	6.5	4.0
06/30/85		1.0	2.0	4.0	0	0	0	7.5	1.5	1.0	4.0	0	0	0	6.5	2.0	0	1.0	1.0	0	0	4.5	3.5	3.5	10	1.5	0	0	19	7.5	6.5	4.5
aver		1.6	2.3	6.7	.03	0	0	11	1.5	1.7	4.0	0	0	0	7.2	1.0	.62	2.2	.23	0	0	4.1	4.1	4.6	13	.27	0	0	22	10.6	7.18	4.08
PCT		15	21	63	0	0	0	100	20	24	56	0	0	0	100	24	15	55	6	0	0	100	19	21	59	1	0	0	100	48	33	19

day shift   evening shift   night shift   all shifts   all levels sonnel throughout the year in order to pick up problems before the end of the fiscal year. She can also compare this table to the scheduled staffing to determine any discrepancies and investigate the cause.

The director of nursing would have a wider scope and would be interested in monthly averages of *all* units. She would focus on the bottom lines of the reports in Figure 4 and 5 to get a global picture of how the units compare to each other. It would be important for her to monitor monthly averages to determine if there are any yearly trends in patient census, patient acuity, or staffing. It could be detrimental, for example, to have a pattern of higher patient census in August, at the same time that patient acuity increased and staffing decreased. The director of nursing would also want to monitor the percentage of care each unit was able to give (based on the hours of care needed and the hours available). If the percentage fell below an acceptable standard, the manager of the unit would have to explain the cause and develop a plan to correct the problem, and the quality of care on that unit would be closely monitored during that time. The director of nursing also utilizes patient classification data over a year to justify the need to maintain or increase the department's budgeted positions.

The hospital administrator would focus on the report shown in Figure 2 to see monthly averages for patient acuity and the need for nursing care per unit and for the hospital as a whole. The emphasis in examining the report illustrated in Figure 3 would be the monthly average for staffing patterns per shift per unit. The hospital administrator would be interested in all the areas the director of nursing reviews and more. For example, if there was a need to develop a specialty unit, the monthly summary would be the resource used to determine where the unit should be placed, based on acuity trends, staffing trends, and specific unit trends. The administrator can use the patient classification data for both long- and short-term planning for the institute.

Ad hoc reports may be generated to supply additional tabulations of data for any of the purposes described or for other management needs. For example, the administration of the Rehabilitation Institute recently wanted to assess the impact of the implementation of diagnosis related groups (DRGs) in acute care on the nursing care requirements of rehabilitation patients. Historical data for the years 1982–85 produced by the patient classification system were reviewed and the annual average amounts of nursing care hours needed by unit and for the hospital as a whole were compared (see Fig. 6). It was expected that the hours needed per patient would increase over this period, especially after implementation of the DRG system. This hypothesis was based on the assumption that patients were being discharged earlier from acute-care facilities to the rehabilitation hospital. Therefore, the average patient at

Figure 6
Yearly Average of Patient Care Hours Needed, per Patient per Day, and Daily Census, by Unit

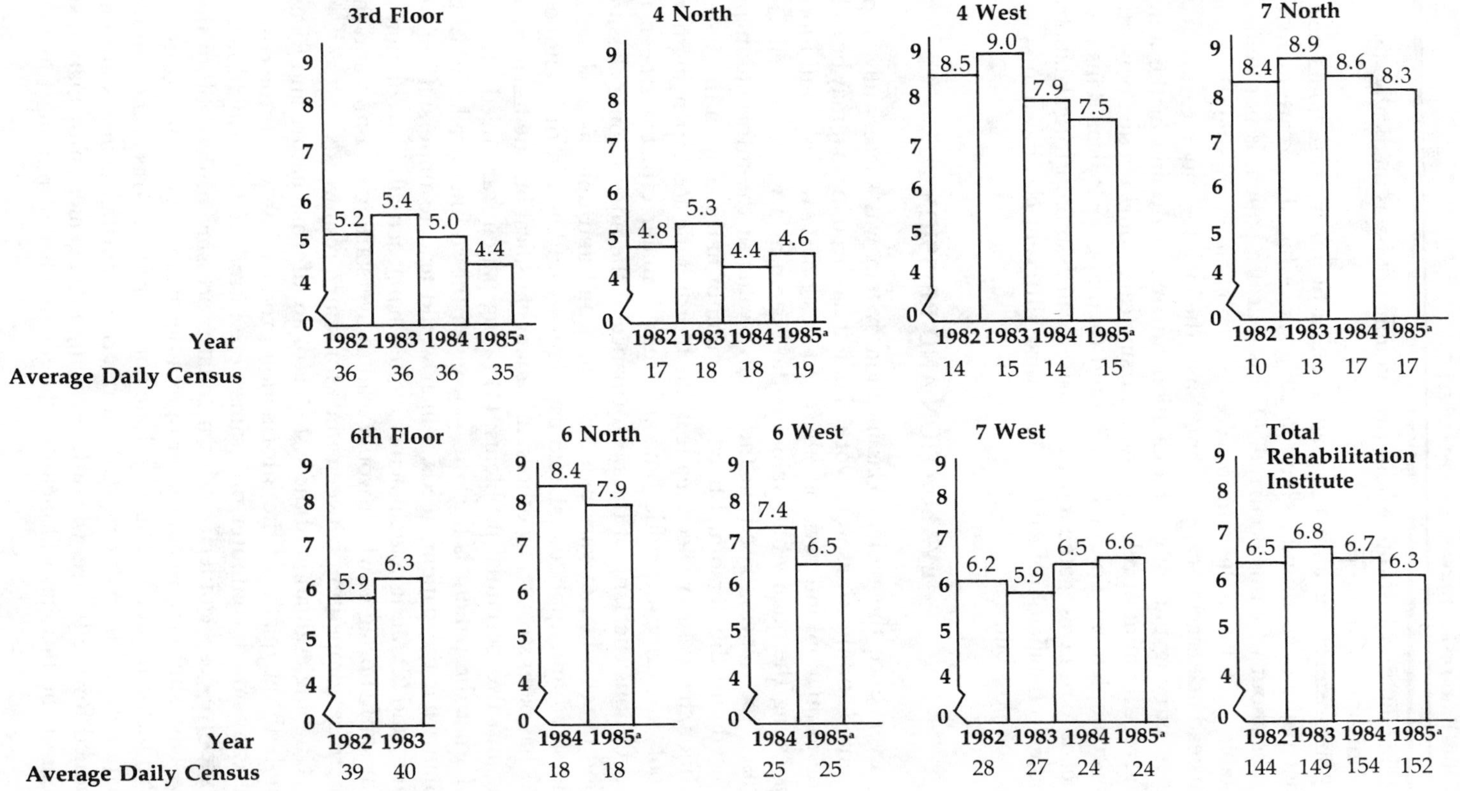

[a]Figures for 1985 are for January through May only.

Rehabilitation Institute would presumably not be as medically stable on admission as in the past.

Surprisingly, the annual average number of nursing care hours needed per patient was found to have *declined* somewhat. There are many theories about why this occurred. One is that if a patient is not medically stable, then he or she can not receive rehabilitation nursing; the patient instead needs acute-care nursing. Since the tool does not measure acute-care nursing but only rehabilitation nursing, a decline in the annual average amount of rehabilitation nursing care hours needed per patient since implementation of DRGs would then appear logical. This theory needs to be investigated more extensively; analysis of historical data from other rehabilitation facilities that utilize different classification systems is one possibility.

EVALUATION AND REVISION

Ever since the patient classification system was successfully implemented and the kinks were worked out, it has been in what may be called the evaluation and revision phase. In this phase, we are continuously assessing the quality and value of the system as a whole as well as its cost-effectiveness, based on the relative value of the information produced and the personnel needed to monitor and maintain the system. Minor changes have been made in the tool and the accompanying handbook to clarify difficulties encountered. A major effort has been the continuous checking of the performance of the nurses doing classification to see whether various nurses on a unit and units as a whole understand and apply the system as originally outlined in the handbook. As has been stressed by others, in patient classification one has to guard against two perennial problems: (1) rating patient care needs in terms of what the patient is likely to get, given the staffing available, rather than what the patient needs, which would lead to understaffing of a unit; and (2) rating patient acuity higher than it actually is to compensate for staff shortages, which would lead to overstaffing of a unit and thus increase competition between units for scarce resources.

Ongoing evaluation of the system is of an informal nature and focuses on both the quality of the information produced as well as the cost. As already noted, computer programs were introduced to bring down the excessive costs connected with manual processing of data. Since then, we have shifted most computer operations from a mainframe computer to a microcomputer. This was done both to reduce costs and to simplify data entry, thus reducing data-entry errors. Further changes are envisioned for the future, when the growing management information system of the hospital will include a larger number of nursing functions.

REHABILITATION NURSING   291

We envision as the ultimate development a system whereby floor nurses classify their patients using a touch-sensitive computer screen on which the tool is presented. Totaling of classification points over units and calculating staff requirements would be an automated function, and the end result would be a report on staffing requirements printed in the nursing administration office. The technology to do these things is available; it is a question of waiting for it to be economically feasible.

If the time it takes to do a specific nursing task depends on such factors as type of patient, physical layout of the hospital, and nursing care delivery approach (Giovannetti, 1979), then a change in any of these factors may result in a need to change one's patient classification system. Since the Rehabilitation Institute system was introduced on all units, we have seen the following changes: introduction of new specialty units for spinal cord injury, geriatrics, chronic pain, and musculoskeletal disorders, with resulting changes in patient mix; some modification in the physical environment, such as satellite therapy areas; and changes in the personnel mix and nursing care delivery approach, often concomitant with the introduction of new specialty units. To determine whether the items on the tool still are the nursing tasks that take up the majority of the staff's time and whether the point values are still realistic, we need to repeat most of the original studies. At the time of writing, we are planning new frequency tallies and observation studies. This is expected to be a major rather than a minor revision of the tool, because we are considering changes in the way teaching and therapeutic communication are handled.

Teaching is currently an item within each of the seven areas of the tool. Therapeutic communication, including spiritual and emotional support, is not an explicit item but is factored into the point value of all teaching items. As part of the revision of the tool, we plan to consider whether these items should be handled in a different way, with a more finely graduated point system.

Teaching performed by nurses in a rehabilitation environment typically is integrated with and done as part of physical care. As such, teaching is generally done in small increments of time each day, rather than in the large blocks the current system assumes; teaching, as a task, typically rates 4 points, or about one hour of care. Also, the current tool does not permit adding points for teaching if an activity with medium point value is checked—for example, "teach medications with complex medications." In practice, this leads to insufficient "reward" in many instances.

We expect that these and similar changes will maintain the relevance of Rehabilitation Institute's patient classification system to the type of patients the institute serves, as well as the nature of the nursing care it provides. The value of the nursing system and its continued acceptance by nursing staff and management depends on such adjustments as well as the cost-effectiveness, reliability, and usefulness of the information produced.

REFERENCES

Audette, L., Carle, J., Simard, A., & Tilquin, G. (1978). *User's guide to the evaluation form of the level of nursing care required by the patient.* Montreal, Quebec, Canada: University of Montreal, Équipe de Recherche Opérationnelle en Santé.

Burgher, D., & Hanson, R. L. (1980, May–June). Patient classification for nurse staffing in rehabilitation. *Association of Rehabilitation Nurses Journal, 5*(3), 16–20.

Cisarik, J. M., Higgerson, N. J., & Van Slyck, A. (1978). *A patient classification system for nursing services.* Phoenix, AZ: St. Luke's Hospital Medical Center.

Giovannetti, P. (1979, February). Understanding patient classification systems. *Journal of Nursing Administration, 9*(2), 4–9.

Jordan, H. S., & McCoy, C. (1984, October). *Time study—Direct patient care using acuity level and disability as variables.* Paper presented at the 61st Annual Session of the American Congress of Rehabilitation Medicine, Boston, MA.

Meyer, D. (1978). *GRASP: A patient information and workload management system.* Morgantown, NC: MCS.

Plummer, J. (1976, May). Patient classification proves staffing needs. *Dimensions in Health Services, 53*(5) 36–38.

Schuster, L. (1984, October). *Patient classification index.* Paper presented at the 61st Annual Session of the American Congress of Rehabilitation Medicine, Boston, MA.

Tilquin, C. Audette, L, Carle, J., & Lambert, P. (1978). *User's guide to the measurement module for staff required on each unit for each work shift.* Montreal, Quebec, Canada: University of Montreal, Equipe de Recherche Opérationnelle en Santé.

Torrez, M. R. (1983, May). Systems approach to staffing. *Nursing Management, 14*(5), 54–58.

A Patient Classification Tool
for Maternity Services

Mary B. Killeen

Patient classification devices play an important part in prospective payment systems and hospital reimbursement. At first glance prospective reimbursement and diagnosis related groups (DRGs) do not appear to have much impact on maternity services because federal legislation affects only Medicare reimbursement. Any lack of impact is only temporary, however, because (1) an increasing number of states are including Medicaid patients in a DRG-type reimbursement formula, and (2) hospitals' financial information systems are increasingly based on DRG data bases. Consequently, a patient classification tool that is reliable and valid is essential to the clinical and fiscal decision making of efficient and effective nurse managers in maternity services as well as elsewhere in the hospital.

The Joint Commission on Accreditation of Hospital's requirement that nursing departments have a patient classification system, as well as the importance placed on these instruments by the hospital industry, provide compelling evidence for all nursing departments, especially specialty services, to examine what they need to do to determine patient care requirements. In the study described in this paper, a maternity patient classification tool was tested for reliability and validity.

Patient classification is defined as the categorization of patients according to an objective assessment of the level of their nursing care requirements (Giovannetti, 1979). Patient classification systems are used to predict staffing needs. Patients are placed in a particular category based on the amount of time their care requires or by descriptive criteria of the acuity of their condition. From the number of patients in each category, the number of nursing care hours required is calculated. These numbers determine the number of staff needed to care for a particular group of patients.

Classification of maternity patients is a unique problem because their nursing care requirements are qualitatively and quantitatively different from those of other patients in the hospital. Maternity services, with essentially well patients, rate low in priority in the acute-care environment of most hospitals. The needs of patients in a maternity service are the opposite of those of medical-surgical patients, because emotional and teaching needs take first priority with new mothers and infants. Medical care needs are minimal, and physical care needs are met largely through self-care with guidance and assistance. Moreover, the "patient" is in reality a family: the mother, her unborn or newborn child, and the significant others. Finally, nursing care needs are complex because in the routine hospital stay the mother is seen in four stages of childbearing, which correspond to the hospital units of antepartum, labor and delivery, postpartum, and nursery.

PATIENT CLASSIFICATION

In a definitive review of nursing staffing methodologies, Aydelotte (1973) reported on 41 patient classification studies. She noted that classification schemes generally are built around the following variables: (1) capabilities of patients for caring for themselves, (2) special characteristics of the patients, (3) acuity of illness, (4) skill level of personnel required in patient care, and (5) placement of the patient. Patient classification techniques developed since 1973 have been similar, mainly providing for computerization of earlier methods. The systems usually classify patients into three or four levels of care, based on physical and psychosocial needs, medical diagnosis, and therapy and teaching-learning requirements. Young, Giovannetti, Lewison, and Thomas (1981) conclude that patient classification devices, while not a panacea, have widespread application and are essential for adequate monitoring of costs.

Many patient classification systems use indicators of physical care alone. These systems assume that the caregiver meets the patient's emotional and teaching needs while providing the technical aspects of care (Giovannetti, 1979). Other systems account for both teaching-learning needs and emotional or psychosocial needs, including those used by Georgette (1970), Holbrook (1972), and Thomas (1971) and the widely used CASH system (DesOrmeaux, 1977).

Patient classification systems that are adaptable to the maternity units of the hospital are rare. Most schemes are devised for use on medical-surgical floors or, infrequently, in pediatrics (Clark, 1971). Warstler (1972) included separate sets of definitions for the medical-surgical patient, the maternity patient, the newborn infant, and the psychiatric patient. All items, however, are based on physical needs only. No patient classifications were found for maternity patients that include assessment of psychological and teaching-learning needs.

MATERNITY PATIENT CLASSIFICATION TOOL

The patient classification instruments for maternity services in this study have evolved over five years through two research studies (Cleland, Marz, & Killeen, 1984; Killeen, 1980) and use in a metropolitan Detroit hospital with a high volume of maternity patients (4,000 deliveries annually).

In a 1979 study to determine the adequacy of nurse staffing on maternity units (Killeen, 1980), five advanced maternity graduate students, including the author, constructed four maternity patient classification tools for antepartum, labor and delivery, postpartum, and newborn patients.[1] The tools were believed to be fairly good indicators of nursing care requirements but were not tested for interrater reliability or validity.

In 1980 the author implemented the four tools in a large maternity service in a suburban Detroit teaching hospital. The criteria statements in all four tools were modified somewhat, initially by expert clinicians in the hospital and later at the time of a six-month evaluation. After one year, nursing hours per patient day were determined for level 1, 2, and 3 patients. These data were used to predict staffing and for budgetary cost forecasting, using the hospital's computerized system.

The resulting Killeen maternity patient classification tool (composed of the four original individual tools) is specific for maternity patients for the following reasons:

1. It reflects the psychosocial and informational needs of these essentially well patients.

2. The care needs are those with which maternity nursing is concerned and are not defined in the language of another discipline.

3. The tool is adaptable to the family-centered care approach using couplet care or traditional nursery-postpartum units.

4. The Killeen tool was designed to reflect regionalization in perinatal care. Careful attention was given to the range and com-

---

[1]The author wishes to acknowledge the contributions of the students, J. French, V. Denniston, L. Thede, and C. Feenstra, to the initial development of the original tools.

plexity of services that level I, II, and III hospitals provide. The categorization that results from the use of the tool can be related to the intensity of care provided by the institution. For example, level III hospitals will have patients representing all three levels of nursing care needs, but level I hospitals should have few level 2 and no level 3 patients if proper patient referrals have been implemented.

The maternity tool was designed to differentiate maternity patients into groups that require different levels of nursing expertise and thus to be related to levels of nurse competency. As with other patient classification tools, it does not reflect all of a patient's nursing needs. The tool's components serve as indicators of a larger grouping of care requirements that differentiate the care needed for different levels of patients.

In the postpartum and infant classification tools, the assessment criteria for differentiating the complexity of a patient's nursing needs across the childbearing stages are grouped into five separate dimensions of nursing care: teaching, counseling, physical care, technical monitoring, and advanced clinical observation and decision making (see Figs. 1 and 2).

The dimension of teaching includes the patient's need for information about infant care and self-care. Counseling refers to assisting the family in developing adaptive mechanisms in their new status. As in other patient classification systems, the physical care dimension refers mainly to the patient's dependency needs. Technical observation-monitoring involves all types of monitoring and often depends on medical orders. Advanced clinical observation and decision making is related to physical and emotional problems of the patient that require independent nursing action and a high level of judgment.

Within each dimension, specific categories of patient care needs are assigned a score of 1 through 3, with 1 indicating least complex and 3 indicating most complex needs. Scores are totaled to give a cumulative score. Patients with a total score of 5 to 7 are classified into level 1, those with scores of 8 to 11 into level 2, and those with scores of 12 to 15 into level 3. The range of scores for each level was independently determined in the earlier study and finalized by group consensus. The higher the level, the more expert the nursing care needed. In general, level 1 patients require normal physical and emotional care and have many informational needs. Level 2 patients have an added potential to be at risk, but with proper monitoring and prevention are maintained with supportive care. They require specialized teaching, prioritization of needs, and technical skills. Level 3 patients require the highest level of care,

Figure 1
Patient Classification—Nursing Criteria
Postpartum
(Baby's needs not considered on this form)

Dimensions	Score	Categories
Teaching (individual needs, family realtionship)	____ 1	Comfortable—realistic concept of normal involution.
	____ 2	Fairly comfortable—needs reinforcement.
	____ 3	Uncomfortable—has multiple teaching needs.
Counseling (individual needs, family relationship)	____ 1	Motivated for self-care; reality acceptance; absence of anxiety.
	____ 2	2–3 areas of psychosocial need; requires guidance; developing awareness of reality; lack of support.
	____ 3	More than 3 areas of psychosocial needs; shock/denial; requires active crisis intervention
Physical care	____ 1	Self-care.
	____ 2	Partial or complete bath.
	____ 3	Complete bath and complex needs.
Technical monitoring (relates to medical care)	____ 1	More than 72 hours after cesarean section; more than 24 hours after vaginal delivery.
	____ 2	Less than 24 hours after vaginal delivery; less than 72 hours after cesarean section.
	____ 3	Medical complication.
Advanced clinical observation and decision making (relates to nursing orders)	____ 1	No variation in postpartum course.
	____ 2	1–2 variations in postpartum course.
	____ 3	Greater than 2 variations in postpartum course.
Total score	____	

Patient classification level	I	II	III
Score	5–7	8–11	12–15

including counseling, guidance, group teaching and reinforcement, and specific nursing interventions.

TESTING THE TOOL

A study conducted by Dr. Virginia Cleland of Wayne State University in Detroit (Cleland, Marz, & Killeen, 1985) provided an opportunity to test the modified postpartum and newborn classification tools for reliability and validity.

Two hospitals (labeled as Hospital A and Hospital B), one urban and one suburban, whose staff were willing to participate, were selected for the study. Both were private, not-for-profit hospitals with over 500 beds, and each had two postpartum and nursery units. Data were gathered one day each week over a five-week period, with a different day selected for each week. The first day of data collection on each unit was utilized

Figure 2
Patient Classification—Nursing Criteria
Infant
(Babies in neonatal intensive care units are excluded)

Dimensions	Score	Categories
Teaching	___ 1	Review of basic information; experienced mom with child under 4 years.
	___ 2	Parents interested in infant care needs; 1–2 areas of new knowledge.
	___ 3	Needs more than two areas of new knowledge.
Counseling	___ 1	Reality acceptance; absence of anxiety; bonding and caretaking established.
	___ 2	Developing awareness of reality; bonding being established; requires guidance.
	___ 3	Shock/denial; bonding not initiated; requires active crisis intervention.
Physical care	___ 1	Minimal needs; e.g., healthy vaginally delivered infant after 12 hours; cesarean section otherwise healthy after 24 hours.
	___ 2	Moderate needs; e.g., vaginal delivery less than 12 hours, cesarean section less than 24 hours; learning to nipple; infant with self-limiting complications such as hyperbilirubinemia with bililite Rx.
	___ 3	Complex needs.
Technical monitoring	___ 1	Healthy neonate; surveillance of normal physiological responses, e.g., healthy vaginally delivered infant over 12 hours; cesarean section otherwise healthy after 24 hours.
	___ 2	Surveillance for regulatory disorders and tolerance to specific treatments, e.g., healthy vaginally delivered infant less than 6 hours; healthy cesarean section less than 12 hours.
	___ 3	Surveillance utilizing monitoring equipment with constant nursing observation.
Advanced clinical observation and decision making	___ 1	Healthy infant: vaginal delivery over 12 hours; cesarean section over 24 hours. Premature infant 36–38 weeks with no other problem, over 12 hours.
	___ 2	Newborn with potential for a regulatory disorder; newborn 6–12 hours old.
	___ 3	Potential for two or more regulatory disorders; babies less than 6 hours; normal appearance with questionable history.
Total score	___	

Patient classification level	I	II	III
Score	5–7	8–11	12–15

as a trial to test procedures regarding the tools and method of collection. Therefore, final analysis consists of four days' data collected over a period of four weeks.

Nine nurse raters were selected by nursing middle managers at each hospital, using education and experience as the criteria. Three external raters were also used at each hospital. Criteria for their selection included an MSN degree with specialization in maternity nursing, a minimum of two years of relevant experience, and general familiarity with patient classification tools. They also had to be currently clinically active. The nine internal and three external raters each classified all subjects on all items of the Killeen tool.

Assessments using the tool were based upon data contained in patients' records and Kardexes. All raters were instructed to base their classifications on patient care requirements, not on nursing actions or lack of actions documented on the chart. Raters assessed a minimum of 20 mothers and 20 infants selected randomly on each unit by project staff. Patients were not interviewed. A patient was scored at the lowest level if documentation was not present. Because of shortages of personnel, some raters at Hospital B had had previous contact with the selected patients. Prior to data collection, all project participants and alternates attended training sessions. Actual patient records and Kardex entries were used in the training program. These practice records never involved patients later assigned as study subjects.

Raters were randomly assigned a time for each day of data collection. First raters began assessments at 10:30 a.m. and later raters were instructed to use 10:30 a.m. as a reference point for a patient's condition. Alternates, who attended the same training sessions, were used as necessary. Each rater required about two hours to read the records and Kardex entries and to then classify the 10 mothers and 10 infants.

DATA ANALYSIS

Reliability

Reliability of the tools was tested by examining the percentage of agreement among the raters on classification of mothers at both Hospital A and Hospital B. The number of agreements on the classification level of each patient was divided by the total possible number of agreements to give a percentage of agreement. The mean of the percentage of agreement on ratings of individual patients on the postpartum and infant tools at each hospital for each day of the study is reported in Tables 1 and 2. On the postpartum tool, Hospital A, with a mean percentage of agreement of 87 percent, had a higher level of interrater reliability than

Table 1
Raters' Percentage of Agreement on Postpartum Patient Classification Tool

Day	Classification Level		Total Classification Score (within one point)	
	Hospital A	Hospital B	Hospital A	Hospital B
1	86	84	74	74
2	87	84	84	68
3	92	84	84	78
4	85	76	75	70
Mean	87	82	79	73

Hospital B, with 82 percent. On the infant tool, Hospital B had the higher mean—84 percent as opposed to 78 percent for Hospital A.

For a more refined look than was possible using classification level, each patient's total score, which could range from 5 to 15, was examined for the percentage of ratings that fell within one point of each other. Again, Hospital A showed a higher level of interrater agreement on the postpartum tool (see Table 1), with a mean of 79 percent agreement compared to 73 percent for Hospital B. Hospital A also had a higher percentage of agreement on the infants' tool using this measure (see Table 2).

The reliability of the maternity patient classification tool was also tested by use of alpha coefficients (see Table 3). Consistency of the 12 raters was demonstrated by alpha coefficients of .66 to .89 for postpartum patients and .50 to .95 for infants. Except for the counseling item on the infants' tool at Hospital B, these alpha coefficients are considered high for a clinical study.

Table 2
Raters' Percentage of Agreement on Infants Classification Tool

Day	Classification Level		Total Classification Score (within one point)	
	Hospital A	Hospital B	Hospital A	Hospital B
1	78	80	83	71
2	84	91	80	74
3	86	82	81	81
4	65	81	67	67
Mean	78	84	78	73

Table 3
Internal Consistency of Items on the Killeen Maternity Classification
Tool (Alpha Coefficients)

Dimensions	Hospital A		Hospital B	
	Postpartum (N = 78)	Infants (N = 75)	Postpartum (N = 78)	Infants (N = 80)
Teaching	.88	.94	.79	.95
Counseling	.74	.75	.78	.50
Physical care	.88	.89	.82	.74
Technical monitoring	.84	.90	.89	.76
Advanced observation and decision making	.66	.87	.82	.73

Content Validity

The content validity of the maternity patient classification tool was established by a group of 12 nurses. This group consisted of the original three external raters, six of the original internal raters, plus three additional external raters. Nine of them had MSN degrees in maternity nursing, and three were maternity staff nurses at the local hospital that had used this tool for several years.

The questionnaire for establishing content validity of the postpartum and infant tools used a variation of the Porter (1962) technique of using stem questions to arrive at discrepancy scores for individual items on an instrument. This questionnaire measured the discrepancy between the extent to which an instrument should summarize the individual nursing care dimensions and the extent to which the instrument actually does summarize the nursing care dimensions. A portion of the questionnaire is shown in Figure 3. Respondents rated each item on a 5-point scale with 1 being "minimal extent"; 3, "moderate extent"; and 5, "large extent." A discrepant score (the rating of the extent to which the tool should summarize the nursing dimension minus the extent to which it does) was calculated for each nursing dimension item. Respondents were asked to rate the Killeen tool along with the maternity patient classification instruments in use for maternity patients at Hospital A and Hospital B. In Hospital A, an inhouse medical-surgical tool was adapted for maternity use, and Hospital B developed its own maternity tool. Neither tool was tested for reliability or validity or gave specific weighted attention to learning or counseling needs. The three tools, labeled tools A, B, and C, were included in the questionnaire to force members of the expert panel to make judgments. The questionnaire also asked respondents for

Circle the appropriate number.

PART I

1. To what extent should an instrument allow you to summarize the learning needs of the mother?

1	2	3	4	5
minimal		moderate		large

2. To what extent should an instrument allow you to summarize the emotional needs of the mother?

1	2	3	4	5
minimal		moderate		large

3. To what extent should an instrument allow you to summarize the care needs of the mother and infant?

1	2	3	4	5
minimal		moderate		large

4. To what extent should an instrument allow you to summarize the medical care needs for monitoring the mother and infant?

1	2	3	4	5
minimal		moderate		large

5. To what extent should an instrument allow you to summarize the nursing care needs for observation and decision making regarding the mother and infant?

1	2	3	4	5
minimal		moderate		large

PART II

Tool A

6. To what extent does this instrument allow you to summarize the learning needs of the mother?

1	2	3	4	5
minimal		moderate		large

7. To what extent does this instrument allow you to summarize the emotional needs of the mother?

1	2	3	4	5
minimal		moderate		large

8. To what extent does this instrument allow you to summarize the physical needs of the mother and infant?

1	2	3	4	5
minimal		moderate		large

9. To what extent does this instrument allow you to summarize the medical care needs for monitoring the mother and infant?

1	2	3	4	5
minimal		moderate		large

10. To what extent does this instrument allow you to summarize the nursing care needs for observation and decision making regarding the mother and infant?

1	2	3	4	5
minimal		moderate		large

comments and suggestions to improve the tools and to suggest items to include that were left out in their opinions.

Table 4 displays the mean discrepant scores of the 12 raters on each dimension of each tool. In addition a total mean score for each tool was calculated. Overall, the Killeen tool showed the lowest discrepant scores, ranging from .33 to .92. Discrepant scores for Tool A ranged from 1.00 to 2.25, and scores for Tool B ranged from .75 to 1.50. In all cases, except for technical monitoring (where Tool B had a lower score), the Killeen tool had the lowest discrepant score, indicating that it was closer to the ratings of what such a tool should cover than the other two tools. Moreover, based on their ratings on the "should" scale, all panelists agreed that counseling and teaching needs were as important or more important than the physical, technical monitoring, or nursing observation and decision making dimensions.

On a two-factor repeated measures analysis of variance, the main effect of type of tool (tool A, B, or C) was significant at the $p < .05$ level (see Table 5). The dimensions of the three tools taken alone were not found to be significant as expected. Discrepant scores varied across dimensions of the three tools ($p < .01$). Examination of the mean type of tool discrepancy rating indicated that the Killeen tool received a lower discrepancy rating than the other two tools.

CONCLUSIONS

The percentages of interrater agreement achieved by the maternity tool were based on four days spent at each institution by staff who were for the most part not assigned to the patients and using patients' records only. Nevertheless, the results would be acceptable to nursing administrators. For internal purposes, the percentage of agreement could be raised by increasing the raters' familiarity with the instrument through continued usage and by using staff actually assigned to the patients as raters. The stability of measurements by the instrument as determined over the four-week period demonstrates consistency. The high internal consistency of the items indicates more than adequate reliability. Content validity was established through the aid of a modified Porter format questionnaire.

As with all instruments, the reliability and validity of this tool is not an inherent property, but rather is established for use under different conditions or with different samples (Polit & Hungler, 1983, p. 386). Therefore, reliability and validity must be checked when instituting any tool in a new setting. The Porter format is helpful in making this task easier.

Finally, the results show the importance of assessing the learning and

Table 4
Content Validity: Mean Discrepant Scores of 12 Nurse Raters

Tool		Dimension			
	Teaching	Counseling	Physical	Technical Monitoring	Advanced Observation and Decision Making	Mean
Tool A	1.75	2.25	1.00	1.00	1.42	1.48
Tool B	1.50	1.25	.92	.75	1.50	1.18
Tool C (Killeen)	.33	.50	.92	.83	.67	.65

Table 5
Analysis of Variance

Source	Sum of Squares	Degrees of Freedom		Mean Squares	F-Ratio	Probability
Raters	98.594		11	8.963		
Tools	21.378	2		10.689	4.067	.031
Tools × Raters	57.822		22	2.628		
Dimensions	5.522	4		1.381	1.618	.187
Dimensions × Raters	37.544		44	0.853		
Tools × Dimensions	16.344	8		2.043	5.023	.001
Tools × Dimensions × Raters	35.790		88	0.407		
		14	154			
			11			

emotional needs of maternity patients and suggest that these needs should be considered essential criteria when evaluating tools used in a maternity service. With increasingly shortened postpartum hospital stays, patients' learning needs will most often be provided for during the prenatal and postnatal periods. While new mothers are hospitalized, patient classification tools that estimate the maternity patients' unique needs are essential.

REFERENCES

Aydelotte, M. K. (1973). *Nurse staffing methodology.* (Publication No. 73-433). Washington, D.C.: U.S. Government Printing Office.

Clark, L. E. (1977). A model of nurse staffing for effective patient care. *Journal of Nursing Administration, 7*(2), 22–27.

Cleland, V., Marz, M. S., & Killeen, M. B. (1985). A nurse staffing evaluation model. *Michigan Hospitals, 21*(2), 13–16.

Cleland, V., Marz, M. S., & Killeen, M. B. (1984). *Methodological studies relating to nurse staffing.* Unpublished manuscript.

DesOrmeaux, S. P. (1977). Implementation of C.A.S.H. patient classification system of staff determination. *Supervisor Nurse, 8*(4), 29–30, 33–35.

Georgette, J. K. (1970). Staffing by patient classification. *Nursing Clinics of North America, 5*(2), 329–339.

Giovannetti, P. (1979). Understanding patient classification systems. *Journal of Nursing Administration, 9*(2), 4–9.

Holbrook, F. K. (1972). Charging by level of nursing care. *Hospitals, 46,* 80–88.

Killeen, M. B. (1980). *Maternity nursing staffing as related to patient classification, unit activity, level of nursing competency and perception of adequacy of care.* Unpublished master's research paper, Wayne State University, Detroit, MI.

Polit, D. F., & Hungler, B. P. (1983). *Nursing research: Principles and methods.* Philadelphia: J. B. Lippincott.

Porter, L. W. (1962). Job attitudes in management. *Journal of Applied Psychology, 46,* 375–384.

Thomas, L. A. (1971). Predicting change in nursing values. *Journal of Nursing Administration, 1*(3), 50–58.

Warstler, M. E. (1972). Some management techniques for nursing service administrators. *Journal of Nursing Administration, 2*(6), 25–34.

Young, J., Giovannetti, P., Lewison, D., & Thomas, M. (1981). *Factors affecting nurse staffing in acute care hospitals: A review and critique of the literature.* Hyattsville, MD: Division of Nursing, U.S. Department of Health and Human Services.

Developing Cost Awareness in Nursing Students

Carole A. Mutzebaugh

The American Nurses' Association's 1980 *Social Policy Statement* on nursing elaborates the social contract between the profession of nursing and
the society in which nursing professionals practice. One of the social
forces that directs nursing today is the financing of health care. Because
of the emphasis on cost containment within the entire health care delivery system, the education of students preparing to enter health professions must include concepts of cost efficiency while maintaining the
effectiveness of care in order to demonstrate social responsibility.

In curricula crowded with knowledge essential for nursing practice,
how can information and values about cost-effective nursing care be
emphasized? What response can we give to employers who demand
greater awareness of these issues from newly graduated nurses? The
clinical exercise described in this paper identifies a method through
which students can become aware of the costs of nursing care and hospitalization.

NEED TO TEACH COST CONTAINMENT

Shortly before the initiation of diagnosis related groups (DRGs) for
Medicare patients in 1983, Davis (1983) predicted that nursing education
would have a reason to incorporate concepts of fiscal management and
cost-effective patient care into curriculum. Less than six months after
the implementation of prospective payment, Hamilton (1984), discussing

DRGs and hospital staffing, wrote: "There is a growing need to document the cost of specific health care services and nursing is no exception."

It is evident that the education of nurses must include an awareness of cost containment in health care to help nurses survive a changing economic system. Yet undergraduate nursing curricula are crowded with the skills and knowledge needed for patient care. These include the biopsychosocial basis for nursing assessment as well as the problem-solving abilities needed to carry out the nursing process. As technology advances, new and revised patterns of care are incorporated into nursing curriculum content. In addition, focus on interpersonal techniques for developing and maintaining communication with patients and peers has increased. Concepts of cost containment recently have been added to courses in nursing management, but the clinical instruction of nursing students continues to emphasize techniques of care and a variety of short-term experiences. Traditional clinical teaching prevails despite the reality that nurses today face patients with shorter hospitalizations and more intense illnesses.

Creativity in clinical instruction can help faculty adjust to teaching in hospitals with decreased resources and declining censuses. Carpenito and Duespohl (1985) state that students are in the clinical setting to learn professional nursing. But professional nursing in the hospital, as in other settings, includes more than hands-on patient care. It is helpful to re-member that patients are hospitalized because of the need for 24-hour nursing care. Otherwise, patients could receive treatment in an outpatient setting with follow-up home care. Students need to be made aware that, as consumers of nursing care, patients (as well as third-party payers) are also concerned with the costs of nursing care.

Implementation of DRGs and the resulting shifts in patterns of patient care related to cost containment have affected the clinical learning of students. In a challenge to nursing educators, a *Journal of Nursing Education* editorial scolds, "We need to analyze the health needs of today, anticipate the needs of tomorrow and prepare nurses to meet these challenges" (Bush, 1985, p. 89). In spite of declining hospital censuses, decreasing availability of clinical resources for students and faculty, and increasingly ill patients who are discharged earlier, little has been pub-lished on how concepts of cost containment can be integrated into stu-dent learning objectives. Grace (1985) views nursing faculty as "too far distanced to have any real ability to become part of the decision-making related to cost effective health care," despite their intellectual interest. Yet, it is these same distant faculty who will stimulate the career goals of the future caregivers and leaders in nursing.

The money issues in health care delivery also translate into issues of professional autonomy. One of the ten megatrends in nursing is "separating nursing costs from other hospital expenses [which] will give nurses greater recognition" (Costra, 1985). It is evident from both published and unpublished institutional research and studies that nurses are indeed identifying and placing a value upon patient care services. (Department of Nursing Services, 1984; Sovie, Tarcinale, VanPutte, & Stunden, 1985; Vail, Norton, & Rimm, 1985).

THE CLINICAL EXERCISE

To develop a method of helping baccalaureate students become aware of the costs of direct nursing care in a patient setting, the author designed a clinical experience that would provide the opportunity for students to assess the cost-effectiveness of nursing care in a primary care delivery system (defined in terms of cost of care and length of hospital stay) as well as to stimulate students' interest in nursing's role in cost containment within a hospital setting. The students who participated in this exercise were 18 seniors in a baccalaureate nursing program. These students who were registered nurses with lengths of experience ranging from 6 months to 10 years, were enrolled in a lecture-clinical course on clinical synthesis. The focus of the course, as the name implies, was to put nursing "all together" in a clinical setting. The objectives of the course were to (1) evaluate the impact of ethical, legal, and social processes on the health care system utilizing a systems perspective as a framework; (2) evaluate personal role and effectiveness as a provider of health care as part of a health care delivery system and individual; and (3) apply principles of management to the planning and implementation of health care delivery. The theory component of the course was structured so that students could function as a group to make guided decisions about the delivery and evaluation of patient care. Decisions made in the classroom were actually implemented later in the clinical setting.

The clinical setting at Parkview Episcopal Medical Center was limited to 11 or 12 patient beds within a 40-bed surgical unit. This patient area was physically separated by a hallway from the mainstream of staff activities. Two full-time university faculty members, the unit head nurse, and an adjunct faculty member employed by the medical center arranged for 24-hour-a-day supervision of the students for 12 consecutive days.

In classroom planning activities, students selected a primary care model for delivery of patient care and designated a student manager to be responsible for communication with staff and problem solving with peers. The class identified student managers for all shifts, and developed a 12-day schedule. Additional clinical time was allotted for evaluation and for other objectives not addressed in this paper.

Table 1
Feeding Activities: University Hospital Patient Classification System

Nursing Activity	Weighted Factors per Shift		
	11 p.m.–7 a.m.	7 a.m.–3 p.m.	3 p.m.–11 p.m.
Independent w/feeding	1	1	1
Assist feeding	3	3	3
Total feeding	11	11	11
Tube feeding	8	8	8
Intake and output	5	5	5
Force fluid nourishment	2	2	2

Source: Department of Nursing Service, University Hospital, *Acuity Record* (Denver: University of Colorado Health Science Center, 1984).

DETERMINING COSTS

All students were familiar with the concept of patient classification systems for staffing purposes. However, few were aware that some systems could be used to identify direct and indirect costs of nursing care. A three-step process was used to determine direct costs of patient care. Although the process is similar to the procedure for determining relative intensity measures (RIMs), individual patient data rather than collective data was the focus.

The first step in determining the cost of care was to calculate the average hourly cost of a nurse employed in the community. This was done by adding the average wage and the cost of employment benefits, including vacation, sick leave, holidays, insurance, workers' compensation, tuition reimbursement programs, educational (but not inservice) programs, reduced meal charges, and special employee benefits common in the community. These benefits cost the employer about 20 percent of the nurse's hourly wage. This step can be presented by the following formula:

$$\overline{PBh} = \text{Mean pay and benefits per hour of nurse}$$

The second step was to determine the time spent in nursing care using a patient classification system that assigns the various activities of nursing care to a specific time framework. These activities are also called weighted factors because each is assigned a value or weight. They can include indirect care time or be limited to actual nursing contact with the patient. The students in this study reviewed two classification systems. In one system (Department of Nursing Service, University Hospital, 1984), the

Table 2
Feeding Activities: Vail, Norton, and Rimm Patient Classification System

Weighted Factors	Nursing Activity
5	Tube feeding (bolus) every 4 hours or 6 times a day
8	Tube feeding (bolus) every 3 hours or 8 times a day
10	Tube feeding (bolus) every 2 hours or 12 times a day
2	Tube feeding (continuous) per bottle change
6	Adult meals, older than 5 years (spoon feed 3 times a day)
10	Child meals, younger than 5 years (spoon feed 3 times a day)
2	Infant/neonate bottle × 1 feeding
12	Infant/neonate bottle every 6 hours or 6 times a day
24	Infant/neonate bottle every 2 hours or 6 times a day

Source: Jame D. Vail, Dena A. Norton, and Elizabeth A. Rimm, *The Workload Management System for Nursing* (Bethesda, Md.: Walter Reed Army Medical Center, 1984).

factors represent direct nursing time only. Table 1 gives an example of weighted factors for one set of nursing activities in this system. The weighted factors are multiplied by a time constant of 6 minutes to give the time for each activity, as well as by a unit constant to account for indirect care.

In the system the students finally selected (Vail, Norton, & Rimm, 1984), time for related activities is incorporated into direct care time. Table 2 shows the weighted factors for the nursing activities involved in feeding in this system. To determine the cost of nursing care to the patient, the weighted factor is multiplied by the time constant in minutes (in this system, 7.5 minutes), and this total is divided by 60 to give the time of care in hours. This procedure is represented by the following formula:

$$HC = \frac{Wf \times Tm}{60}$$

where HC represents hours of care, Wf represents the weighted factor for the nursing activity, and Tm is the time constant in minutes.

Calculate cost of nursing care by combining steps 1 and 2 as follows:

$$\text{Cost of nursing care} = \frac{Wf \times Tm \times \overline{PBh}}{60}$$
$$= HC \times \overline{PBh}$$

Table 3
Nursing Care Activities Following a Cholecystectomy

Postoperative Day 1		Postoperative Day 2	
Weighted Factor	Nursing Activity	Weighted Factor	Nursing Activity
6	Postoperative vitals	2	Vital signs every 4 hours for 6 assessments
2	Intake and output every 8 hours	2	Intake and output every 8 hours
6	Assisted care—positions self	6	Assisted care
0	Feeding	0	Feeding
6	IV simple	6	IV simple
2	Enema		
2	Simple dressing	2	Simple dressing
2	Medications every 3 to 8 hours	2	Medications every 3 to 8 hours
2	Assist out of bed to bathroom	2	Assist out of bed to bathroom
2	Assist out of bed to walk	2	Assist out of bed to walk
2	Incentive spirometer, cough and deep breathing	2	Incentive spirometer, cough and deep breathing
4	Postoperative teaching		
36		26	

For example, to calculate the cost of nursing care over 48 hours for a patient following a cholecystectomy, the students recorded the nursing activities shown in Table 3, along with the weighted factor for each. First, the hours of nursing care are calculated, using the total weighted factors for each day and the time factor (Tm), 7.5 minutes:

$$\frac{36 \times 7.5}{60} = 4.50 \text{ hours} \qquad \frac{26 \times 7.5}{60} = 3.25 \text{ hours}$$

Then the cost of nursing care is calculated using the total hours of care (4.50 + 3.25 = 7.75) and the nurse's average wage and benefits (PBh):

$$\text{Cost of nursing care} = 7.75 \times \$16$$
$$= \$124 \text{ for 48 hours}$$

To practice use of the cost formula, each student functioned as the primary nurse for at least one patient. In addition to planning, imple-

Table 4
Nursing Care Activities for a Colostomy Revision

Admission		Day of Surgery	
Weighted Factor	Nursing Activity	Weighted Factor	Nursing Activity
12	Admission data	2	Preoperative injection
4	Preoperative teaching	2	Vital signs
2	Vital signs		Postoperative
2	Colostomy care—readjustment of colostomy bag only	4	Vital signs every 2 hours
		4	Assist to turn, cough, and deep breath every 2 hours
		2	Up at bedside 3 times a day
		6	IV therapy
		6	Activities of daily living
		2	Simple dressing 2 times
		2	Medication for pain 3 times
—		2	Intake and output every eight hours
20		32	

menting, and coordinating patient care for the hospitalization of the patient, the student was required to use the patient classification system selected in the classroom to determine the cost of one patient's care for a continuous 48-hour period. This meant that the primary student nurse considered all nursing activities involving a specific patient, whether performed by the primary or associate student nurse.

Table 4 shows the nursing activities that students found represented the nursing care given to a patient with a colostomy revision upon admission and the day of surgery. The following calculations give the cost of nursing for the day of admission:

$$\text{Cost of nursing care} = \frac{20 \times 7.5}{60} \times \$16$$
$$= \$40$$

Nursing costs for the day of surgery are as follows:

$$\frac{32 \times 7.5}{60} \times \$16 = 64$$

Table 5
Cost for 48 Hours of Nursing Care for Selected Diagnoses

Medical Diagnosis	Units of Care	Hours of Care	Cost (at $16 per Hour)
Osteoarthritis	46	5.75	$ 91.00
Tonsillectomy	20	2.50	40.00
Laminectomy	60	7.50	120.00
Epistaxis	103	12.90[a]	206.00
Mastectomy	83	10.40[a]	166.00
Cholecystectomy	28	3.50	56.00
Cholecystectomy	94	11.75	188.00
Cholecystectomy	62	7.75	124.00
Total hip replacement	190	23.75	380.00
Epididymitis	60	7.50	120.00
Parotidectomy	88	11.00	176.00
Repair diaphragmatic hernia	116	14.50	232.00

[a]Rounded to nearest tenth.

EVALUATING THE COSTS OF CARE

To evaluate the cost of nursing care, the students compared the total charges for the hospital stay with the allowable costs under Medicare. For example, a student noted that the total hospital reimbursement for a cholecystectomy patient under that DRG was $4,440.45, compared to actual hospital charges for that student's patient of $2,704.00.

Summary data from selected patients indicate that direct nursing care costs could be measured. The data in Table 5 represent the students' calculations of the costs of nursing care for selected medical diagnoses based on the time spent in direct nursing services for 48 hours and an average nursing cost (wages and benefits of $16 per hour).

Examining cost-effectiveness, as measured by the difference between the actual length of hospitalization and the length of hospital stay allowable under DRGs pointed out to students that health care costs could be contained. Table 6 shows data on allowed and actual length of stay for several patients. The inclusion of three patients with the same diagnosis, cholecystectomy, points out the individuality of patient response to treatment, including nursing care. The amount of direct care given over a 48-hour period varied among these patients from 3.5 hours to 11.75 hours. The care was cost-effective in all three cases since the patients were all discharged before the allowable time elapsed, even though the time of discharge ranged from seven to two days earlier than allowed.

Table 6
Length of Stay for Selected Diagnoses

Medical Diagnosis	Allowed Stay under DRG[a]	Actual Stay
Tonsillectomy	48 hours	27 hours
Laminectomy	13 days	3 days
Epistaxis	3 days	5 days
Mastectomy	9 days	4 days
Cholecystectomy	11 days	6 days
Cholecystectomy	11 days	4 days
Cholecystectomy	10 days	8 days

[a]Data from *The Physician's DRG Working Guidebook* (Louisville, KY: St. Anthony Hospital, 1984).

RESULTS OF THE EXERCISE

After participating in the clinical exercise, students became more aware of the need to have planned goals for patient care in order to have a basis for determining patient outcomes at discharge. The realization that each patient contact could carry a price tag made students review the nature of the time they spent with patients. Finally, comparing the costs of care to the hospital with the reimbursements allowed under Medicare helped students appreciate the value of effective nursing care in cost containment.

The realization that time spent in nursing activities can be documented and fixed to a dollar amount surprised students. One student, an experienced nurse, commented, "Unless I figured the cost of this case wrong, I think that it is really cheap!" The added realization that practicing nurses are responsible for many patients further demonstrated to students that nursing service can actually generate revenue for the hospital.

DISCUSSION

As an exploration into methods of teaching cost containment in overall care of patients, the process described here can be incorporated into any clinical setting. The history of events leading to efforts at cost containment in health care and the directions for using factors and patient classification systems can be covered in the classroom. The time involved can be limited to as little as two to three hours without sacrificing existing content objectives. In the clinical setting, the use of the formula to calculate the cost of nursing care is easily incorporated into the recording activities for patient care. Additional clinical time for the students to contact the DRG reviewer or accounting office to obtain information about the hospital's DRG allowances is negligible.

Although all the students in this class were registered nurses, none was familiar with the practice of identifying actual costs for direct patient care. Consequently, the content presented was at a basic level suitable for the beginning baccalaureate student.

Frequently the affective domain of learning is given less attention in clinical areas than cognitive or psychomotor objectives (Field, Gallman, Nicholson, 1984). The three levels of the affective domain can be addressed through the clinical exercise described. These levels are *receiving*—a simple awareness or attention to phenomena; *responding*—self-initiated participation in an activity; and *valuing*—appreciation and acceptance of a belief (Krathwohl, Bloom, & Masia, 1956). To facilitate *awareness* of cost-containment factors, the faculty can ensure that methods to calculate cost of nursing care and the cost of hospitalization are presented to students. *Responding* to the economics of health care is guided through assignments that require students to compare projected costs (DRG allowances) with actual costs and to calculate costs of nursing care using a patient classification system. *Valuing*, while more difficult to address adequately in a short time, can be facilitated through group discussions in which students identify preferences or by encouraging students to initiate investigations into prices and charges for health care.

Although the particular clinical experience described here was an intensive synthesis of previous nursing and support courses, cost awareness can be included at any level in the curriculum and as an ongoing feature of clinical learning that begins with campus laboratories. One way to develop this awareness early in the educational process is to place a current market price on all equipment that students use in practice laboratories, including thermometers, bed linen, disposable trays, and intravenous solutions and tubing as well as specialty equipment. Community health nurses have documented time spent in client activities for years. Students in community-based agencies can do the same. Faculty can use each clinical setting to foster attitudes and values about the economies of nursing care and cost containment in the health care system. The concept of cost can be integrated throughout the curriculum, just as the concept of the nursing process is.

If new applications of clinical cost management are going to work, students must have opportunities to understand and practice cost containment in patient care settings. For too long, nurse educators have left the methods and concepts of health care finances to graduate programs in administration. To prepare for the future, baccalaureate students need information on which to build as practicing nurses.

REFERENCES

American Nurses' Association (1980). *Nursing: A Social Policy Statement.* Kansas City, MO: American Nurses' Association.

Bush, J. (1985, March). DRGs challenge nursing curricula (Editorial). *Journal of Nursing Education,* p. 89.

Carpentino, L. J., & Duespohl, T. A. (1985). A guide for effective clinical instruction. Rockville, MD: Aspen Systems Corp.

Costra, T. D. (1985, May/June). Megatrends in nursing. *Nursing Life,* pp. 17–21.

Davis, C. K. (1983, Summer). Nursing and the health care debates (Editorial). *Image,* p. 67.

Department of Nursing Service, University Hospital (1984). *Acuity record.* Unpublished record form. Denver, CO: University of Colorado Health Science Center.

Field, W. E., Jr., Gallman, L. V., Nicholson, R., & Dreher, M. (1984, September). Clinical competencies of baccalaureate students. *Journal of Nursing Education,* pp. 284–288.

Grace, H. K. (1985). Can health care costs be contained? Nursing's responsibility. In J. C. McClosky & H. K. Grace (Eds.), *Current issues in nursing* (pp. 744–751). Boston: Blackwell Scientific Publications.

Hamilton, J. M. (1984). Nursing and DRGs: Proactive responses to prospective reimbursement. In F. A. Shaffer (Ed.), *DRGs: Changes and challenges* (pp. 99–107). New York: National League for Nursing.

Krathwohl, D. R., Bloom, B. S., & Masia, B. R. (1956). *Taxonomy of education objectives.* New York: David McKay Co.

The physicians' DRG working guidebook (1984). Louisville, KY: St. Anthony Hospital.

Sovie, M. D., Tarcinale, M. A., VanPutte, A. W., & Stunden, A. (1985, March). Amalgam of nursing acuity, DRGs and costs. *Nursing Management,* pp. 2–42. Reprinted in this volume, pp. 121–148.

Vail, J. D., Norton, D. A., & Rimm, E. A. (1984). *The workload management system for nursing.* Bethesda, MD: Walter Reed Army Medical Center.

Development of a Patient Classification System for Home Health Nursing

Vivian Hayes Churness, Dorothy Kleffel,
Joan Jacobson, and Marlene Onodera

In light of the move toward cost containment, early discharge from the acute-care setting has become a fact of life. Home health agencies report they are caring for patients who are more acutely ill than ever before. Many patient visits require more than two or three hours instead of the standard 45 minutes. With such a great variation in patients' needs, a fixed fee per visit is no longer equitable. In addition, the usual practice of assigning nurses to visit a fixed number of patients each day does not allow for optimal scheduling.

To address these concerns, the staff of the Visiting Nurse Association of Los Angeles, Inc. (VNA–LA), a voluntary nonprofit home health agency, and faculty members of the Department of Nursing of the University of Southern California (USC) have developed a patient classification instrument that reflects the amount of skilled nursing care required by patients receiving in-home services. Once reliability and validity have been established, the tool can be used to (1) allocate charges for home visits according to the amount of nursing time used, (2) set objective nursing productivity standards, (3) schedule visits according to the patients' requirements for nursing care, and (4) project costs of nursing for a prospective payment system.

EXISTING CLASSIFICATION SYSTEMS IN HOME HEALTH CARE

Various patient classification systems that define requirements for nursing care are currently used in acute-care hospital settings throughout the country. As recently as 1978, however, there were virtually no

319

applications of patient classification systems in the area of home health nursing (Giovannetti, 1978). Since that time, several classification systems for patients receiving nursing care at home have been reported in the literature. These few systems have been used to guide health professionals in assessing patients, diagnosing problems, and planning nursing interventions. They have also been useful in formulating outcome criteria by which progress toward goals can be met. Some have been used to measure nursing needs and costs.

Daubert (1979) describes a classification system used by the VNA of New Haven, Connecticut, which is based on the rehabilitation potential of patients admitted to the agency. The method of classification is a prototype evaluation model which describes typical cases representing increasing need for nursing services. Patients are matched to one of five categories, based on simultaneous consideration of a number of characteristics. The categories range from Group I, representing patients with acute illnesses who are expected to return to normal functioning, to Group V, which includes patients with end-stage disease for whom the outcome criterion is the maintenance of comfort and dignity. The system has been useful in quality-assurance programs and for developing service goals for individual patients. The system also has the potential for measuring requirements for nursing time and the actual cost of services.

Harris, Santoferraro, and Silva (1985) adapted the New Haven classification system to collect patient outcome data at the VNA of Eastern Montgomery County, Pennsylvania. Costs per case by discipline were computed for each of 33 patients classified into five groups according to potential for rehabilitation. Costs were also computed according to nine major disease categories of the ninth revision of the International Classification of Diseases (ICD-9). Although there were marked differences in costs by health care provider (nurse, home health aide, occupational therapist, physical therapist, medical social worker, or speech therapist), the average costs per case were similar when classified according to either system. Monitoring of costs by use of more than one classification system, as was done in this study, is desirable as a basis for testing alternative methods for reimbursement of home health services.

The VNA of Omaha, Nebraska, has developed and validated a classification scheme for client problems or nursing diagnoses in community health nursing. The system consists of 38 problem labels in the areas of environmental, psychosocial, and physiological problems and health behaviors. Using this scheme of standard nomenclature, staff are able to sort and organize assessment data, increase efficiency of documentation, and improve communication among nurses (A Classification Scheme, 1980; Martin, 1982). Plans are now being made to modify this system as a basis for predicting patient requirements for nursing.

The caseload/workload analysis system, in use in community health settings since 1979, utilizes an instrument-based classification of cases according to degree of difficulty (Allen, Easley, & Storfjell, 1985, 1986). Difficulty is based on clinical judgment, teaching needs, physical care, psychosocial needs, number of agencies involved, and number and severity of problems. These ratings, along with other information, are used to diagnose problems in caseload management and to project staffing needs.

These classification schemes categorize patients according to potential for rehabilitation and patients' problems or degree of difficulty, but not according to the amount and level of skill required. A need thus exists for a reliable and valid tool to assess the amount of nursing time required for home visits.

VNA–LA STUDY

The present study was designed to develop a patient classification system that accurately reflects the amount of skilled nursing care required by patients receiving professional nursing services. Development and testing of a patient classification instrument was followed by evaluation of the instrument as a management tool. The first phase of the study, that of instrument development, is reported here.

The study was carried out by the VNA–LA, the largest home health agency in the West, which covers over 3,000 square miles in the city and county of Los Angeles. Staff in six area offices make a total of over 200,000 visits a year. Data were collected from 158 home visits and included all VNA–LA programs and areas (except for a desert area 80 miles away). Data collected from repeat visits to the same patient were not included in the analysis.

Data Collection

To achieve content validity, it was necessary to determine what activities constitute a typical home visit. The information was readily obtainable because documentation of what occurs during a home visit is routinely recorded in the nurse progress notes of the VNA–LA medical record (see Fig. 1), which are completed for each home visit. The progress notes include a list of 85 nursing activities grouped into 22 categories. This list of nursing activities was originally developed by the Visiting Nurse Association of Orange County, California, and adapted by the VNA–LA to facilitate the recording of skilled nursing activities and to save time in documenting the home visit. According to agency protocol, the home health nurse circles the code number for each activity and makes comments in the space provided below. Although the categories may

Figure 1
THE VISITING NURSE ASSOCIATION OF LOS ANGELES, INC.
NURSE PROGRESS NOTES

PATIENT NAME	M.R. #

1. BLADDER CARE:
- a. insertion of indwelling catheter
- b. irrigation of indwelling catheter
- c. instruction of non-medical person re catheter care
- d. instruction of non-medical person re catheter irrigation
- e. instruction of non-medical person re bladder training
- f. instruction regarding use of external catheter
- g. application of external catheter

2. COLOSTOMY/ILEOSTOMY/ILEOCONSUIT CARE:
- a. colostomy irrigation
- b. appliance/bag application
- c. instruct non-medical person regarding:
  1. colostomy care
  2. ileostomy care
  3. ileoconduit care

3. DECUBITUS CARE: a. treatment of decubitus   b. instruction regarding decubitus care

4. DIABETIC INSTRUCTIONS REGARDING:
- a. urine testing
- b. insulin preparation/administration
- c. skin care/foot care
- d. hypo/hyperglycemic reactions
- e. diet

5. WOUND CARE:
- a. assessment/evaluation of wound
- b. application of non-sterile dressing
- c. application of sterile dressing
- d. application of dressing with prescribed medication
- e. instruction of non-medical person re wound care
- f. bagging of fistula/draining wound

6. EYE CARE: c. instruction to non-medical person re:
- a. eye dressing
- b. adm of eye medication
  1. eye medication
  2. eye dressing
  3. S/S of complications

7. BOWEL CARE: a. manual removal of fecal impaction   b. enema administration   c. instruction in establishing bowel program

8. HOME HEALTH AIDE: a. instruction   b. supervision

9. IPPB: a. administer treatment   b. instruction regarding use of IPPB equipment   c. evaluate/supervise use of IPPB

10. MEDICATIONS:
- a. review purpose, dosage, schedule, side effects & refills
- b. administer IM medication
- c. administer SQ medication
- d. prefill syringes
- e. administer IV fluids/medications
- f. teach non-medical person injection technique
- g. apply topical medication

11. MENTAL HEALTH: a. counseling   b. mental health teaching   c. emotional support

12. FEEDING TUBES:
- a. insertion/reinsertion NG tube
- b. reinsertion of gastrostomy tube
- c. instruction regarding:
  1. preparation of feeding
  2. administration of feedings
  3. obtaining formulas
  4. care of equipment

13. NUTRITION: a. instruct regarding diet   b. supervision regarding diet   c. instruct-force fluids   d. instruct-limit fluids

14. OXYGEN: a. instruct re administration of O_2 b. instruct re use of O_2 & equipment   c. evaluate/supervise use of O_2 & equipment

15. RANGE OF MOTION: a. instruct regarding ROM   b. perform ROM

16. SKIN CARE: a. instruct re skin care   b. instruct regarding patient positioning

17. TERMINALLY ILL: a. instruct regarding care   b. anticipatory grief counseling   c. funeral arrangement counselling   d. bereavement

18. PAIN / SYMPTOM CONTROL: a. evaluation of pain and symptom control   b. instruct pain and symptom control

19. TRACHEOSTOMY CARE: a. instruct re care   b. instruct re suctioning   c. change trach   d. suction trach

20. INSTRUCTION IN DISEASE PROCESS   **21. LAB SPECIMENS OBTAINED**

22. ACTIVITY:
- a. instruct regarding amount/type activity
- b. instruct regarding energy conservation
- c. instruct regarding safety in the home
- d. instruct regarding use of equipment

NARRATIVE NOTES   Use code numbers/letters for activities listed above.
Indicate results, patient's response, degree of learning, plans, etc.

	SIGNATURE
	DATE

TIME: FROM_____ TO_____ SOURCE OF FEE_____ RETURN HV DATE_____

VNA-LA   227W

sometimes overlap, the list has consistently proved useful in assuring accurate documentation.

This nursing activities list was modified for use in the present study to include a space to enter the amount of time in minutes utilized for each activity. The activities were timed by an observer during the visit and estimated by the nurse after the visit. Time spent by the nurse in previsit and postvisit activities was also recorded. Previsit activities consisted of telephone calls to patients, consultation with physicians and other members of the health team, planning, recording, and travel. Postvisit activities included telephoning, planning, recording, and in-house team conferences. In addition, the observer collected demographic information on each patient, including medical diagnosis, and noted such factors as limited mobility and visual or auditory limitations. Copies of the problem list and treatment plan were obtained for every patient.

Procedure

Two licensed vocational nurses were trained to observe home visits and collect data. The area director in each area office identified nurses who were willing to be accompanied on home visits by the designated observer who collected the data. An attempt was made to include as many of the VNA–LA specialty programs as possible. The data collector usually accompanied each participating nurse for an entire day, allowing a sample of a typical caseload of patients to be obtained.

Before leaving the office, the nurse discussed the day's assignment with the data collector, including demographic information about the patients and their problem list and treatment plan from the chart. The data collector also observed the nurse planning, recording, making telephone calls, conferring with other team members, and gathering supplies. The data collector then accompanied the nurse to each patient's home and, with the patient's prior permission, observed, timed, and recorded the various nursing activities. After the visit, the nurse independently recorded her estimate of the time involved in carrying out the various components of the visit. The nurse was instructed by the data collector to record all postvisit activities on a form that was provided.

ANALYSIS AND RESULTS

Data were analyzed using descriptive statistics. A total of 158 home visits were included in the study, 22 to 40 visits from each of the five area offices. Five programs were represented: medical-surgical (101 visits), hospice (20 visits), enterostomal therapy (15 visits), infusion therapy

(12 visits), and pediatrics (10 visits). The majority of visits (134) were routine or continuing, 17 were new admission or assessment visits, 4 were discharge visits, and 3 were reassessment visits.

Patients range in age from 3 weeks to 97 years, with 65 percent of the sample age 65 or older. Sixty percent of the sample were women. Twelve sources of fee payment were identified, the major source being Medicare (109 visits). The second most frequent source of payment was Medi-Cal (17 visits), the California version of the federal Medicaid program.

Time spent by the nurse in the home ranged from 10 minutes to 2 hours, with a mean time of 36 minutes. Historically, the VNA–LA has estimated a typical visit to last 45 minutes, and results of this study indicated that 75 percent of the visits took 45 minutes or less. The mean previsit time, excluding travel, was 12 minutes, and the mean postvisit time was 29 minutes. Cross tabulation of direct and indirect nursing time by program and type of visit is displayed in Table 1.

All categories of nursing activities were sampled except intermittent positive pressure breathing (IPPB) and range-of-motion exercises. The maximum time observed for any one activity was 92 minutes to administer intravenous therapy. The minimum time noted for many activities was one minute. However, because many activities occured simultaneously or in conjunction with other activities, minimum times can be misleading.

A more detailed analysis of the data observed for three of the major categories is reported in Table 2. In this table first and third quartile points are reported for each activity. For example, 50 percent of the time a colostomy appliance or bag was applied, it took the nurse from 7 to 26 minutes. The maximum time utilized was 40 minutes, and 1 minute was the minimum time for any activity.

All data collection instruments were reviewed carefully, and an estimate of interrater reliability was determined. Written comments were considered, as were activities that occurred simultaneously. There was a high level of agreement between the nurses' estimates and the data collectors' records in the amount of time spent in directly observable activities, such as giving injections and teaching colostomy care. However, time estimates for activities such as counseling and emotional support were inconsistent. In many instances, the nurse and data collector both noted that teaching occurred but had differing perceptions of what was being taught. For instance, one data collector identified as separate activities many functions that nurses viewed as a whole. In bladder care, as an example, nurses tended to group a number of activities and label them "instruction in catheter care," whereas the data collector identified insertion of indwelling catheter, irrigation of catheter, and instruction

Table 1
Time of Home Visit, by Program

Program	Number of Visits	Time (in minutes)	
		Mean	Standard Deviation
Medical-Surgical ($N = 101$)			
Assessment	11	50.2	26.2
Reassessment	2	26.0	1.4
Continuing	84	28.8	14.2
Discharge	4	26.8	5.6
Hospice ($N = 20$)			
Assessment	1	75.0	—
Reassessment	0	—	—
Continuing	19	38.0	14.2
Discharge	0	—	—
Infusion Therapy ($N = 12$)			
Assessment	1	112.0	—
Reassessment	0	—	—
Continuing	11	34.8	18.1
Discharge	0	—	—
Pediatrics ($N = 10$)			
Assessment	1	54.0	—
Reassessment	1	33.0	—
Continuing	8	30.3	13.2
Discharge	0	—	—
Enterostomal Therapy ($N = 15$)			
Assessment	3	56.0	23.3
Reassessment	0	—	—
Continuing	12	58.7	18.2
Discharge	0	—	—

in catheter care as separate activities. This suggests that nurses tend to view certain activities as a whole rather than as discrete elements.

Although teaching often occurs simultaneously with other activities, enough teaching occurs independently to justify including "instruction" as a distinct activity. An example of this is the teaching of a diabetic patient.

Written comments on the instruments by both nurses and data collectors indicated that nurses tended to spend more time with patients who lived alone, had limited mobility, or were very anxious. Contrary to what might be expected, many seriously ill patients required less time for the nurse's visits because of the presence of a caregiver or family members.

Table 2
Observed Duration of Selected Nursing Activities

Nursing Activity	Frequency	Time (in minutes)			
		Mean	Range	Range of 25th to 75th Percentile[a]	Median
Colostomy Care					
Colostomy irrigation	0	—	—	—	—
Appliance/bag application	7	19	1–40	1–26	7
Instruction regarding colostomy care	8	18	2–52	9–40	9
Instruction regarding ileostomy care	1	3	3–3	3–3	3
Instruction regarding ileoconduit care	3	16	1–26	1–26	20
Decubitus Care					
Treatment of decubitus	8	20	2–50	10–29	16
Instruction regarding decubitus care	6	10	4–27	5–14	7
Wound Care					
Assessment of wound	39	2	1–5	1–3	2
Application of nonsterile dressing	5	3	4–10	5–10	5
Application of sterile dressing	19	6	1–15	3–10	6
Application of dressing/medication	21	7	1–20	3–13	6
Instruction regarding wound care	9	6	2–15	3–9	5
Bagging of fistula	2	2	1–2	1–2	2

[a]First to third quartile, or middle 50 percent of sample.

PATIENT CLASSIFICATION INSTRUMENT

The results of data analysis were used to design a patient classification instrument for field testing. A factor evaluation instrument design was selected for use because of its potential for high interrater reliability. Because the instrument is based on observable nursing activities that are normally documented in the patient's medical record, concurrent and retrospective audits of classification ratings can be readily accomplished by independent raters. With a factor evaluation model instrument, specific aspects or elements of patient care are considered one at a time. The elements, or factors, that best predict the amount of time required for the entire visits are noted and assigned a weight according to their relative time requirements. From these weights, a total score is computed for each home visit. On the basis of these scores, home visits can be classified into five levels on an ordinal scale, with the higher-ranked visits requiring more nursing time. For example, a patient with a total score of from 1 to 19 would be classified into level I. It is estimated that patients at this level will require an average of 30 minutes of nursing time for each home visit. Patients with scores of 20 to 29 would be designated as level II, requiring about 45 minutes of nursing time, and so on. Factor weights for various categories of activities were determined by noting the amount of time required for 75 percent of the observations (the third quartile point) of each activity. In instances where categories of activities were changed from those used in the study, an estimate was used. An instrument format is used that allows either manual or computer scoring.

In designing the instrument, overlapping categories of nursing activities were combined. For example, decubitus care and wound care appeared as separate activities on the data collection form. Because raters disagreed as to whether the nursing intervention for patients with large decubitus ulcers should be recorded as decubitis care, wound care, or both, it was decided that these activities could best be combined into one category. All data collection forms were reviewed and the frequency with which each activity occurred was noted as well as comments about which activities occurred simultaneously. Categories of activities infrequently encountered were eliminated. An "other" category was added with instructions to specify the activity and the amount of time it consumed. The following are the final categories or factors that were designated:

1. Bladder/catheter care
2. Bowel care
3. Colostomy care

Figure 2
VNA–LA/USC Patient Classification Instrument

NURSING ACTIVITY CHECKLIST

Instructions: Please check the column which best describes the nursing service required. Check all that apply.

Category	Nursing Activity			Score
1. Colostomy care	Assessment/ instruction if patient familiar with colostomy A. ☐	Appliance/bag application B. ☐	Colostomy irrigation/care/ instruction if new patient C. ☐	1. __ __
2. Decubitus/ wound care	Assessment/ instruction A. ☐	Dressing/ med application B. ☐	Wound soak or complex dressing C. ☐	Multiple sites (over 30 minutes) D. ☐	2. __ __

Note: Scoring of the instrument is described in Figure 3.

   4. Decubitus/wound care
   5. Diabetic instruction
   6. Feeding tube
   7. Health assessment
   8. Laboratory specimen
   9. Oral medications and injections
  10. Intravenous fluids or total parenteral nutrition
  11. Mental health
  12. Oxygen therapy
  13. Other

Any patient teaching that is not a component of any of the designated categories is also recorded, as is the presence of certain modifying factors such as impairment of vision or mobility. Plans have been made to pilot test the instrument and revise categories as needed based on interrater agreement and subjective judgment.

An example of the patient classification index showing two patient care categories is presented in Figure 2. Nurses using the instrument are directed to check all activities that are applicable to the patient visit. After they fill out the instrument, clerical personnel score it, using the list of factor weights for the items checked. After assigning the weights

Figure 3
Proposed Factor Weights for Two Nursing Activity Categories
in Patient Classification Instrument

NURSING ACTIVITY CHECKLIST

Category	Nursing Activity				Score[a]
1. Colostomy care	Assessment/ instruction if patient familiar with colostomy A. 10 ☑	Appliance/bag application B. 26 ☑	Colostomy irrigation/care/ instruction if new to patient C. 40 ☐		1. *B 26*
2. Decubitus/ wound care	Assessment/ instruction A. 9 ☑	Dressing/ med application B. 13 ☑	Wound soak or complex dressing C. 29 ☑	Multiple sites (over 30 minutes) D. 35[b] ☐	2. *C 29*

Total Score ____ *55*

[a]Enter highest number checked for category in this column. Letters will be assigned to the designated factor weight by clerical personnel. This can be done manually or with computer assistance.
[b]If amount of time recorded is greater than or equal to 45 minutes, record that number. Otherwise, enter 35, as indicated.

for each item, they compute a total score for each patient, with higher scores designating patients requiring more nursing time. (A portion of a checklist, completed and scored for two categories, with the factor weights and scoring guide, can be seen in Figure 3). If the scores are found to correlate highly with the amount of time actually required for patient visits, the instrument will have predictive validity.

Testing for interrater reliability is currently being conducted. It is anticipated that appropriate revisions in the instrument will be made periodically until there is a substantial percentage of agreement among raters as well as a high degree of predictive validity.

CONCLUSIONS AND RECOMMENDATIONS

The proposed patient classification instrument for home health nursing is based on time requirements for various activities observed during actual home visits. Whether these activities are the critical indicators of time required is yet to be validated.

Interrater reliability of the instrument will be difficult to determine in a home health setting; however, this can be accomplished by asking a number of nurses to independently rate a videotaped home visit using the new tool. Visits can also be rated independently by nurses using patient medical records.

No attempt has been made to measure quality of nursing care delivered. The instrument proposed for use is intended to measure only the amount and level of care actually given, not the care that should be given.

REFERENCES

Allen, C. E., Easley, C., & Storfjell, J. I. (1985, October 15). A system for caseload/ workload analysis. Paper presented at the 4th Annual Meeting of the National Association for Home Care, Las Vegas, Nevada.

Allen, C. E., Easley, C., & Storfjell, J. I. (1986). Cost management through caseload/workload analysis. In this volume, pp. 331–346.

A classification scheme for client problems in community health nursing (1980). (DHHS Publication No. HRA 80-16 HRP-0501501.) Washington, D.C.: U.S. Department of Health and Human Services.

Daubert, E. A. (1979). A patient classification system and outcome criteria. Nursing Outlook, 6, 450–454.

Giovannetti, P. (1978). Patient classification in nursing: A description and analysis (DHEW Publication No. HRA 78-22 HRP-0500501). Springfield, VA: National Technical Information Service.

Harris, M.D., Santoferraro, C., & Silva, S. (1985). A patient classification system in home health care. Nursing Economics, 3 (October), 276–282.

Martin, K. (1982). A client classification system adaptable for computerization. Nursing Outlook, 11/12, 515–517.

Cost Management through Caseload/ Workload Analysis

Carol Easley Allen, Cheryl E. Easley, and Judith I. Storfjell

Management of health care costs in today's hospital encompasses more than inpatient care. The introduction of a prospective payment system that rewards early discharge of patients has resulted in the provision of home care services for patients by an increasing number of hospitals. Nurses are the largest professional group staffing such programs. Thus, in addition to concern with the costs of care in the acute-care setting, nursing must develop rational strategies for cost-effective management of the caseloads and workloads of nurses in home care programs.

The purposes of this discussion are to describe a patient classification system that is appropriate for home care nursing, involving both caseload and workload assessment, and to discuss the implications of such a system for cost-effective management of health care. The federal regulations and reimbursement mechanisms that constrain the contemporary home care delivery system will be reviewed and the home care market will be described, especially in regard to programs affiliated with hospitals. The discussion will then focus on the application of a set of instruments designed to collect and tabulate data on caseload and workloads in home care nursing and their uses and implications for fiscal management.

THE HOME CARE SCENE

By the late 1800s in both the United States and Great Britain, skilled nursing care was available to the sick in their homes under the auspices of organizations existing for this purpose. Public and private funding led to the rapid growth of both public and voluntary home nursing agencies in the early 1900s. Typically, such agencies were termed public health nursing agencies, visiting nurse associations, or community nursing services (Knollmueller, 1983).

The introduction of Medicare, Medicaid, and Title XX funding for homemaker, chore, and companion services in the 1970s led most home care agencies to tailor the services they provided to those reimbursable under federal guidelines (Reif, 1984). Concomitantly, with the geometric growth in the federal outlay for institutional care, home care began to be viewed as a cost-reducing alternative. Changes in federal policy were implemented to encourage the substitution of home care for inpatient care. The 1980 Omnibus Reconciliation Act liberalized home care coverage by (1) eliminating the 100-visit limitation on Medicare Parts A and B; (2) removing the three-day prior hospitalization requirement for home care eligibility under Part A; and (3) eliminating the $60 deductible prior to eligibility for home care under Part B.

The 1981 Omnibus Reconciliation Act lifted some of the restrictions on Medicaid funding for home care by permitting the waiver of some constraints on benefits and reimbursing a wider array of services, provided such services were lower in cost than, and could be substituted for, long-term care in an institutional setting (Reif, 1984; Wood & Estes, 1984).

The demand for home care services increased dramatically following the enactment of the Tax Equity and Fiscal Responsibility Act (TEFRA) in 1982 and the 1983 Social Security Amendments. The combined effect of these two legislative initiatives for institutional cost containment, through limitation of reimbursement and the enactment of prospective payment, has been a partial shifting of emphasis from hospital care to home care. The incentive for early discharge that is built into the prospective payment system has propelled home care services into an attractive position in the health care market.

However, federal cost-containment efforts have had restrictive as well as encouraging effects on home care funding in recent years. The government, as well as private health care insurers, want to be sure that reimbursed home care actually represents an alternative to hospital or institutional care and not an additional service. They are also concerned that no new client groups be created as the beneficiaries of home care services. Reif (1984) notes that although reimbursement for home care was liberalized in 1980, significant restrictions on eligibility and benefits remain. The most important of these restrictions stipulates that the beneficiary must be homebound and must require skilled nursing service. Certain Medicaid home care benefits are available only to patients who would otherwise be placed in nursing homes. Various strategies were implemented to increase competition in the home care market, thereby reducing charges.

The government has also acted to reduce expenditures for programs that fund home care. Examples of cost-containment measures that have severely constrained patients' access to home care services include stringent review of claims prior to authorization, restrictive eligibility requirements, setting of cost ceilings on reimbursement rates, and placing Title XX within a block grant while reducing funding (Reif, 1984). The restrictions on Medicaid eligibility and reimbursement in some states have had a particularly detrimental impact on visiting nurse associations and the lower-income clients that such agencies traditionally serve (Hartley & McKibbin, 1983). According to Wood and Estes (1984):

> It would appear that federal policy is encouraging the provision of home health through Medicare, but perhaps the unanticipated result of this policy in conjunction with Medicaid contractions is a treatment system for the non-poor and an increasing exclusion of coverage for the low-income population. There is a growing reluctance on the part of home health agencies to treat Medicaid patients, according to their reports [p. 60].

It is notable that with the expansion currently taking place in home care, Medicare and Medicaid expenditures for home care have remained low. In 1974, home care costs accounted for 1.2 percent of Medicare and 0.3 percent of Medicaid expenditures. By 1982, these percentages had increased to 2.3 percent and 1.7 percent, respectively (Reif, 1984). However, the growth of the home care market is better indicated by the $9.1 billion it generated in 1985 and the $16.3 billion that is projected for it for 1990 (Mershon & Wesolowski, 1985).

HOSPITAL-AFFILIATED HOME CARE

Hospitals are being urged, in a variety of ways and for a number of reasons, to develop home care programs. Home care facilitates the early discharge that is demanded by the prospective payment system. Thus, as a hospital increases its home care potential, its profitability is enhanced. Since there is still cost reimbursement for home care, revenue-producing hospital-affiliated agencies can be reimbursed for some of the hospitals' overhead, thus alleviating a share of the burden of non-revenue-producing departments.

Hospitals can control home care referrals. (Christy & Frasca, 1983; Lorenz, 1984). Provided antitrust and freedom-of-choice issues are adequately addressed (Pyles, 1984), a hospital-affiliated agency commands significant access to all patients discharged from the hospital. As competition in the home care market increases, control of referrals may well predict an agency's viability. The rapid growth of the home care industry, presently assessed at 20 percent annually (Kuntz, 1984), is another incentive for the development of hospital-affiliated home care, especially in view of the large profits being realized by many of the giant national health care corporations.

A number of advantages derive from the affiliation of home care agencies with hospitals. Although the hospital serves as a referral source for the home care program, the reverse situation is also possible; the home care program may funnel patients into the diagnostic and treatment services of the hospital (Christy & Frasca, 1983; Wodniak & Kirk, 1984). Thus, the hospital system maintains more comprehensive control over the total patient care package, with all the advantages of coordination, quality assurance, and revenue production that such control implies. It has been argued that hospital-affiliated home care programs are able to care for more acutely ill patients, since such programs have more access to the clinical resources of the hospital and its professional staff (Christy & Fracas, 1983). Other advantages relate to the planning, fiscal, and management systems already in place in the hospital and the support services, such as dietary, pharmacy, and rehabilitation services, that would be available to the hospital-affiliated program. In addition, Wodniak and Kirk (1984) note that "a home health program is essential if the hospital plans to develop an HMO, a PPO (preferred provider organization) or a MeSH (medical staff and hospital) organization" (p. 58).

In spite of the rapid expansion in the home care market, there are some reasons for caution. These include factors that may either inhibit the development of hospital-affiliated home care programs or significantly curtail their financial robustness over time, with potentially serious implications for home care nursing. There is no hard evidence that home care actually reduces health care costs. Although some analysts are equivocal on this issue (Louden, 1983; "What Experts Are Saying," 1984), others are positive that the costs of home care will be high, although no one is urging that home care be abandoned as a major component of the health care system for this reason ("What Experts Are Saying," 1984). At present, adequate evidence does not exist on which to base a comparison of home care with other types of care (Spiegels & Domanowski, 1983; Thomas, 1984). We have already noted the rise in costs of home care, with the resultant tightening of federal reimbursement mechanisms, and the reluctance of the government and private insurers to create new client populations or drastically expand expenditures for home care. Based on this combination of factors, one might reasonably predict that within the near future public and private payers will act to significantly limit or reduce spending on home care.

Many observers expect that a prospective payment system will be implemented eventually in federal home care funding (Lorenz, 1984). Private insurers are likely to institute prospective payment mechanisms for hospital care shortly, and it is likely that they will also follow the federal lead in placing their home care benefits in such a reimbursement system. Challenging the conventional wisdom that prospective reimbursement will be implemented in home health care by the end of the decade, Bridges (1984) foresees such a system in home care within the next two years. Factors favoring his prediction include the pressure exerted on Congress by the budget deficit and the growing demand from within the home care industry for a payment system that rewards efficiency. The Health Care Financing Administration is presently funding a five-year demonstration project to explore the feasibility of prospective reimbursement in home care.

The other major reason for caution in relationship to home care is the possibility that growth will slow in the home care market. A number of sponsors are entering the business, while the utilization of home care services is not commensurate with the decrease in length of hospital stay. The new type of home care patient, who is released from the hospital needing only a few days of recovery care, does not generate the demand for home care of the traditional long-term chronic patient (Kuntz, 1984). Private insurers indicate that their home care options are underutilized (Thomas, 1984). While this may denote a demand for home care that could be developed, the fact that physicians are failing to prescribe home care services does not augur well. As an indication of the difficulties in the home care business, Kuntz (1984) cites one national home care corporation that incurred such large financial losses as a result of restrictions on reimbursement for enteral therapy that funding fell below projections.

NURSING AND HOME CARE

Nurses are the major group of professionals working in the home care system. It is likely that more and more nurses will be employed in home care settings as some hospital nursing positions are terminated in the fallout from prospective reimbursement at the same time that new nursing positions are being created in the home care arena. As patients are discharged earlier from hospitals, increasing numbers of them have need of specialized and high technology nursing care at home. The population of home care patients is expanding to include more infants, children, and young adults than ever before. Nurses with the advanced technological clinical expertise developed in the hospital and those with specialized clinical skills, such as the care of children or high-risk infants, are increasingly being courted for the home care setting.

This situation holds both a promise and a challenge for professional nursing. It is encouraging that home care nursing provides employment for nurses that promises the opportunity for the enactment of a highly autonomous model of practice. On the other hand, the influx of new nurses into the home care arena makes it incumbent on those of us with a vested interest in the perpetuation of the "public health ideal" in community nursing care to transmit this philosophy to agencies and practitioners so that it is not lost in the shuffle.

Home health nurses have a unique opportunity to clearly demonstrate the cost-effectiveness of the care that they give, since their services represent a separate budget item. Hospital nurses, as we all are aware, are attempting to separate the costing of their services from the room rate. In home care, nursing services can be costed out and related directly to the agency's profitability. It is extremely important that the package of nursing services offered to the home care patient is not only profitable from the agency's viewpoint, but is truly comprehensive with reference to a professional standard of nursing care. As prospective reimbursement comes closer to becoming a reality in home care, the issue of patient classification is becoming critical.

Whatever prospective payment system is finally enacted for home care will be based on some sort of patient classification and case-mix system. We maintain that a system based on patient diagnosis, such as diagnosis related groups (DRGs), is not adequate for home care nursing. The variation in home care nursing requirements is not dependent on medical diagnoses. Nurses can and must have a part in the process through which a classification system for home care is chosen, both now and in any future prospective reimbursement arrangement. Only in this way can professional nursing care be assured the place it deserves in home care. The patient classification system we have developed was designed to reflect this nursing viewpoint.

CASELOAD/WORKLOAD ANALYSIS

The Easley-Storfjell Instruments for Caseload/Workload Analysis in Community Health Nursing (CL/WLA) were developed as a pragmatic response to a request from a group of community nursing supervisors in southwestern Michigan. Home care supervisors and administrators are increasingly being required to document both the quality and quantity of care being provided by nurses. Comprehensive management data is also needed on which to base evaluation and planning in home care agencies. At present there is a paucity of adequate tools available for effective and efficient collection, interpretation, and comparison of data regarding sevices provided in caseload fashion. There is a concomitant need for adequate systems to classify home care patients.

The Easley-Storfjell Instruments meet the following objectives:

1. To provide a summary description of a staff's caseload and workload, both individually and collectively.

2. To serve as a basis for case assignment through determination of the acuity and time demand of individual cases, analysis of case mix for the individual nurse, identification of significant types of nursing skill required by each case, and provision of a rationale for assignment of cases to the appropriate level of nurse or nursing assistant.

3. To assist in diagnosis of problems in caseload management.

4. To provide data on which to base evaluation of cost management.

Although these instruments were originally designed for manual use, a format for microcomputer application of the system has been developed.

The system consists of two components: caseload analysis and workload analysis. These terms may be defined as follows:

Caseload analysis: A summary of the characteristics of cases carried by a particular professional nurse, technical nurse, or nursing assistant.

Workload analysis: A summary of all activities required of a community health agency nursing employee, including caseload responsibilities.

Several considerations governed the development of the instruments:

- They were designed as a supervisory tool. It was envisioned that the nursing supervisor would perform the ratings with each staff nurse initially and periodically. In this way caseload/workload analysis could be combined easily with case review and other joint activities of the supervisor and staff nurse.

- The tools were also designed for simplicity and ease of use. A disadvantage of some patient classification systems devised for community nursing setting, such as home care, is that they contain too many variables or require lengthy analysis (Senzilet, 1983). Although we realized that more elaborate systems would provide more data than CL/WLA, we also recognized that too much complexity might discourage adequate use of the tools and could possibly affect their reliability.

- CL/WLA was developed to reflect and account for the team nurs-

Figure 1
Caseload Analysis Guidelines

TIME DETERMINATION

1. Monthly or less; only one visit.
2. Biweekly.
3. 1–2 times per week.
4. 3–5 times per week.

Note: For extensive follow-up or lengthy visits (over 1½ hours) add one time level. For brief visits (under ½ hour) subtract one time level.

DIFFICULTY DETERMINATION

Assign the highest numerical categorical rating (most difficult) in which the case meets two or more of the criteria, based on:

A. Clinical judgment
B. Teaching needs
C. Physical care
D. Psychosocial needs
E. Multi-agency involvement
F. Number and severity of problems

1. Minimal
A. Requires limited judgment, use of common sense, observation of fairly predictable change in patient status.
B. Requires basic health teaching.
C. Requires none or simple maintenance care.
D. Requires ability to relate to patients and families.
E. Requires limited involvement of only one other agency/provider.
F. Few or uncomplicated problems.

2. Moderate
A. Requires use of basic problem-solving techniques, ability to make limited patient assessments.
B. Requires teaching related to common health problems.
C. Requires basic rehabilitation or use of uncomplicated technical skills.
D. Requires use of basic interpersonal relationship skills.
E. Requires limited involvement of two other agencies/providers.
F. Several problems with limited complexity.

3. Great
A. Requires use of well-developed problem-solving skills enhanced by comprehensive knowledge of physical and social sciences, ability to make patient and family assessments.
B. Requires teaching related to illness, complications, and/or comprehensive health supervision.
C. Requires use of complicated technical skills.
D. Requires professional insight and intervention skills in coping with psychosocial needs.
E. Requires extensive involvement of at least one other agency/provider or coordination of several agencies/providers.
F. Several complicated problems.

4. Very great
A. Requires use of creativity, ability to initiate and coordinate plan for patient or family care, use of additional resources and increased supervisory support, ability to make comprehensive patient and family assessment.
B. Requires teaching related to unusual health problems or teaching/learning difficulties.

**Figure 1
(cont.)**

C. Requires knowledge of scientific rationales which underlie techniques and ability to modify care in response to patient/family need.
D. Requires ability to intervene in severe psychosocial problems.
E. Requires extensive coordination of multiple agencies/providers.
F. Numerous or complicated problems requiring augmentation of the knowledge base.

---

ing approach that frequently characterizes community nursing service. However, the tools are equally applicable to a nurse who carries a caseload singly.

- Finally, the CL/WLA instruments were designed to be utilized in conjunction with other analyses commonly used in community nursing, such as as time and cost studies.

It is crucial to meaningful caseload analysis to understand that assigning caseloads to nurses by equal numbers of patients does not ensure equality in assignment. The 20 cases assigned to one nurse may require a considerable difference in expertise and time than the 20 cases assigned to another. Appropriate comparison of caseload demand requires an assessment of the level of nursing service needed by each patient or family in the caseload and the time required to render the necessary care, as well as the number of cases or families being visited. Thus, time required and difficulty were determined to be the two most important factors in the grouping of cases for CL/WLA. The tools were devised to allow separate and combined assessments in both areas.

Time was operationalized according to a four-point scale based on the number of home visits that a particular case requires over a period of time (see Fig. 1). The ratings range from 1, cases requiring home visits monthly or less frequently, to 4, cases requiring visits three to five times per week. The actual requirements associated with the rating levels can be adjusted to provide a realistic assessment of the home visiting patterns that prevail in a particular agency. Such adjustments have been made by some of the agencies currently using the instruments.

Difficulty is determined on the basis of the overall demand for nursing resources presented by a particular patient or family. Although intensity or acuity of the case is included in the difficulty rating, other factors that typically influence the nursing care requirements in community nursing settings are also reflected. Cases are assigned to one of four difficulty ratings, ranging from minimal (1) to very great (4), based on six criteria: clinical judgment, teaching needs, physical care, psychosocial needs, multiagency involvement, and number and severity of problems. Descriptions of the nursing care requirements for the six criterion for each level of difficulty are shown in Figure 1. The difficulty levels may be easily correlated to the levels of nursing practice and ancillary nursing support frequently available in community nursing settings.

The Easley-Storfjell Instruments were designed as supervisory tools. The supervisor and the staff nurse should confer on the ratings of time and difficulty for each new case that is added to the nurses's caseload. The ratings should be assigned following the initial assessment of the case. If CL/WLA is being initiated with a caseload that already exists, the ratings may be made during a supervisor-nurse conference. The client's health record, the assessment of the case by the nurse, and the professional judgment of the nurse and the supervisor are the bases for the ratings of time and difficulty. Data from the caseload analysis, such as the number of visits required by the nurse each month, are combined with workload information that is specific to the agency and to the nurse's particular responsibilities to complete the workload analysis. This is also performed as a joint activity by the supervisor and the nurse.

Caseload analysis begins by listing all patients in the caseload on a caseload analysis roster showing the number of weeks the case has been open, the priority, program, or diagnosis of the case, and the time and difficulty rating for each case. The total of time and difficulty ratings may be included; however we have not as yet been able to ascertain a use for this number, in spite of several creative suggestions from agencies using CL/WLA.

The time and difficulty ratings then are charted on the caseload analysis graph (see Figure 2) for a graphic representation of the caseload. This instrument is designed to facilitate calculation of the number of visits required each month in order to meet caseload demands. It also depicts the pattern of difficulty in a particular caseload.

A description of caseload requirements, in terms of numbers of home visits, addresses only a portion of a nurse's responsibility, however. Other activities, assignments, and time adjustments constrain the amount of time that can be devoted to direct patient care. Through an analysis of the nurse's total workload, the actual time that is available for direct care may be ascertained. A time allocation worksheet allows a calculation of the time needed for the range of activities and time adjustments that characterize the nurse's total workload. Personal time, supportive activities, special assignments, and community service activities are addressed. Typical community nursing categories have been included, such as supervisor-nurse conferences, hospital liaison, and clinic supervision. In keeping with the flexibility designed into the system, we have encouraged agencies to modify this tool to provide a realistic representation of actual components of the agency's workload.

Figure 2
Easley-Storfjell Instruments for Caseload/Workload Analysis

CASELOAD ANALYSIS GRAPH

Name _____ Position _____ Date _____

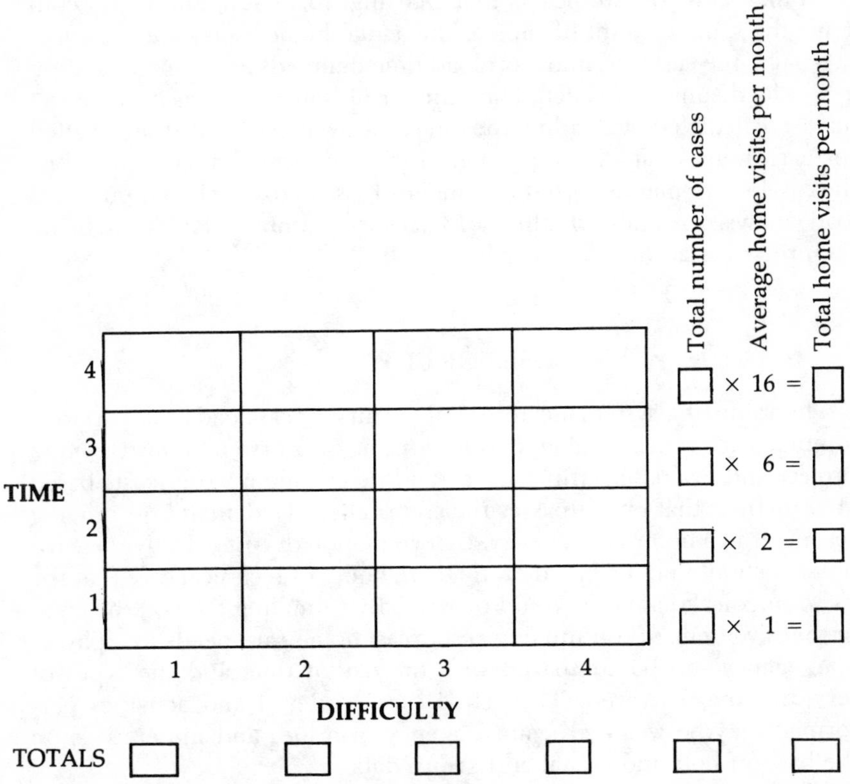

CODES

Time	Difficulty	Based On:
1. Monthly; one visit	1. Minimal	A. Clinical judgment
2. Biweekly	2. Moderate	B. Teaching needs
3. One–two times per week	3. Great	C. Physical care
4. Three–five times per week	4. Very great	D. Psychosocial needs
		E. Multi-agency involvement
		F. Number and severity of problem

Subtracting the time needed for scheduled activities from the total time available indicates the time that may be devoted to home visits. Home visiting time includes the time actually spent in the home, travel, charting, and follow-up activities. The rule of thumb, based on averages from time and cost studies, is that charting, follow-up, and travel consume the same amount of time as the actual home visit.

Finally, the caseload and workload time demands are summarized on a workload summary sheet. The number of home visits each nurse can make is calculated by dividing the total time available by the time needed for each home visit. A comparison of the number of visits required by the caseload demands with the number of visits possible based on workload analysis, reveals whether an excessive number of visits is being required or if additional visits are possible.

USES OF CL/WLA

The value of a systematic appraisal of nursing caseload and workload in home care is inestimable. It is important for nurse administrators to project and evaluate staffing needs and determine nursing costs based on a method that encompasses the comprehensive demand on nursing resources in a home care agency. Determination of cost-effectiveness for nursing should not be based on the bare bones of technical care that the use of medical diagnosis would provide. By compiling data on the comprehensive demand on nursing resources, home care needs in a particular agency can be compared with the use of time and the types of service being delivered. The actual care rendered and activities performed may be weighed against agency priorities and imperatives on the basis of both individual and group data.

Through repeated analyses over time, trends in service delivery may be ascertained. As analysis reveals the specific nature of nursing care requirements that contribute to the difficulty of particular caseloads, needs of individuals and groups for staff development may be projected. Data provided by workload trends for the entire agency may be used to justify requests for budgetary adjustments to increase the nursing staff.

The use of CL/WLA allows nursing supervisors and administrators to base staffing decisions on projections of the nursing care demands of the agency's caseload. The difficulty profile of a caseload may reveal a need for staffing adjustments, thus indicating the level of nursing staff adequate to provide appropriate care, while avoiding underutilization of the skills and educational preparation of any individuals on the nursing team. In this way, nursing costs are managed effectively, and the nurse administrator has hard data with which to justify the budgetary requirements of a nursing staff mix based on the agency's comprehensive demand for nursing resources.

In supervision of individual members of the nursing staff, CL/WLA has proved useful in defining realistic caseload and workload goals. A concentration of highly difficult cases in one nurse's caseload may signal a need for additional supervisory support, while a caseload difficulty rating lower than a nurse's skills warrant may be the key to restlessness or low morale. The average length of time cases are open should alert the supervisor to nurses who either carry cases too long or close them too quickly. The length of time a case is open is also a cost factor. Cost-effectiveness must be pursued while necessary and comprehensive nursing care needs continue to be met.

The CL/WLA may be especially valuable when transferring cases from one nurse to another or orienting new staff. As home care agencies move toward lengthening the extent of service provision to a 24-hour-a-day, weeklong schedule and increase their use of part-time staff, the time and difficulty ratings provide a readily available method of allocating cases among a varying group of nursing staff at any given time. The ratings will also facilitate handling of student nurses' assignments.

CL/WLA IN USE

Although the Easley-Storfjell Instruments have not as yet been stringently tested for reliability and validity, a number of community health and home care agencies in the United States and Canada, as well as the U.S. Army, are currently using these tools. Nursing supervisors and administrators have been pleased with the opportunity to obtain a clearer picture of agency caseloads and workloads for planning, staffing, and budgeting purposes. The systematic analysis allows nurses to organize activities, streamline caseloads, and obtain a realistic overview of workload demands, all of which leads to greater efficiency, more appropriate utilization of time, and increased cost-effectiveness. The ability to document nursing staffing needs to support agency programs has been frequently cited as a valuable outcome of the use of this system. The positive feedback we have received encouraged us to develop the microcomputer application already mentioned and to modify the instruments for use in social casework.

Although the Easley-Storfjell Instruments were developed in 1977, it is interesting to compare this system to the guidelines for workload measurement recently developed by the Management Information Systems Project in Canada to ensure that the necessary components for effective information management were available in any of the many systems being utilized throughout that country (Senzilet, 1984; St. Germain & Meijers, 1984). The CL/WLA tools adhere closely to the requirements cited in the guidelines. In brief, the CL/WLA system

- Is flexible enough to allow modification based on agency philosophies, goals, and standards.
- Accounts for the unique blend of nursing care requirements of each case.
- Associates each element of care required with the workload.
- Includes identification of acuity but bases weighting on the workload.
- Describes components of the workload in sufficient detail.
- Reflects the time required to deliver care according to established standards.
- Allows for selective revision and updating.
- Encompasses personnel who provide direct patient care and excludes management and support personnel.
- Is functional with manual input but amenable to computerization.
- Is flexible.
- Allows extraction of data for categories of work by occupational level.
- Provides managers with information that will assist in the assignment of workloads to personnel.
- Provides for the extraction of data to support the preparation of the budget and for planning and control at all levels of management.

In addition, the CL/WLA system allows for a testing process to monitor the accuracy of assessment, interrater reliability, and validity of the system.

CONCLUSION

Nursing as a profession has the right to define its domain and establish standards for nursing care based on professional ideals and goals. The model of care that will be recognized in home care nursing will be critically influenced by the patient classification system that is adopted and the overall dimensions of the method of workload determination that is deemed appropriate by the public and private agencies that fund home care activities. In this time of change and cost containment, nursing must seize the opportunity to determine the shape of the reimbursement mechanism that will define nursing care in the real world of dollars and cents. The development of systematic models such as the Easley-Storfjell Instruments provides home care nursing administrators with the hard data necessary to rationalize comprehensive demand for nursing resources while demonstrating efficiency in management of personnel and budgets.

REFERENCES

Bridges, R., (1984, February). Planning ahead for home care DRGs. *Caring 3*, 30.

Christy, M. W., & Frasca, C. (1983, December). The benefits of hospital sponsored home care programs. *Journal of Nursing Administration, 13*.

Hartley, S. S., & McKibbin, R. C. (1983). *Hospital payment mechanisms, patient classification systems, and nursing: Relationships and implications*. Kansas City, MO: American Nurses' Association.

Knollmueller, R. N. (1983, March). Funding home care in a climate of cost containment. *Public Health Nursing, 1*, 17.

Kuntz, E. F. (1984, May 15). For-profits adding home health care to aid bottom lines. *Modern Health Care, 14*, 170.

Lorenz, B. R. (1984, February). Prospective reimbursement in health care and related problems and opportunities for home health agencies. *Caring, 3*, 27.

Louden, T. L. (1983, December). Opportunities—and competition—in home health care are on the rise. *Modern Health Care, 13*, 109.

Mershon, K., & Wesolowski, M. (1985, January). Strategic planning for the business of community health and home care. *Nursing & Health Care, 6*, 33–35.

Pyles, J. C., (1984, February). Referral arrangements between hospitals and home health agencies. *Caring, 3*, 55–56.

Reif, L. (1984, November–December). Making dollars and sense of home health policy. *Nursing Economics, 2*.

St. Germain, D., & Meijers, A. (1984, May). Nursing workload measurement: An expanded future role. *Dimensions in Health Service, 61*, 18–20.

Senzilet, L. D. (1983, July). Workload measurement systems: A management tool. *Dimensions in Health Service, 60*, 38–40.

Senzilet, L. D. (1984, July). Workload measurement systems: Three recording methods. *Dimensions in Health Service, 61*, 32–33.

Spiegels, A. D., & Domanowski, G. F. (1983, May). Does home care cost less? A review and assessment. *Caring, 2*, 31.

Thomas, D. R. (1984, June). Trends in insurance coverage for home health care. *Caring, 3*, 54.

What experts are saying about DRGs and home care (1984, February). *Caring, 3*, 33.

Wodniak, J. S., & Kirk, J. (1984, February). Trend: Hospitals' entry into home health. *Caring*, *3*, 57.

Wood, J. B., & Estes. C. L. (1984, June). Home health care under the policies of new federalism. *Caring*, *3*, 58–59.

Part 4
Afterword

Where Do We Go from Here?

Phyllis Giovannetti

In this paper I will explicate the contributions of the previous papers in *Patients and Purse Strings* to our understanding and knowledge of the costs of nursing care and of fiscal management and control in nursing. In fulfilling this task, I have focused my comments on what I believe are the major impediments to the generation of new knowledge in this area. To date, a variety of patient classification schemes have formed the framework for the costing out of nursing care. I believe that it is the *misunderstandings* that surround the concepts of patient classification, along with those of patient acuity and severity of illness, as well as specific procedures and practices related to nurse staffing determination and costing that are the major impediments to new knowledge in this area. It is imperative that we come to some common understanding of that about which we speak. Only when understanding is present can we proceed with agreement and disagreement—the prerequisites to real debate and the impetus for new knowledge.

PATIENT CLASSIFICATION

Patient classification is a generic term referring to the process of grouping patients into mutually exclusive categories. The term by itself conveys very little information. It derives meaning only when it is accompanied by a statement of purpose—for example, the classification of patients according to their perceived requirements for nursing care for the purpose of nursing personnel determination and allocation, or the classi-

349

fication of patients according to total hospital resource consumption for the purpose of prospective payment. The first example describes many of the instruments germane to nurse staffing methods. The second example describes the DRG system. Clearly, they are different. The objective of the first is to predict nursing care time requirements for some future time period, such as the next shift or the next 24 hours; the objective of the second is to establish a price per hospital stay. There is no reason to believe that one can replace the other, or that there is a direct relationship between the two.

Several of the papers in this volume, notably those by Atwood, Hinshaw, and Chance; Martin and Kelly; and Sovie, Tarcinale, VanPutte, and Stunden provide evidence that while DRGs may be fairly homogeneous with respect to total hospital resource consumption, they are not homogeneous with respect to nursing personnel resource consumption. As Atwood, Hinshaw, and Chance clearly point out, DRGs alone do not provide a firm basis for the management of nursing personnel. They do not predict the complexity of nursing care, the amount of nurse staffing needed, or the amount to charge the patient for nursing care.

There are many opportunities for classifying or grouping patients. The paper by Young, Carson, and Lander introduces another classification scheme referred to as patient management categories. The categories define clinically specific patient types, each requiring distinct diagnostic and treatment strategies, for the purpose of measuring nursing costs and productivity. We can and have classified patients according to age, sex, blood type, diagnosis, and problems, to name but a few possibilities. In spite of the thousands of opportunities for patient classification, the term has been used almost exclusively to refer to the classification systems available for grouping patients according to their perceived requirements for nursing care for the purpose of nursing staff determination and deployment. Such exclusivity has led many to speak of patient classification in terms of a universal purpose. Continued use of the generic term in the absence of a clear statement of purpose, is misleading and inappropriate.

PATIENT ACUITY AND SEVERITY

Two other terms that are highly susceptible to misunderstanding are *patient acuity* and *severity of illness*. When these terms are used by nurses in the context of nurse staffing, it is assumed that they refer to the intensity of nursing workload. When employed by non-nursing personnel, they may take on quite different meanings. The medical connotation of acuity and severity refer to comorbidities, or the seriousness of the patient's illness. Furthermore, within the medical context, patient acuity and severity of illness levels do not necessarily correlate with nursing workload intensity.

We need to explore these terms more thoroughly and guard against the common practice of assuming that patient acuity and severity of illness can serve as proxy measures of nursing care time or nursing intensity. There are many patients who require extensive amounts of nursing care time and yet are not considered to be acutely or severely ill. As clearly illustrated in the paper by Lucke and Lucke, severity of illness and nursing intensity are represented by two distinct classification schemes. While the two measures may be highly correlated, especially when tested on samples of critical care patients, they are not interchangeable. Lucke and Lucke found that the addition of a nursing intensity measure improved the prediction of overall resource utilization by critical care patients over that of DRG and severity-of-illness predictors.

CLASSIFICATION TYPES

Within the context of patient classification, considerable confusion and misunderstanding surrounds the various designs or types of classification instruments. The patient classification instruments commonly utilized for nurse staffing decisions are generally considered to belong to one of two types—prototype or factor evaluations. Prototype instruments are hierarchial in design and are characterized by a selection of descriptors or profiles that represent the nursing care requirements of a typical patient in each category. The characteristics of the actual patient are compared with those described in the profiles or prototypes, and the patient is classified into the category of care whose description he or she most closely matches. The classification instrument illustrated in the paper by Allen, Easley, and Storfjell represents an example of prototype evaluation.

The second type of classification instrument, factor evaluations, is also based on selected patient characteristics or elements of care. As with the prototype design, the selection of characteristics or care elements is generally limited to those items found to have explanatory power as predictors of nursing care time. The selected items are typically referred to as "critical indicators of care" and include at minimum, the predictors of nursing care time identified by Connor and his associates at the Johns Hopkins Hospital in the late 1950s and early 1960s (Connor, 1961a, 1961b). These predictors largely relate to patients' abilities to function independently in the areas of feeding, bathing, and ambulation—the activities of daily living—and to their coping skills and knowledge requirements. To my knowledge, the inclusion of a variety of additional indicators or factors has not been shown to add to the statistical validity of these classification schemes, although they are often thought to be important in terms of users' subjective perceptions. Both prototype and factor evaluation instruments can be true classification schemes in that they group patients into mutually exclusive groups. Examples of the factor evaluation type of classification instrument are found in the papers by Churness, Kleffel, Jacobson, and Onodera; Killeen; Paradise, Dijkers, and Maxwell; and Sovie et al.

It is interesting to note the variety of critical indicators, both in scope and number, that make up each of these instruments. Some indicators represent patient states, such as "complete immobility," while others represent nursing care activities, such as "tube feed q4h." Thus, some critical indicators may be described as predictors of care activities, while others represent actual care practices. Knowledge of these distinctions is important. The use of actual care practices (e.g., tube feed q4h) in contrast to patient characteristics (e.g., complete immobility) have implications for both the ease with which the systems can be manipulated and for the quality of care. Potentially, a patient can be elevated to a higher category by selecting additional care practices or those that have higher weights. Furthermore, staff may be rewarded by keeping patients in more dependent states for longer periods than necessary—an issue of quality.

A third category, nursing care task documents, is suggested as a term that more accurately describes some of the instruments that are neither prototype nor factor evaluations. Nursing task documents use a listing of most if not all of the nursing care tasks or activities that may be required by patients. Generally, each task or activity is associated with a value representing the "actual" or "standard" time or a relative weight representing the time required to carry out or complete the task. Some tasking documents do result in mutually exclusive groups and thus can be considered classification instruments. For others, the unique care requirements of each patient are individually calculated, thereby eliminating the designation of categories. The paper by Heyrman and Nelson provides a good example of this latter case. It is interesting to note that while the writers advise that patients are never classified, they nevertheless have decided to refer to their instrument as a patient classification system.

Awareness and understanding of the differences among the various types of classification instruments is important. The type of instrument is central to the question of comparability of classification information between facilities and in many cases between units within a facility. Some types are more amenable to the determination of skill level, while others may be more useful in terms of patient placement. Some are considered to be more appropriate within the realm of independent professional nursing practice. Others are thought to perpetuate a view of nursing that is limited to the carrying out of tasks. Failure to understand the design differences in classification types has not infrequently resulted in unjustified rejection of a particular instrument. The development of a unique classification instrument may be a useful exercise; the purpose, however, should be fully recognized and not attributed to lack of available instruments.

QUANTIFICATION TECHNIQUES

The various methods of quantifying the patient classification instruments used for nurse staffing offer another area of potential confusion. To highlight the issues related to quantification, it is helpful to distinguish between the processes used to designate the categories of care, referred to as phase 1, from those used to convert categorical information into hours of nursing care or staffing coefficients, phase 2. The application of a true factor or prototype evaluation instrument yields nothing more than a category of care. That is, individual patients are identified as belonging to one of a number of possible groups. This designation into groups is not unlike that used in the DRG classification system, where patients belong to a specific DRG. At the completion of phase 1, classification instruments that have the same purpose and the same number of categories (assuming acceptable levels of interrater reliability), are capable of providing comparable data within and between hospitals with similar patient populations.

The classification of a patient into a specific category, however, provides insufficient information for determining nurse staffing levels or, in the case of DRGs, total hospital resource consumption. Thus, a second computation involving the designation of appropriate weights must be made. In the case of the nursing instruments, the weights or coefficients are generally represented in terms of nursing care. This second function, frequently referred to as the "quantification phase," involves the assignment of weights reflecting the magnitude of the nursing care time required to care for patients within each of the categories. In some cases, the quantification may be limited to direct care time, and additional calculations are required to produce a total care time. In other cases, the quantification may initially reflect total care time.

The extent to which care times are comparable among like categories, both within and between institutions, depends on the procedures used for identifying the time coefficients. If the coefficients are derived from unit-based observational studies or unit-based negotiations, it is likely that the resulting coefficients will differ among units within a hospital as well as among hospitals. Kaspar's paper highlights some of the definitions and problems related to quantification.

Given the many factors that affect nursing care time over and above the care requirements of patients, it is not surprising that quantification studies typically yield both direct care and total care times that differ across different nursing units. For example, a category 3 patient on an orthopedic unit may require more hours of care than a category 3 patient on a short-term surgical unit—a function not only of the normal variances within a patient category, but also of the potential variances due to such additional factors as differences in the expertise and levels of nurses, physical layout and design of the units, physician practices, leadership skills of the head nurses, and standards of care, to name just a few. If, as is the case in many institutions, the indicators for classification are unique to each nursing unit, this provides a further reason for the lack of comparability among classifications.

It should be emphasized that the "standardized" nurse staffing classification instruments offered by many proprietary firms do not necessarily resolve the question of comparability. The weights used to correspond to each of the critical indicators of care are not to be confused with staffing coefficients. The weights attached to the indicators are relative values only and are used in the factor evaluation type instruments as decision rules for specifying which combinations of indicators define a particular category. Furthermore, implementation of these systems in most instances involves modifications in the selection of indicators and their weighting to meet the individual desires and demands of the user institutions.

The comparability of classifications is not necessarily a problem given the purpose of the instruments. Since the major force behind the development and implementation of classification instruments based on patients' requirements for nursing care has been to assist individual institutions and units with the complex task of nurse staffing, there has been little incentive to ensure universal comparability. On the contrary, dissatisfaction with global staffing standards has no doubt served as a prime incentive to avoid universality. The problems of lack of comparability surface, however, when the same instruments are used as a basis for determining the costs of nursing care within the framework of DRGs, which represent a universal system yielding comparable data. The data representing the costs of nursing care within specific DRGs that have currently been amassed, including the substantial number of studies reported elsewhere in this publication, provide evidence. With rare exception, the investigators have acknowledged the absence of generalizability resulting from noncomparable data bases. The implications of noncomparability may not be serious if the object is to determine real costs. They may be extremely serious if the object is charges on the basis of costs. Questions of productivity and quality will take on new meaning.

JUDGING CLASSIFICATION INSTRUMENTS

There are established rules for judging and evaluating a patient classification instrument. The rules include, but are not limited to, measuring the instrument's degree of homogeneity, reliability, and validity in terms of its explicit purpose. Criticism of a particular classification instrument ought to be made on the grounds of its failure to meet essential evaluation criteria. Unfortunately, many of the published accounts of patient classification instruments fail, in the first instance, by not explicating their purpose and, in the second, by neglecting to provide evidence of their degree of homogeneity, reliability, and validity. Happily, this is not the case for most of the papers in this volume. Equally unfortunate is the quickness with which many instruments are judged to be inadequate. In the face of uncertainty, we ought to withhold judgment and await or inquire for further information. To agree or disagree in the absence of understanding is inane.

The proliferation of patient classification instruments designed for nurse staffing is, in my opinion, largely due to our failure to understand them or to inquire as to their performance on essential evaluation criteria such as reliability and validity. Some credit for the proliferation must also be given to proprietary vendors, who in order to successfully "vend" must make a case for a unique product. While I do not devalue the learning and internal commitment that comes with the developmental process, I believe there are other and better ways of learning and other and better means to achieve internal commitment.

The application of many patient classification instruments used for nurse staffing determination and deployment require an element of prediction. That is, patients' current characteristics are used as a basis for determining future care requirements, for example, for the following shift or 24-hour period. Thus, at any one point in time, patients' predicted category of care might not equal their actual category of care. The difference is less likely to be a function of a nurse's ability to use professional judgment in the task of prediction than a function of an "unpredictable" change in a patient's requirement for care.

A somewhat related problem is that patients might not receive the amount of nursing care commensurate with their category. This becomes a real possibility when actual staffing levels are not matched to the levels suggested by the classification instrument or when nursing personnel fail to deliver the amount of care specified for each patient category. Although appropriate validity testing attempts to resolve in part some of these potential discrepancies, the problem is not resolved when classification information is used to determine the costs of nursing care. As previously noted, most patient classification instruments in nursing were designed to group patients according to their perceived care requirements for the purpose of staff determination and allocation. How well they group patients according to the nursing care actually provided is yet another question. One ought not to discredit a classification instrument because it does not do what it was never designed to do. If criticism is in order, it must rest upon the users of the instrument who employ it for purposes other than its original ones.

QUALITY IMPLICATIONS

A final issue related to the application of classification instruments in nursing, and one that affects their application as both staffing methods and costing methods, is that of the quality of nursing care. While a thorough discussion of quality would no doubt require a document the size of this book, a few comments are necessary. First, it is recognized that the realm of quality assurance in nursing is vast. Second, quality is multidimensional and thus unlikely to be adequately assessed on the basis of one measuring tool. Third, evidence of acceptable reliability and validity values is lacking for the vast majority of instruments that assess quality of nursing care. These represent serious limitations with respect to the measurement of quality. While I believe that, in many instances, heroic efforts are made in the interest of ensuring that staffing coefficients assigned to the categories of patient classification instruments are in keeping with our best professional judgment of quality care, the fact is that we fall short of supportive evidence.

We cannot assume that the staffing coefficients attached to patient classification instruments always result in the highest quality of care delivered in the most efficient manner. The scholarly paper prepared by Edwardson addresses these concerns. Given the extent to which users rely on staffing coefficients, their derivation is indeed an onerous responsibility. The responsibility is further heightened when patients are charged on the basis of these coefficients. Perhaps the greatest research need is the development and testing of quality measures.

CONCLUSION

Many of the papers in this volume are outstanding. Yet I believe they contribute incrementally rather than exponentially to the expansion of knowledge. Claim for the latter must await evidence of understanding of the meaning of terms, the explicitness of purpose, and the identification of procedures. The prerequisites to real debate, the impetus for new knowledge, is that understanding. In the absence of clearly defined terms, explicitness of purpose, and identifiable procedures, understanding is thwarted and so too is our knowledge.

The absence of new knowledge is not the only loss incurred. Without true understanding, we risk spending valuable time and resources on activities that lead to nothing more than what is commonly referred to as "reinventing the wheel." Perhaps more costly is the risk we take that while engaged in nonsensical debate, the answers to the questions we seek will come to us from another source. We may be awakened, and not so gently, I fear, by the realization that the magic figures for that which we search have been given to us, or more likely, imposed upon us. The scenario could be rather like that which occurred with the legislation of DRGs. For nursing, it might be the designation of a single and universal nursing care cost or time coefficient. Even the designation of several universal nursing care cost or time coefficients, representing each of several categories or groups of patients, would not lessen the impact.

Whatever the case, I have little difficulty envisioning that we would spend decades struggling to practice as professional nurses within a system that drives our practice and within a system we are powerless to affect. Nurses represent the only group of health care providers that are consistently and significantly influenced by factors largely outside their control. It behooves us to obtain some control over this system and to direct it to safeguarding the welfare of patients. Nurses need to ensure that the goals of the health care system are directed toward the needs of the patients and not, as it so often appears, the needs of the institutions, their sponsors, their directors, and their employees.

The prospective payment system implemented on the basis of DRGs has served to awaken within nursing the need to pursue the identification of the costs of nursing care. The paper by Mutzebaugh provides a plan to ensure that nurses have the necessary fiscal management skills to identify these costs. I believe that we can proceed with new and heightened levels of awareness, cooperation, and collaboration. We can broaden our thinking from that of nursing problems to health care problems.

Many nurses were horrified by the news of the legislation of DRGs just a few years ago. We were frightened that nursing would be shortchanged and that decisions would be made that would place professional nursing practice in jeopardy. The nursing profession responded to this news and responded rather well. In particular, a great many studies were conducted that demonstrated that DRGs were not homogeneous with respect to nursing care. There is little debate about that question today. Many of the studies that were conducted to provide such evidence paid attention to the problems of distinguishing between costs based on care rendered and costs based on care required.

As we proceed with defining and extracting the true costs of nursing care, we will come closer to defining our product. This exercise, I believe is the most exciting and holds the greatest promise for professional nursing practice. It will endeavor to unfold the nature, object, and scope of nursing. We must and will come to terms with what nursing is, what is unique about nursing, and what contributions nursing makes to the good life. At this point we will no longer be powerless; we will be able to effect the changes that are necessary to ensure the delivery of quality nursing care, no matter what the setting.

REFERENCES

Connor, R. J. (1961a, May). Effective use of nursing resources: A research report. *Hospitals, 35*, 30–39.

Connor, R. J. (1961b, May). A work sampling study of variations in nursing workload. *Hospitals, 35*, 40–41.

Contributors

Carol Easley Allen, PhD., RN, is Associate Professor, Department of Nursing, California State University, Los Angeles.

Jan R. Atwood, PhD, RN, FAAN, is Professor, College of Nursing, University of Arizona, Tucson.

Janet S. Bailie, MSN, RN, CCRN, is Director of Quality Assurance/ Utilization Management, West Florida Regional Medical Center, Pensacola, Florida.

Elizabeth A. Buck, MSN, RN, is Instructor, School of Nursing, Southern Illinois University at Edwardsville.

Marlene S. Carson, RN, is Nurse Research Analyst, Pittsburgh Research Institute, Center for Health Services Research, Pittsburgh, Pennsylvania.

Helen C. Chance, MS, RN, was formerly Director of Nursing and Associate Administrator, University Medical Center, Tucson, Arizona.

Lynne H. Cheatwood, BSN, RN, is Computing Resource Coordinator, Miami Valley Hospital, Dayton, Ohio.

Vivian Hayes Churness, DNSc, RN, is Assistant Professor, Department of Nursing, University of Southern California, Los Angeles.

Marcel Dijkers, PhD, is Director of Research, Rehabilitation Institute, Detroit, Michigan.

Cheryl E. Easley, AM, RN, is Interim Assistant Dean for Undergraduate Studies, School of Nursing, University of Michigan, Ann Arbor.

Sandra R. Edwardson, PhD, RN, is Associate Professor, School of Nursing, University of Minnesota, Twin Cities, Minnesota, and Senior Consultant, Health Management Systems Associates, Minneapolis, Minnesota.

Phyllis Giovannetti, ScD, RN, is Professor and Director, Research Facilitation Office, Faculty of Nursing, University of Alberta, Edmonton, Alberta, Canada.

Lois Grau, PhD, RN, is Associate Director, Brookdale Research Institute for Aging, Third Age Center, Fordham University, New York, New York.

Joanne S. Harrell, PhD, RN, is Assistant Professor, School of Nursing, University of North Carolina at Chapel Hill.

Karole Schafer Heyrman, MA, RN, is Patient Classification Project Coordinator, Department of Nursing, University of Illinois Hospital and Clinics, Chicago.

Ada Sue Hinshaw, PhD, RN, FAAN, is Professor and Director of Nursing Research Center, College of Nursing, University of Arizona, and Director of Nursing Research, Nursing Department, University Medical Center, Tucson.

Joan Jacobson, MSN, RN, is Assistant Professor, Department of Nursing, University of Southern California, Los Angeles.

Deborah Kaspar, MSN, RN, is Senior Consultant, Health Management Systems Associates, Minneapolis, Minnesota.

Patricia A. Kelly, MS, CCRN, was, at the time of the study, Education Coordinator, Department of Nursing Education and Resources, Miami Valley Hospital, Dayton, Ohio, and is a doctoral student at Francis Payne Bolton School of Nursing, Case Western Reserve University, Cleveland, Ohio.

Mary B. Killeen, MSN, RN, C, is Clinical Nurse Specialist, Sinai Hospital of Detroit, and a doctoral student at Wayne State University, Detroit, Michigan.

Dorothy Kleffel, MPH, RN, is Director of Research and Education, Visiting Nurse Association of Los Angeles, Los Angeles, California.

Chris Kovner, PhD, RN, is Assistant Professor, Division of Nursing, School of Education, Health, Nursing, and Arts Professions, New York University, New York, New York.

Susan A. Lander, RN, is Nurse Research Analyst, Pittsburgh Research Institute, Center for Health Services Research, Pittsburgh, Pennsylvania.

Linda K. Lesic, BSN, RN, is Director, Nursing Management and Information Systems, Shadyside Hospital, Pittsburgh, Pennsylvania.

Joseph Lucke, PhD, is Research Methodologist, Research and Publication Support Service, Lehigh Valley Hospital Center, Allentown, Pennsylvania.

Kathleen Lucke, MSN, RN, CCRN, is Director, Teacher-Practitioner-Researcher Program, Allentown, Pennsylvania, and was, at the time of the study, Project Coordinator for Critical Care, Wishard Memorial Hospital, Indiana University Medical Center, Indianapolis.

Patricia A. Martin, MS, RN, is Nurse Researcher, Miami Valley Hospital, and faculty member, Wright State University–Miami Valley School of Nursing, Dayton, Ohio, and a doctoral student at Francis Payne Bolton School Nursing, Case Western Reserve University, Cleveland, Ohio.

Marylou Maxwell, MSN, RN, is Clinical Nurse Specialist, Rehabilitation Institute, Detroit, Michigan.

Carole A. Mutzebaugh, EdD, RN, is Associate Professor, University of Southern Colorado, Pueblo.

Kathleen M. Nelson, BSN, RN, is Patient Classification Project Coordinator, Department of Nursing, University of Illinois Hospital and Clinics, Chicago.

Marlene Onodera, MS, MPA, is Research Analyst, Visiting Nurse Association of Los Angeles, Los Angeles, California.

Teri Paradise, RN, C, is Nursing Outreach Coordinator, Rehabilitation Institute, Detroit, Michigan.

Franklin A. Shaffer, EdD, RN, is Deputy Director, National League for Nursing, New York, New York.

Margaret D. Sovie, PhD, RN, FAAN, is Professor of Nursing and Associate Dean for Nursing Practice, School of Nursing, University of Rochester, and Associate Director for Nursing, Strong Memorial Hospital, University of Rochester Medical Center, Rochester, New York.

Judith I. Storfjell, MS, RN, is President, Health Care at Home Management Corporation, St. Joseph, Michigan.

Ann Stunden, BA, is Associate Director, University Computing Center, University of Rochester, Rochester, New York.

Michael A. Tarcinale, PhD, RN, is Assistant Professor, School of Nursing, University of Rochester, and Instructor in Staff Development, Strong Memorial Hospital, University of Rochester Medical Center, Rochester, New York.

Alison VanPutte, MS, RN, is Assistant Professor of Nursing and Pediatrics, School of Nursing, University of Rochester, and Clinical Chief for Pediatric Nursing, Strong Memorial Hospital, University of Rochester Medical Center, Rochester, New York.

Gail A. Wolf, DNS, RN, is Vice President for Nursing, Shadyside Hospital, Pittsburgh, Pennsylvania.

Jonelle E. Wright, PhD, RN, is Assistant Professor, School of Nursing, University of Maryland, Baltimore.

Wanda W. Young, ScD, is Vice President, Health Care Research, Blue Cross of Western Pennsylvania, and President, Pittsburgh Research Institute, Center for Health Services Research, Pittsburgh, Pennsylvania.